The Dao De Jing

A Qigong Interpretation

道德經氣功解

Lao Tzu
Translation and Commentary by
Dr. Yang, Jwing-Ming

YMAA Publication Center
Wolfeboro, NH USA

YMAA Publication Center, Inc.
PO Box 480
Wolfeboro, New Hampshire, 03894
1-800-669-8892 • info@ymaa.com • www.ymaa.com

ISBN: 9781594396199 (print) • ISBN: 9781594396205 (ebook)

Managing Editor: T. G. LaFredo

Copy Editors: Dorin Hunter and Leslie Takao

Cover design by Axie Breen

This book typeset in Electra LT

Illustrations courtesy of the the author unless otherwise noted.

10   9   8   7   6   5   4   3   2   1

Publisher's Cataloging in Publication

Names: Laozi, author. | Yang, Jwing-Ming, 1946- translator, author of added commentary.
Title: The dao de jing : a qigong interpretation / Lao Tzu ; translation and commentary
    by Dr. Yang, Jwing-Ming.
Description: Wolfeboro, NH USA : YMAA Publication Center, [2018] | Includes
    bibliographical references.
Identifiers: ISBN: 9781594396199 | 9781594396205 (ebook) | LCCN: 2018945774
Subjects: LCSH: Laozi. Dao de jing. | Laozi--Criticism and interpretation. | Taoism. |
    Taoist philosophy. | Philosophy, Chinese. | Qi gong. | Mind and body. | Meditation. |
    Well-being. | Qi (Chinese philosphy) | Medicine, Chinese. | BISAC: PHILOSOPHY /
    Taoist. | BODY, MIND & SPIRIT / I Ching. | HEALTH & FITNESS / Alternative
    Therapies.
Classification: LCC: BL1900.L3 E5 2018 | DDC: 299.5/1482--dc23

NOTE TO READERS
The practice, treatments, and methods described in this book should not be used
as an alternative to professional medical diagnosis or treatment. The author and
publisher of this book are NOT RESPONSIBLE in any manner whatsoever for any
injury or negative effects that may occur through following the instructions and
advice contained herein.

It is recommended that before beginning any treatment or exercise program, you
consult your medical professional to determine whether you should undertake this
course of practice.

The use of 《these brackets》 in Chinese text denotes a book title.

Printed in Canada

I dedicate this book to my mother, Ms. Xie-Jin, Yang
(楊謝盡女士). Without her, I would not be able to offer
this book to you. Without her love and education,
I would not have reached the level of understanding
about life that I have today.

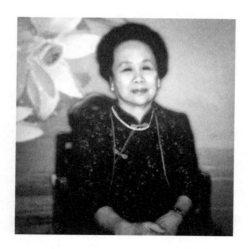

Table of Contents

Dao Jing (Dao Classic)—Chapter 1 to 37

Foreword

Thomas G. Gutheil, MD

When the mind is steady, then you can acquire calmness. When you are calm, then you find peace. When you are at peace, then you are able to ponder. When you are able to ponder, then you gain. All objects have their initiation and termination, and all matters have a beginning and expiration. If one knows the beginning and the end, then one is closer to the Dao.

—Li Ji

I am deeply honored by the invitation to write this preface to Dr. Yang's meticulously crafted book; yet I am also humbled by the task of trying to introduce a work of such depth and complexity. Some time ago, in the twenty years or so during which I had the exhilarating experience of studying Shaolin Gongfu under his tutelage, I gradually discovered his interests in Eastern scholarship beyond the practical martial arts. One of the fruits of that scholarship is before you now. Be sure, however, that the connections and associations I derive are entirely my own, as are any errors or misunderstandings.

Dr. Yang appropriately begins with, and repeatedly addresses, the obstacles that both Eastern and Western readers encounter in grappling with the concepts in this book. He outlines the various levels of obstacles. First, in attempting to deal with ancient texts there are challenges of meaning, especially given the inherent redundancy of much of the Chinese language, where the same character or word may have different meanings based on context and tone. Second, there is the Chinese cultural worldview, which must affect this discussion. Third is the use of metaphor and analogy—what Western readers perceive as a colorful language not usually used to discuss serious principles, where anatomic/physical and symbolic usages coexist comfortably. For example, water is used as an image of desirable humility: water humbly reaches the lowest level (we say "water seeks its own level") without complaint. Indeed, this preface is intended as a first step in surmounting those same obstacles by attempting to place these traditional ideas in a modern context accessible to today's readers.

Finally, there is the use of paradoxes; for example, *wuwei* can be translated as "the doing of not doing." Somewhat similar to the *koan* in Buddhist thought, the paradox forces the reader's mind into a new channel. In this connection, martial arts students may recall Bruce Lee's description of his art in *Enter the Dragon* as "fighting without fighting." Paradoxically as well, the purpose of study, concentration, and effort is to achieve "emptiness" that can be filled by new ideas and to recover the innocence of childhood. Elsewhere in this text, reference is made to a "semisleeping" state, itself a parallel to Buddhist themes such as zazen meditation.

Understanding the Dao is certainly made challenging in itself, since it is described as without shape and color—indeed, without explicit or concrete description. It thus resembles—in its formlessness and ubiquitous permeation of all things—God, Nature, and even "the Force" used by the Jedi in the Star Wars universe. Lest readers feel this is far-fetched, Dr. Yang observes later in this book: "Dao is always in a state of high alertness so it can sense any disorder in this universe and respond to the changes." Note how this closely parallels the notion of a "disturbance in the Force." The "De"—the manifest universe—is described as an expression of the Dao.

One of the ways in which Dr. Yang takes on the challenges noted above is by frequently quoting other authors and scholars as they comment on the same material; this is helpful to the student, since reading any one description of a subject may confuse a reader, but other phrasings, other images, may clarify the point.

Dr. Yang ranges freely among such relatively familiar concepts as qi, body meridians, the *Yi Jing*, yin and yang, and the third eye. More expansively, he relates those basics to such widely separated fields as scientific research into the tiny particles composing matter and the theory of the subconscious, most elaborately introduced in Europe by Dr. Sigmund Freud. In fact, Dr. Yang calls on his audience to develop a scientific approach to spirit, and professes no conflict between these two ideas.

One important concept about the Dao, among many, is the generalization from the person's self (a "small universe") and the person's body, to the family, then to the natural world at large and to governments; this potential application is captured by the familiar expression, "the body politic." Running through the discussion is the notion of achieving a calm and peaceful mind by using the "wisdom mind" to govern the "emotional mind"—to achieve, among other goals, a union of body and spirit and a deep connection to the natural world. The wuji state, described as neutral mind without thoughts, echoes modern conceptions of meditation and mindfulness: a personal peace should lead eventually to a society at peace.

How does the health practice called qigong apply to these ideas? In chapter 13, Dr. Yang summarizes with a military metaphor:

Qigong practice can be compared to a battle against sickness and aging. If you compare your body to a battlefield, then your mind is like the general who generates ideas and controls the situation, and your breathing is his strategy. Your qi is like the soldiers who are led to various places on the battlefield. Your essence is like the quality of the soldiers, such as educational background and the skills of combat, etc. Finally, your spirit is the morale of the army.

This paragraph captures and summarizes the unity among the themes described in this book—themes such as the concept of qi, the central importance of breathing and the centrality of notions about spirit.

Because this book is highly detailed, it requires close attention, but the repetitions and clarifications make understanding easier for the serious student. This book joins a series from Dr. Yang, which, in all, make available to the Western reader some of the most important elements of Eastern thought, including lost documents otherwise unavailable.

Dr. Thomas G. Gutheil
Harvard Medical School
January 1, 2017

Foreword

Mr. Charles Green

For a student of life, there is perhaps no single better text—certainly of its length—than the *Dao De Jing*. Its simplicity contrasts simultaneously with its profundity, two sides of an infinitely valuable coin. As with all great works of human civilization, we can return again and again to contemplate it during our lives, gaining new insights into ourselves and the world around us each time. This is because it shares—as best as it can, within the constraints of the construct of human language—universal truths about the nature of existence and our place in it, as seen from an ancient yet ever-fresh perspective.

This new work by Dr. Yang, Jwing-Ming is a considered and humble—yet at the same time bold—attempt to add yet another layer of profundity to our understanding of Lao Zi's ancient classic, being a systematic treatment of its relevance for meditation and qigong. For Western minds unaccustomed to traditional Chinese methods of layering multiple meanings in arts and practice, this may appear to be a somewhat radical reinterpretation of the original work. It is more correct, however, to see it as revealing yet another layer of understanding of the root of Daoist practices, which holistically consider a person and their place within the universe, rather than focusing on individual acts in isolation from the greater picture. Indeed, a fundamental point of qigong meditation and practice is to align ourselves better with the natural way or direction (Dao) of the universe, essentially by definition the healthiest path available for both body and mind.

Even a surface treatment of the basic concepts contained in the *Dao De Jing* can bring rewards to a practitioner of life. Above all, the idea that some of the deepest truth and understanding we can obtain is fundamentally experiential in nature, rather than to be found in a fixed set of "facts"—a very modern lesson, as we are forced to revise our understanding of the world periodically with new developments across all of the sciences. The notion of the experiential layer of life as being most profound plays directly into Dr. Yang's deep investigation of the original text's relevance for mental, spiritual, and physical health practices, many of which are expressed primarily internally and rely upon our mind's direction. These practices, if followed consistently, could be considered a lifestyle; however, they go beyond that and also encompass one's basic orientation toward the universe, as part of the more mundane actions of daily life. Again, this parallels modern concepts of the central importance of our personal attitude toward life and how the *quality* of our thinking can have a profound impact on everything from our physical health to the success we are likely to have in life.

I am honored to be able to write these words, not as a master of Daoist philosophy and history, but from the perspective of a perpetual student who seeks to make what progress he can at life's arts. Reading, contemplating, and practicing (however imperfectly) Dr. Yang's other works on taijiquan and qigong theory and practice have led to significant positive changes in my own life over the past twelve years. This includes being able to rely on qigong practice instead of prescription medication to successfully control hypertension, a condition that surfaced at a relatively young age for me after the experience of serving my country in a time of war. Perhaps even more important, however, has been the integration of multilayered practices that encourage—in reality, require—one to adopt a centered, calm contemplation of events in the perpetual present, which is the only time that we can truly experience between the past and future. It is in such contemplation of events that we are able to discern the Dao and move more easily with its current, rather than attempting to paddle upstream. In that spirit, I look forward to further contemplation of this new work, as a treasure that can be inexhaustibly mined over a lifetime.

Charles Green
January 31, 2017

Foreword

Dr. Robert J. Woodbine

I first met Dr. Yang, Jwing-Ming sixteen years ago in New York City when he taught a qigong workshop at the Open Center. I had recently returned to New York after devoting the previous eight years in Portland, Oregon, to earning my doctorate in naturopathic medicine and masters in Chinese medicine and acupuncture. Having studied and practiced qigong with a variety of qigong and taiji teachers since 1985, it was propitious that Dr. Yang was teaching in New York and I was able to attend his workshop since he was headquartered in Massachusetts at the time.

I found him to be quite knowledgeable, competent, straightforward, and, most importantly, genuinely humble. I chose to study with him and made the biannual treks to Massachusetts to attend his weekend workshops from 2001 through 2007. I would bring along the students I taught so they could experience the wealth of knowledge Dr. Yang offered. In that brief period of time, I observed another admirable character trait—his ardent commitment to truth and clarity.

As an example, when I first learned the taijiquan long form sequence from Dr. Yang and his senior students, the single whip pattern was executed a particular way. Over the years, this was modified and refined, not whimsically, but rather because of Dr. Yang's ceaseless devotion to pondering the deeper meaning of form and application. To him, taijiquan is a living art with an inherent responsibility between teacher and student to adhere to its principles as a living foundation from which to understand and create credible refinements. His commitment to the truth and his ability to change speaks highly of his personal integrity and moral character.

In the world of martial arts and healing, Dr. Yang, Jwing-Ming is highly respected and regarded. His body of work is voluminous. He is a prolific writer, publisher, and producer of books and DVDs regarding the theories and practical applications of Shaolin, White Crane, taijiquan, and qigong. With over fifty-five years of experience in his field,

Dr. Yang has numerous Yang Martial Arts Association (YMAA) schools in various countries throughout the world. His most recent achievement is the creation of the YMAA Retreat Center in the mountains of Northern California to preserve and disseminate the traditional training methods of Chinese martial arts and culture.

Throughout the history of mankind and in every culture, there have been those rare individuals who are compelled to be of service to the rest of us. They have no choice in the matter, as this is an internal calling they are driven to fulfill. As a trained physicist, Dr. Yang's keen intellect and heightened curiosity have driven him to translate the Chinese qigong and taijiquan classics, not for his personal gain, but to share these insights with the world to uplift humanity. This unique interpretation of the classic *Dao De Jing* through the lens of qigong is Dr. Yang's offering to mankind.

Man's inhumanity to man throughout recorded history is nothing new, unfortunately. However, what seems unique to me about our modern culture is the accelerated and pervasive pace at which we seem to be disconnected not just from nature, but from one another. I believe the pendulum has swung quite far in the direction of materialism and consumerism to the extent that there is a profound hollowing out of the spirit. This empty space cannot be fulfilled with what we can acquire or consume.

Dr. Yang's qigong interpretation of the *Dao De Jing* is an answer to contemplate, digest, and then execute. Its power is in the repeated simplicity of Lao Zi's words throughout the eighty-one chapters of the *Dao De Jing*. Its gift is in the clear method (embryonic breathing) that Dr. Yang shares with the reader. He provides a key with which to unlock the pantry to nourish that hollow space and learn to once again commune with nature and each other truthfully and honestly.

For me, qigong training is an invaluable means by which to consciously cultivate one's body, mind, and spirit while promoting self-reliance and self-sufficiency. Far too often, it was my clinical experience with patients that the root of their chronic ailments rested in unresolved emotional tensions and an inculcated adherence to dependency models with healthcare providers. The notion that much of the healing they sought was within and not external to themselves was often foreign but empowering.

The uniqueness and value of Dr. Yang's interpretation of the *Dao De Jing* is that it provides a formulary through which one can be in the world but not of it. Through embryonic breathing meditation, one can gradually quiet the conscious mind and its imbalanced focus on the material world. His thesis that, through embryonic breathing meditation, one can gradually cultivate the awakening of the subconscious mind and its association with the Source of all that exists, is reasonable. What remains for you to consider is doing the practice. As an African proverb states, "First you pray to God, but then you move your feet."

Dr. Robert J. Woodbine
Miranda, California
January 20, 2017

Preface

I have worked on an interpretation of the *Dao De Jing* from a qigong point of view for the last twenty years, and it has been a challenge. I encountered many difficulties and obstacles, and I think it would be helpful to your understanding if you were aware of these issues.

1. **I am afraid my understanding of qigong is still too shallow to be qualified to interpret the Dao De Jing.** I have studied and practiced qigong for more than fifty-four years (since I was sixteen) as of this writing. Despite my years of training and research, I believe my understanding of qigong is still shallow. Nonetheless I think it is important to begin a discussion of the *Dao De Jing* using the qigong theories I feel are the basis of this treatise.

2. **The Dao De Jing was written two thousand five hundred years ago.** Ancient writing is very different from today's writing. In order to interpret this ancient classic, one must know ancient Chinese literature at a profound level. It takes time and energy, study and research in order to begin to understand the meaning of every word.

3. **It is difficult to translate this ancient Chinese language into English without losing some of the meaning.** There are many Chinese words that are difficult to translate into English. The Chinese cultural background is so different from the Western, and the feeling developed from these different backgrounds generates different modes of language and meaning. This difference makes it a challenge to find a correct and exact equivalent English word that adequately conveys the original feeling of the word being translated.

4. **Often, the exact same Chinese character will have several different meanings.** Quite often, a Chinese word has different meanings, depending on where you place

it, how you pronounce it, and how you use it. Whoever interprets the word must consider which meaning to choose based on the context.

5. **Many spiritual qigong terms are hard to translate.** It is often difficult to find the English equivalent for many qigong terms. This is especially true for the *Dao De Jing* since most of it was written from a spiritual viewpoint, often centered on feeling, that is still beyond our current western scientific point of view and understanding. The human science we have developed is still in its infancy, especially in the spiritual sciences. Thus, we cannot yet use our limited science to verify or interpret the existence or phenomena of the spiritual world.

6. **Lack of the same feeling as Lao Zi.** To interpret the *Dao De Jing* accurately, I need to have the same feeling as Lao Zi, the root of his spirit, and this is nearly impossible. I spent countless hours reading, pondering, and meditating, reaching into his feeling to perceive his original meaning and yet I am still concerned about my interpretation. Although many past scholars have interpreted the *Dao De Jing*, most were not qigong practitioners and, unfortunately, they interpreted the *Dao De Jing* from a scholarly point of view. Naturally, though these ancient interpretations have provided us some level of understanding, it is not deep and clear enough, and is missing a qigong perspective. I have found only one book, *Dao De Jing and Qigong*, that tried to interpret the *Dao De Jing* from a qigong point of view.[1] Unfortunately, this book only interprets some chapters that are obviously related to qigong practice.

There is a story about Confucius learning zither from Shi, Xiang-Zi (師襄子)[2]: Shi, Xiang-Zi taught Confucius to play a piece of music on the zither. After learning the piece of music for a period of time, Shi, Xiang-Zi said to Confucius: "You have now learned this piece of music; today you are ready to advance to another piece of music." Confucius replied: "But I have not yet mastered the skills of this music."

After a period of time, Shi, Xiang-Zi said: "Now, you have mastered the skills of this music; you may advance to another." Confucius replied: "But I have not grasped the feeling of the music yet." Again, after a period of time, Confucius was able to play the music with deep feeling. Shi, Xiang-Zi again said: "Now, you are able play the music with feeling; you may advance to another." However, Confucius said: "But, I still don't know the composer's feeling yet." Confucius continued his practice and put his feeling into the composer's feeling. After a period of time, with profound thought, Confucius experienced an epiphany, as if he stood on the high ground and gazed far ahead, and said: "Now, I know who the composer of this music is. This person has dark skin and a tall body, with a wide-open heart and farsighted vision that is able to spread everywhere. If this was not composed by King Wen (文王), who else was able to do so?" Shi, Xiang-Zi left his seat, stood up, saluted Confucius, and said: "The gentleman you are talking about is a sage. This music was passed from him to us, called 'King Wen's Practice.'"

This story illustrates my point. In order to have a perfectly accurate interpretation of the *Dao De Jing*, one needs to have the same feeling and spiritual cultivation as Lao Zi. Naturally, this is improbable. In this book, I have tried my best to interpret it through my understanding and feeling. Please keep your mind open and question everything I have said.

Dr. Yang, Jwing-Ming
YMAA CA Retreat Center
May 1st, 2016

1. 《道德經與氣功》，丁辛百、潘明環編著。安徽科學技術出版社，1996. Ding Xin Bai and Pan Minghuan, *Dao De Jing and Qigong* (Fengyang, China: Anhui Science and Technology Press, 1996).

2. 孔子學琴於師襄子，襄子曰：「吾雖以擊磬為官，然能於琴。今子於琴已習，可以益矣。」孔子曰：「丘未得其數也。」有間，曰：「已習其數，可以益矣。」孔子曰：「丘未得其志也。」有間，曰：「已習其志，可以益矣。」孔子曰：「丘未得其為人也。」有間，孔子有所謬然思焉，有所睪然高望而遠眺。曰：「丘迨得其為人矣。近黮而黑，頎然長，曠如望羊，奄有四方，非文王其孰能為此？」師襄子避席葉拱而對曰：「君子，聖人也，其傳曰《文王操》。」（《孔子家語·辨樂解第三十五》）

About Lao Zi (Lao Tzu)

老子生平

The details of Lao Zi's personal life are a mystery, though there are many legends about him. The most reliable biography about him appears in "History Record" (史記) by historian Si, Ma-Qian (司馬遷) (154–90 BCE) during the West Han (西漢) Dynasty (202–8 BCE).

Lao Zi was born in the sixth century BCE during the Chinese Spring and Autumn Period (春秋) (770–476 BCE) in the Ku county (苦縣) of the state of Chu (楚). His birth name is Li Er (李耳) and he had several nicknames such as Bo Yang (伯陽), Lao Dan (老聃), and Chong Er (重耳).

He worked as a curator of the library (守藏史) at the capital (Luo Yi, 洛邑) of East Zhou's (東周) royal court. Confucius went to see him to ask about proprieties in the ninth year of Lu Ding Gong (Duke Ding of Lu) (魯定公九年) (周敬王十九年) (501 BCE). Confucius was fifty-one years old at that time. After he left Zhou, Confucius told his students: "Birds, I know they can fly. Fish, I know they can swim. Animals, I know they can walk. Those that walk can be caught by traps. Those that swim can be captured by fishing thread. Those that fly can be seized by arrows. As to dragons, I don't know how to handle them since they are able to fly to the sky following the wind and clouds. Lao Zi, whom I saw today, isn't he just like a dragon?"[1]

Later, when the Zhou dynasty was on the verge of collapse, Lao Zi decided to embark on a voyage to the west. As he traveled to the Hangu Pass (函谷關) to enter the state of Qin (秦), he met the guardian of the pass (the official in charge of the border), Yin, Xi (尹喜), who came to admire him. At the request of Yin, Xi, Lao Zi wrote down his teachings, which became the *Dao De Jing*. After he finished, legend has it he rode away on a green bull and was never seen again.

When did he die or how long did he live? No one knows. We only have legends. Some say he lived more than 160 years and others say more than 200.

Whatever the details may be, it is undeniable that the *Dao De Jing* has influenced Chinese culture and philosophy for more than two thousand years. His main philosophy about life cultivation that he shared with the rulers of the era emphasizes wuwei (doing nothing). In qigong training, he is the first ancestor and creator of scholar Daoism who advocated the dual cultivation of the physical body and the temperament.[2] He promoted the importance of being natural and adhering to the Dao. He emphasized keeping the mind in an "insubstantial" state (a higher spiritual state, with the consciousness focused at the third eye) and the body in a serene and calm state.

1. 孔子去，謂弟子曰："鳥，吾知其能飛；魚吾知其能游；獸吾知其能走。走者可以為罔，游者可以為綸，飛者可以為矰。至於龍，吾不能知其乘風雲而上天。吾今日見老子，其猶龍邪！"
2. "性命雙修。"

Introduction/Foundation

The *Dao De Jing* (《道德經》) was written from Lao Zi's (老子) personal understanding of the Dao (道) and the De (德). For this reason, it is important to understand the influences that shaped his point of view. In order to know Lao Zi's motivation in writing the *Dao De Jing*, you need to put yourself in his place during China's long warring period (Chun Qiu Zhan Guo, 春秋戰國) (770–221 BCE). Many kingdoms with various rulers with corrupt officers had occupied all of China. This caused people immeasurable suffering and pain; society was in chaos.

Think about his situation. Since Lao Zi was not a ruler at that time, how was he able to share his opinions or experience with rulers about how to rule a country? Was most of his writing from his imagination or based only on his personal understanding? How was he able to acquire those concepts or knowledge for his writing?

Many chapters in the *Dao De Jing* are purely about qigong, especially the practices of regulating the body (tiao shen, 調身), regulating the breathing (tiao xi, 調息), regulating the mind (tiao xin, 調心), regulating the qi (tiao qi, 調氣), and regulating the spirit (tiao shen, 調神). Therefore, in order to understand these chapters, you should have the foundation of a basic understanding of qigong.

I have summarized those basic concepts in this introduction section. This introduction/foundation will be divided into four parts: "Preliminaries," "Foundations—Basic Understanding," "About the *Dao De Jing*," and "*Dao De Jing* and Humanity's Future." I believe these concepts will help you understand my point of view in interpreting the *Dao De Jing* from a qigong perspective.

Preliminaries

1. Lao Zi was born Chinese and grew up with a Chinese cultural influence. No human artifact can be understood

apart from its cultural background. Therefore, in order to interpret and understand the *Dao De Jing* clearly, you must also have a clear idea of Chinese culture. Without a solid understanding of Chinese concepts, one's understanding of the *Dao De Jing* will be shallow and vague. Naturally, if one uses a non-Chinese cultural background to interpret the *Dao De Jing*, the accuracy of the interpretation will be questionable.

2. When the *Dao De Jing* was written by Lao Zi about two thousand five hundred years ago (476–221 BCE), *The Book of Changes* (《*Yi Jing*, 易經》) had already existed for at least seven hundred years. *The Book of Changes* has been considered the preeminent document of all ancient Chinese classics (Qun Jing Zhi Shou, 群經之首) (The Leader of All Classics) in Chinese history and since then has influenced Chinese culture heavily. Naturally, Lao Zi's mind was also influenced by this classic. Therefore, it is important to understand the basic concepts from *The Book of Changes* of how the yin and yang spaces (yin jian/yang jian, 陰間/陽間) are coexisting and related to each other. Without knowing these basic concepts, you will have difficulty in understanding some of the chapters.

3. Lao Zi was not a politician. He was appointed to the office of shi (zhou chao shou zang shi, 周朝守藏史) (historian) at the royal court of the Zhou dynasty (c. 1046–256 BCE). The shi were scholars specializing in matters such as astrology and divination and also were in charge of sacred books. It is likely Lao Zi had no experience in governing or ruling a country. Therefore, all his writings about the way of governing the countries for those rulers or monarchs were based on his personal understanding through his inner cultivation.

4. From the *Dao De Jing*, it is obvious Lao Zi was a qigong practitioner, a sage, a philosopher, and a teacher who comprehended life and achieved a profound level of

spiritual cultivation. The *Dao De Jing* was written based on Lao Zi's personal understanding about the Dao and the De through his personal qigong practice, especially spiritual cultivation. Since the Dao of managing the body is similar to the Dao of managing a country, Lao Zi was able to incorporate his understanding into his writing that offered moral guidance to historical Chinese rulers. This is because once you have comprehended and mastered the principles and natural rules of the Dao, you will be able to apply them to other fields without too much difficulty. Confucius also said: "My Dao, use the one to thread through (i.e., comprehend) others."[1] This can be seen clearly in chapter 54 of *Dao De Jing*. In this chapter, Lao Zi applied the same Dao for self-cultivation, family, village, nation, and the world. It is recognized that although the theory and the rules of the Dao are simple, they are very difficult to understand and follow.

5. In qigong history, many new qigong theories and practices were developed after Lao Zi. In my twenty years of analyzing and studying the *Dao De Jing* I feel there is no doubt that some of these new developments were derived or influenced from the *Dao De Jing*. For example, there were not many documents on embryonic breathing qigong practice before Lao Zi. Of the more than 150 documents about embryonic breathing meditation written after Lao Zi wrote the *Dao De Jing*, most of the discussions in these documents follow the same theory and practice of the *Dao De Jing*.

6. The Great Nature has simple rules, and from these rules, myriad objects are born, raised, nourished, and then perish. If we follow the rules, we will be able to cultivate our lives within the rules and maintain our health and extend our lives. From following the Dao and the De, we are able to comprehend the meaning of life.

7. Before reading the *Dao De Jing*, first recognize that scholar Dao (Dao xue, 道學) is not religious Dao (Dao jiao, 道教). Scholar Dao is the study of the Dao's philosophy from the *Dao De Jing* written by Lao Zi. Later, during Eastern Han Dynasty (Dong Han, 東漢) (25–220 CE), Zhang, Dao-Ling (張道陵) combined the Daoist and Buddhist philosophies together and created a religious Dao. Therefore, when we study Daoism, we should distinguish the differences between scholar Daoism and religious Daoism.

Foundations—Basic Understanding

1. There is no correct way or perfect set of words to translate the Dao into any language. Even in Chinese society, the Dao remains a mystery and cannot be defined. The Dao is the way of Nature. All we know is that the Dao created all objects in this Nature. Although we don't know the Dao, and cannot see, hear, or touch it, all of us can feel it and know it exists. It may be equivalent to the ideas of God defined by the Western world. When the Dao is manifested, it is the world we see and is called the De. Thus, the De is the manifestation of the Dao.

2. *The Book of Changes* (Yi Jing, 《易經》) describes this Great Nature as having two polarities that balance each other. Though there are two polarities, these two are two faces of the same thing. These two polarities are two spaces or dimensions, called yin space (yin jian, 陰間) and yang space (yang jian, 陽間). Yin space is the spiritual space while yang space is the material space. Yin space is the Dao (道) while the yang space, the manifestation of the Dao, is the De (德). These two cannot be separated and coexist simultaneously. They mutually communicate, correspond, and influence each

other. Therefore, there are two spaces, but in function, they are one. The spiritual energy of the yin space can be considered the mother (female) of myriad objects in the yang space. Since humans, as well as all other entities, are formed and generated from these two spaces, a human being includes both a spiritual and material life. Since we don't actually know what the Dao (i.e., Natural Spirit) is, we also don't know what the human spirit is.

3. The Chinese have always considered the Great Nature to be the "grand universe" or "grand nature" (da tian di, 大天地). In this grand universe, all lives are considered as cells of this universe and are all recycling. Since we, humans, are formed and produced in this Grand Universe, we will naturally copy the same energy pattern or structure. The human body is considered as a small universe or small nature (xiao tian di, 小天地). The head is the heaven (tian ling gai, 天靈蓋) and the perineum is the sea bottom (hai di, 海底). All the cells in our bodies are recycling. In the grand universe, the Dao or the natural spirit is the master. In the small universe, the human spirit (related to our minds) is the master of life. This human spirit is considered as the Dao while the physical manifestation or actions are the De. The Chinese word for morality is "Dao-De" (道德) reflecting that in Chinese culture morality is considered to be related to thinking and behavior.

4. There are two kinds of mind in the human body. The emotional mind is called xin (心) (heart). It is also called heart since it is believed that the heart is related to our emotions. The other is called yi (意) (wisdom mind) and is rational, logical, calm, and wise. In Chinese society, it is said that xin is like a monkey and the yi is like a horse (xin yuan yi ma, 心猿意馬). This is because the emotional mind is just like a monkey: not powerful, but annoying and disturbing. The wisdom mind, by

contrast, is like a horse: powerful, calm, steady, and controllable. Thus, in qigong cultivation, a practitioner will learn how to use the wisdom mind to govern the emotional mind.

5. There are, again, two other different categories of the mind, the conscious mind (yi shi, 意識) and the subconscious mind (qian yi shi, 潛意識). The conscious mind is generated from brain cells located at the cerebrum while the subconscious mind is generated from the limbic system at the center of the head. The conscious mind thinks and has memory while the subconscious does not think but has memory. The conscious mind is related to the type of thoughts and behavior humans typically exhibit after they're born and socialized: emotional, playing tricks, and not truthful. The subconscious mind is related to the natural instinct that we are born with and is more truthful. We live in a duplicitous society, and we all lie and have a mask on our face. From a Chinese qigong understanding, it is believed that the spirit resides at the limbic system and connects to our subconscious mind. The limbic system is called the "spirit dwelling" (shen shi, 神室) or Mud Pill Palace (Ni Wan Gong, 泥丸宮) in Chinese qigong society. It is believed that, in order to reconnect with the natural spirit, we must downplay our conscious mind to allow the subconscious mind to wake up and grow. In order to reconnect to the natural spirit, we must reopen our third eye. The third eye is called "heaven eye" (tian yan/tian mu, 天眼／天目), and through it we are able to connect with Nature (figure I-1).

6. Western science explains there are two polarities in the human body. Each single cell has two polarities and a human's growth is completed through cell division (mitosis) from a single cell. Scientists have also confirmed that we have two brains, one in the head and

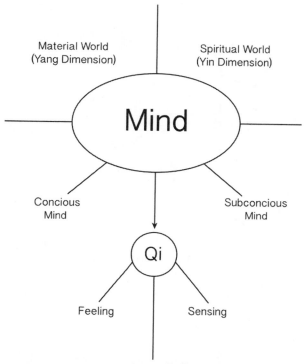

Figure I-1. Yin/Yang Worlds and Mind

the other in the guts. The top brain housed in the skull thinks and has memory, and the lower brain has memory but does not think. These two brains are connected through the spinal cord. Highly conductive tissues construct the spinal cord, and there is no signal delay between the two brains. Therefore, while there are two brains physically, actually, they are only one in function since they synchronize with each other simultaneously (figure I-2). In Chinese qigong, the upper brain is considered as the upper dan tian (shang dan tian, 上丹田) (upper elixir field) while the lower brain located at the center of gravity is considered as the real lower dan tian (zhen xia dan tian, 真下丹田) (real lower elixir field). Elixir means the qi that is able to extend life. These two

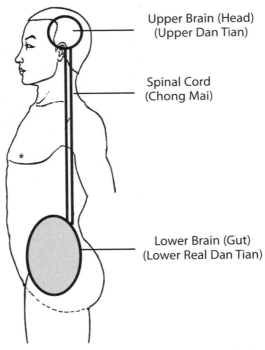

Upper Brain (Head)
(Upper Dan Tian)

Spinal Cord
(Chong Mai)

Lower Brain (Gut)
(Lower Real Dan Tian)

Figure I-2. Two Polarities (Brains) of a Human Body

places are considered as fields since they are able to store and produce qi. The spinal cord is called "thrusting vessel" (chong mai, 衝脈) in Chinese medicine since the qi can thrust through without delay.

7. To begin to understand qigong, you must first know about the human body's qi network. According to Chinese medicine, the body has twelve primary qi channels (i.e. meridians) (shi er jing, 十二經), countless secondary qi channels (luo, 絡), eight vessels (ba mai, 八脈), and one real dan tian (zhen dan tian, 真丹田). The twelve primary channels are likened to twelve main rivers that circulate the qi to the entire body while those secondary channels are considered as streams that branch out from the rivers so the qi can be distributed everywhere in the body. The eight vessels are the qi

reservoirs (qi ba, 氣壩) like lakes, swamps, or dams that accumulate the qi and regulate the qi's quantity in the rivers. The real dan tian is where the battery of the qi is. It produces and stores the qi to abundant levels. The real dan tian is situated at the center of gravity (guts) and is called "qi residence" (qi she, 氣舍). If you are interested in knowing more about the twelve channels and their functions, you should refer to Chinese medical books. Due to limited space here, we will not discuss this further.

8. Another important part of the qi network is the eight vessels. They include four pairs of yin-yang corresponding vessels. That means there are four yin vessels and four yang vessels. The conception vessel (yin vessel) (ren mai, 任脈) runs from the mouth area down the front side of the torso to the perineum where it connects to the governing vessel (yang vessel) (du mai, 督脈). The governing vessel runs upward from the perineum along the center of the back, passing the crown and finally connects with the conception vessel at the mouth area (figures I-3 to I-8). The conception vessel is responsible for the qi's status of the six yin primary channels while the governing vessel governs the qi's condition of the six yang primary channels. There is one vessel that connects the upper brain or upper dan tian to the lower brain or real dan tian. This vessel is the thrusting vessel (chong mai, 衝脈) (spinal cord). This vessel is the most yin among the eight vessels. This vessel corresponds with the most yang vessel among the eight, the girdle vessel (dai mai, 帶脈). Each of the above four vessels exists singularly. There are two pairs of vessels that run through each of the legs, yin heel (yin qiao mai, 陰蹻脈) and yin linking (yin wei mai, 陰維脈) vessels and yang heel (yang qiao mai, 陽蹻脈) and yang linking (yang wei mai, 陽維脈) vessels.

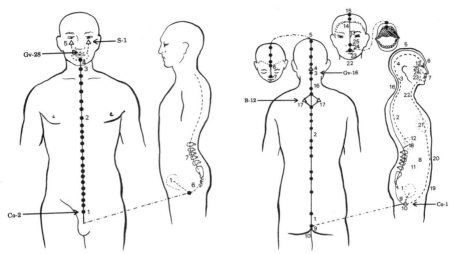

Figure I-3. The Conception Vessel (Ren Mai)

Figure I-4. The Governing Vessel (Du Mai)

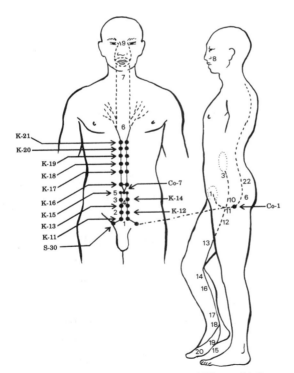

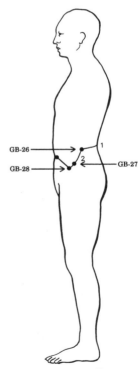

Figure I-5. The Thrusting Vessel (Chong Mai)

Figure I-6. The Girdle Vessel
(Dai Mai)

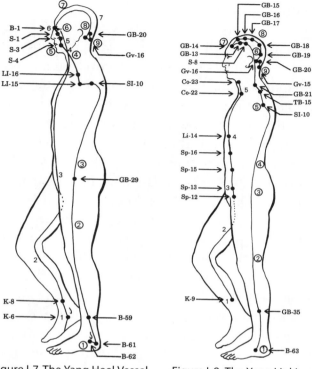

Figure I-7. The Yang Heel Vessel
(Yangqiao Mai) and the Yin Heel
Vessel (Yinqiao Mai)

Figure I-8. The Yang Linking
Vessel (Yangwei Mai) and
the Yin Linking Vessel
(Yinwei Mai)

9. The conception and governing vessels regulate the status of the qi in the twelve primary qi channels. The yin
heel and yin linking and also the yang heel and yang
linking vessels supply and regulate the qi to the legs.
The thrusting vessel connects two polarities, the spiritual center and physical center. The girdle vessel
enhances the qi on the skin, called guardian qi (wei qi,
衛氣) to maintain the strength of the immune system.
The real lower dan tian builds up and stores the qi and
functions as a battery. From this battery, all eight vessels
(reservoirs) receive qi.

10. When the qi storage at the real dan tian is abundant, the qi in the girdle vessel is also abundant. Therefore, the guardian qi will be strong, making the functioning of the immune system more effective. From this, we can see the function of the girdle vessel (extreme yang) is to manifest the qi so the physical body can be strong. When the qi is led upward to nourish the brain (upper dan tian) from the real dan tian, more brain cells will be activated and the functioning of the brain cells will be improved. Through embryonic breathing meditation, the qi stored at the brain can be focused at the spiritual residence (limbic system) and then led forward through the spiritual valley (space between two lobes of the brain) to reopen the third eye. The thrusting vessel keeps your mental and physical body at the centerline while the girdle vessel expands qi horizontally to maintain your mental and physical balance. When you are centered, you have balance and when you have balance, you will be centered. That is why the thrusting vessel and girdle vessel, though they are two physically, in function are actually only one. Together they build a so-called "spiritual triangle" (figure I-9). When the qi in your real dan tian is abundant, your guardian qi will be able to expand further, your immune system will be stronger, and you will be more balanced and stronger physically. Consequently, your physical life will be strong. Furthermore, if you lead the qi up to activate more brain cells and know how to focus the qi forward, you may reopen the third eye so you are able to reconnect with the natural spirit. This is the stage of "unification of heaven and human" (tian ren he yi, 天人合一).

11. In order to reopen the third eye, you will need a great amount of qi to activate more of your brain cells. You will also need to know how to focus the qi like a lens

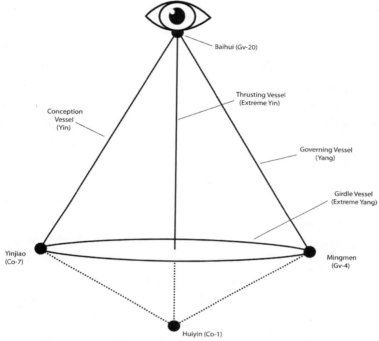

Figure I-9. Spiritual Triangle

collecting sunbeams. When this focused beam of strong qi is led forward, the third eye can be reopened. The way to achieve these goals is through embryonic breathing meditation. From this practice, you learn how to embrace singularity (bao yi, 抱一) (shou yi, 守一). This is mentioned twice in the *Dao De Jing* (chapters 10 and 22) and discussed many times in the ancient documents about the *Dao De Jing*.

12. There are two goals of embryonic breathing practice. One is learning to produce more qi and conserve the qi's consumption so the qi can be stored at an abundant level. The other is to cultivate the mind and learn to lead the qi from brain cells to the limbic system (spiritual residence). In order to do this, you must be calm and downplay your conscious mind. Through correct

breathing techniques, the qi trapped in the brain cells can be led to the center of the head, the limbic system (figure I-10). This will allow you to focus the qi and condense it to a very strong level. Without these two elements—quantity of qi and quality of qi's manifestation—your third eye will not be reopened.

13. There are four stages of spiritual cultivation: self-recognition (zi shi, 自識), self-awareness (zi jue, 自覺), self-awakening (zi wu/zi xing, 自悟／自醒), and freeing your spirit from spiritual bondage (jie tuo, 解脫). The first step is to remove the mask on your face and recognize who and what you really are. This is the stage of facing the truth about yourself. The second step is to be aware of your position or role as a human being in this world and the environment around you. The third step is to awaken your spirit through pondering and feeling. The final step is to set yourself free from spiritual bondage. In order to have eternal spiritual life (unification of heaven and human), we have to set ourselves free from all bondage, especially those spiritual dogmas that have

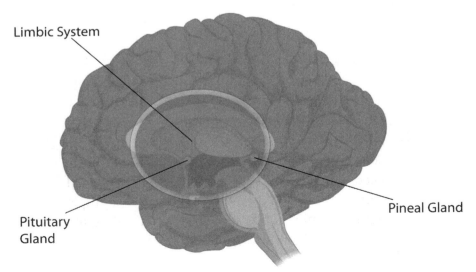

Figure I-10. Limbic System

been established in human history and also those human emotions that continue to hinder and affect our spiritual growth.

About the *Dao De Jing*

1. The *Dao De Jing* is also referred to as the *Lao Zi*. It has been interpreted mostly by scholars instead of qigong practitioners. However, it is evident that the entire book was written based on Lao Zi's personal qigong experience, especially spiritual cultivation. In order to acquire the real essence of the *Dao De Jing*, we must interpret it from a qigong point of view. Only then we will see the origin of Lao Zi's thinking. Since the Dao of managing the body and spirit is the same as managing a country, Lao Zi was able to use his understanding and experience and apply them to the governing of a country. This is because the principles and rules of the Dao remains the same when it is used for self-cultivation (xiu shen, 修身), managing a family (qi jia, 齊家), ruling a country (zhi guo, 治國), or harmonizing the world (ping tian-xia, 平天下).

2. In qigong, we talk about the five regulatings (wu tiao, 五調) that include: regulating the body (tiao shen, 調身), regulating the breathing (tiao xi, 調息), regulating the emotional mind (tiao xin, 調心), regulating the qi (tiao qi, 調氣), and finally, regulating the spirit (tiao shen, 調神). Breathing is considered to be a strategy in qigong practice. When the breathing is correct, the qi can be regulated smoothly. When we apply these qigong self-cultivation principles to other fields—for example, managing a family, ruling a country, or engaging in a battle—we can compare them as follows:

Qigong (修身)	Managing Family (齊家)	Ruling Country (治國)	Battle (作戰)
Body (身)	Homestead (家園)	Country (國家)	Battlefield (戰場)
Breathing (息)	Budget (財經)	Policies (政策)	Strategies (戰略)
Mind (心)	Head of Household (家長)	Monarch (君主)	Commander (主帥)
Qi (氣)	Family Members (家員)	People (百姓)	Soldiers (士兵)
Spirit (神)	Love (慈愛)	Moralities (民氣)	Morale (士氣)

When the *Dao De Jing* talks about the monarch or rulers, it actually refers to the mind. The country is the body, the political policies are breathing, the people are the qi, and people's morality or morale is the spirit. When you read the text with these concepts in mind, you will see how the text can actually talk about qigong. When the rulers are able to follow the Dao, the country will be ruled with peace and harmony. This means when your mind (related to the spirit) is able to follow the Dao, your qi's circulation will be smooth and harmonious.

3. The mind (or spirit)—the ruler of the body just like a monarch governing a country—is the key to both self-cultivation in qigong and to ruling a kingdom. For this reason, the mind has been the major subject in discussions of the *Dao De Jing*. Remember, the spirit (related to the subconscious mind) is the Dao and from this Dao the De is manifested.

4. Since we don't know the Dao, we will not be able to discuss it clearly. However, from observation and under-

standing of the Dao's manifestation, the De, we will be able to trace back to the origin or the very beginning of life and may acquire some clues about the Dao (以德觀道) (Use the De to Observe the Dao). This is no different from those scientists who are looking for the most basic forms of matter, the fundamental particles in the material world. In fact, we can conclude that those material scientists who are looking for the most fundamental particles are approaching the goal from the De (manifestation of the Dao) while those Daoists who are searching for the origin and meaning of the spiritual world are approaching the goal from the Dao (origin of the material manifestation or creation). One approach is through scientific observation and the other through pondering and feeling. One is material science (物質科學) and the other is spiritual science (精神科學). One is searching for the truth of the yang world and the other the truth of the yin world.

5. The *Dao De Jing* covers eight various qigong cultivations that include:
   A. Cultivating the physical body or physical life (regulating the body) (修身) (調身)
   B. Cultivating breathing (regulating the breathing) (修息) (調息)
   C. Cultivating the emotional mind (regulating the heart) (修心) (調心)
   D. Cultivating the temperament (修性)
   E. Cultivating qi (regulating the qi) (修氣) (調氣)
   F. Cultivating the spirit (regulating the spirit) (修神) (調神)
   G. Cultivating hun (cultivating the soul) (修魂)
   H. Cultivating po (cultivating the vitality) (修魄)

   The *Dao De Jing* emphasizes cultivating the mind (related to the Dao/spirit) to nourish the De (deeds) and cultivating the temperament to sustain physical life.[2] In practice, it stresses the level of wuwei (無為) (doing nothing), the stage of "regulating of no regulating"(調而無調). That means things happen naturally and automatically without thinking or intention. In theory, Lao Zi believes it is the spirit (shen, 神) that governs the energy (qi, 氣), and finally manifests into good deeds (De, 德).[3]

In order to cultivate the spirit, we must deemphasize the seven emotions (qi qing, 七情) and the six desires (liu yu, 六慾). The seven emotions are happiness (xi, 喜), anger (nu, 怒), sorrow (ai, 哀), joy (le, 樂), love (ai, 愛), hate (hen, 恨), and lust (yu, 慾). The desires are generated from the six roots that are the eyes, ears, nose, tongue, body, and mind (xin, 心). We must also drop the mask covering our face so we can be truthful with others and ourselves. Without the truth of our inner feeling, we will continue to hinder reopening the third eye. In addition, in order to cultivate our spirits to a higher level, we should accumulate many good deeds (the De). The more we have built up our good deeds, the more powerful our spirit will grow.

6. Through my research and practice of embryonic breathing meditation, I have come to see that the *Dao De Jing* is derived from this spiritual cultivation and applies the principles from various angles. For example, chapter 16 of the *Dao De Jing* talks about two polarities: "Attain the ultimate insubstantiality and maintain the serenity sincerely."[4] In this phrase insubstantiality refers to cultivating your mind (upper brain or dan tian) and serenity refers to maintaining your physical body's (lower brain or real lower dan tian). These two cultivations of mind and body are the beginning stage of embryonic breathing. In order to understand spiritual cultivation to reopen the third eye, you must know what are the spiritual valley (shen gu, 神谷) and valley spirit (gu shen, 谷神) referred to in chapter 6. The spiritual valley is the space between the two lobes of the brain. The way to reach the final stage of embryonic breathing is through wuwei

(無為) (regulating of no regulating), embracing singularity (bao yi, 抱一) referred to in chapter 10, and keeping the mind and the qi at the center (shou zhong, 守中) as referred to in chapter 5. Wuwei means you are doing it without having to think about it—subconsciously. All of these are crucial keys of embryonic breathing meditation.

7. The final goal of spiritual cultivation is to reopen the third eye (tian men, 天門) (chapter 10) and reunite the human spirit with the spirit of Nature (tian ren he yi, 天人合一). To reach this goal, we must cultivate our subconscious mind, recognize and awaken our spirit, and cultivate it. These steps will reopen the third eye and finally reunite our spirit with the spirit of Nature. In doing so, we will have become part of the Dao again.

We can summarize that the focus of the entire *Dao De Jing* book is about two essential concepts: the Dao (mind) and the De (behavior). Lao Zi used different angles and many examples throughout various chapters to repeatedly lead us to these two important roots. Through this strategy of repetition, I believe he hoped readers would be able to comprehend and, eventually, embody these two roots. Though the Dao and De may be easy to understand, living them is hard. The final goal of spiritual cultivation is reaching the goal of "wuwei," the mind of doing without doing or the regulating of no regulating (subconsciously).

Dao De Jing and Humanity's Future—Questions to Ponder

1. The *Dao De Jing* offers us an opportunity to explore the spiritual world. It has inspired us to study, research, and further understand the meaning of spirit. I believe that, while the twentieth century's focus was material science, the twenty-first century should be the century for spiritual science. Now is the time for us to develop spiritual science to further understand the meaning of our lives. After all, we cannot deny that, though material

science has led us to a material life of luxury, we still do not have a clear idea of what the spiritual world is. Half of the science is still missing, and we are still confused and unhappy about our lives.

2. When we are alive, our material and spiritual lives are united in a physical form. When we die, they are separated. If it is true that our physical lives belong to the yang world and our spiritual lives belong to the yin world, then the boundary of our existence is life and death. According to religious qigong, our physical bodies will be recycled (they will return to the dust) while our spiritual life reincarnates into a different and new life in a physical form. As we develop our understanding of spiritual science in the twenty-first century, will we be able to literally travel in the spiritual (yin) world using spiritual energy and consciously reform our life to return to the physical (yang) world? What role does our understanding of gravity and antigravity play in this? Is this possibly the boundry between the two dimensions, the yin and yang spaces of the spiritual and physical worlds respectively? Both the *Yi Jing* (*Book of Changes*) and the *Dao De Jing* have offered us many ideas to ponder.

3. We cannot deny that spirit governs our physical lives. However, how can we develop our spirit scientifically? If the spiritual world (the Dao or yin world) is the mother of the material world (the De or yang world) and both worlds are mutually influencing each other, how can we consciously reach the yin world? Is this what the *Dao De Jing* is referring to? In order to reach the yin world, we have to resist emotional temptations, meditate to wake up the subconscious mind, return to the purity of infancy, maintain righteous thoughts and deeds, keep simplicity of mind, be truthful with ourselves and others, and have a heart of benevolence. Can we cultivate these until the wuwei stage?

There are so many questions remaining to be answered. Will we be able to reveal the secret of the spiritual world scientifically in this century?

Note:

If you are interested in knowing more about spiritual qigong practice, please refer to the following books and DVDs:

A.   *The Root of Chinese Qigong* (Book)
B.   *Qigong Meditation—Embryonic Breathing* (Book)
C.   *Qigong—Secret of Youth* (Book)
D.   *Understanding Qigong 1–6* (DVDs)

You can find these books and DVDs from YMAA Publication Center (www.ymaa.com).

1. 孔子曰：“吾道一以貫之。”
2. 修心養德、 修行養命。
3. 神—氣—德
4. “致虛極，守靜篤。”

Dao Jing (Dao Classic)—Chapters 1 to 37

Note:

The first subtitles of most of the chapters were given by a Tiantai Mountain (天台山) Daoist hermit, He Shang Gong (河上公). Little is known about his personal background such as his place of origin and exactly when he was born. However, his interpretation of the *Dao De Jing*, known as "He Shang Gong's Chapters of Lao Zi (老子) (*Dao De Jing*)" (《老子河上公章句》) written during the Western Han Dynasty (西漢) (228 BCE–8 CE), has significantly influenced Chinese scholars' studies about the *Dao De Jing*. The second set of subtitles for all of the chapters were given by the author of this book, Dr. Yang, Jwing-Ming (楊俊敏) based on his understanding from a qigong point of view.

CHAPTER I
Comprehending the Embodiment of the Dao—The Entrance of Dao

第一章
體道—道門

「道」可道，非常『道』；
名可名，非常『名』。
『無』，名天地之始；
『有』，名萬物之母。
　　　故
常『無』，欲以觀其妙；
常『有』，欲以觀其徼。
此兩者，
同出而異名，同謂之玄。
玄之又玄，眾妙之門。

The Dao that can be described is not the eternal Dao.
The Name that can be named is not the eternal name.
Nothingness can be named as the initiator of heaven and earth
    (i.e., Nature);
having can be named as the mother of myriad objects.
    Therefore,
Always (maintain) nothingness, wish to observe its marvelousness.
Always (maintain) having, wish to observe its returning (i.e., recycling).
    These two,
are commenced from the same origin but named differently, both
    are marvelous and profound.
Profundity within profundities, it is the gate of all marvelousness
    (i.e., variations).

General Interpretation

This first chapter is the root or foundation of the entire *Dao De Jing*. It is from this root that all the discussions in the following chapters are derived. Therefore, it is the most important chapter if one wants to accurately extract and apply concepts from this book. Fan, Ying-Yuan (范應元) said: "(This chapter) is the door of entering the 'Dao' and the foundation of establishing 'De' (i.e., Dao's manifestation). It is the total conclusion of this classic (i.e., Dao De Jing)."[1]

Dao (道) is the way of nature that cannot be described or interpreted by words. The work *Guan Zi* (《管子·內業》) says: "What is the Dao? The mouth cannot describe it, the eyes cannot see it, and the ears cannot listen to it."[2] The Daoist book, *Can Tong Qi* (《參同契》) says: "The Great Dao does not have sound and is without odor and has no color and no emptiness. (Then), what can we say about it? It is because there is yin and yang hidden within this no sound and no odor. And there is a creation and derivations contained in this no color and no emptiness."[3]

From these two sayings, we can see the Dao itself does not have any colors, physical forms, sounds, odors, or anything humans can describe. Though it cannot be sensed or seen, it is there and existing. Its power is great and it gives birth to all lives and objects.

The Daoist script, *Qing Jing Jing* (《清靜經》) say: "The Great Dao does not have shape (i.e., is not visible), but it gives birth to heaven and earth (i.e., the universe). The Great Dao does not have compassion, but it moves the sun and moon. The Great Dao has no name, but it grows and nourishes myriad objects. I don't know what its name is, but if forced to name it, call it 'Dao.'"[4] Fan, Ying-Yuan (范應元) concluded: "The long-lasting and natural Dao exists, but without shape; though shapeless, there is an essence (i.e., content). It is so big that there is no external boundary; thus, there is nothing not included within. It is so tiny without an internal boundary; thus, there is no tiny place that cannot be entered. Therefore, there is nowhere it cannot permeate (i.e., reach)."[5]

This means the Dao is everywhere and there is no boundary, no limitation of time or space. It is something that, though it reaches everywhere, cannot be described. The reason for this is simply because the

Dao is so profound and marvelous that it cannot be described by the limited human knowledge and concepts we have discovered or defined. If we use this limited knowledge to explain the Dao, the Dao will have been distorted and will not be the original natural Dao anymore. For example, the Dao is truthful and does not lie. However, we all lie and play tricks on each other. Consequently, we all have a mask on our faces. The Dao does not have emotions, colors, good or bad, glory, dignity, honor, pride, or any other desires created by humans. We humans are truly in a deep bondage to the matrix of all of these human emotions. Therefore, if we use our emotional and untruthful mind to judge the truth of the Great Nature, then the interpretation of the Dao will not be truthful.

The Great Nature does not have a name or give a name to anything. Therefore, all of the myriad objects do not have names. It was we humans who gave names. Once these names are given and defined, the natural truth is again distorted and becomes misleading. Therefore, once we have given the names to those objects or feelings around us, we have created a matrix (masked society) that is not the natural Dao but a human Dao. That means, again, we have defined Nature or the Dao through our limited mind.

Relatively speaking, nothingness can be considered as yin (陰) that initiates the millions of things (having). Having is the manifestation of nothingness (yin) and is considered as yang (陽). Nothingness is called the wuji state (無極) (no extremity, no polarities). From this wuji state, through taiji (太極) or Dao (道), the "having" is initiated. "Nothingness" and "having" are two aspects of the same "Dao"; even though there are two, actually, it is one; though it is one, actually, there are two. From "having," yin and yang's two poles (or polarities) are derived. From this, you can see that yin and yang's two poles are "the having" of the myriad objects, which is relative to nothingness (figure 1-1). From these two poles, the millions of objects can be derived.

Wang, An-Shi (王安石) said: "The origin of the Dao is from 'nothingness.' Therefore, when (one) always keeps 'nothingness,' the marvelousness (of the Dao) can be observed. The application of the Dao belongs to 'having.' Thus, when (one) always has 'having,' the natural recycling can be seen (i.e., comprehended)."[6] Gui, Jing-Yu (龜井昱) also

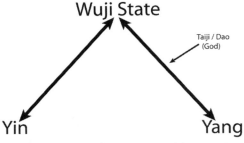

Figure 1-1. Yin and Yang Derived from Wuji
(Nothingness)

said: "To always keep 'nothingness' is to observe (the Dao's) marvelousness in initiating objects. To always keep 'having' is to observe the object's returning at the end."[7] Finally, Teng, Yun-Shan (滕雲山) said: "Always 'nothingness' means the Dao itself. It is marvelous to initiate 'having' from 'nothingness.' Always 'having,' the movements (i.e., actions) are generated from calmness. What is 'jiao' (徼)? It means the ending of objects, from 'having' returning to 'nothingness.'"[8] "Jiao" (徼) means the border or the ultimate end.

Qigong Interpretation:

In qigong practice, through a few thousand years of pondering and practice, the Chinese people have been trying to understand the grand universe (da tian di, 大天地), the small universe (xiao tian di, 小天地), and their mutual relationship. From this understanding, they hope to live long and to comprehend the meaning of life. Since *The Book of Changes (Yi Jing, 《易經》)*, the Chinese have believed there are two dimensions coexisting in this universe. These two dimensions are called "yin space" (yin jian, 陰間) and "yang space" (yang jian, 陽間). Yin jian is the spiritual world that cannot be seen while yang jian is the material world we live in. When we are alive, our physical body is in the material world with a spirit living within. However, after we die, the physical body reenters the recycling process while the spirit will be reincarnated.

Traditionally, the Chinese considered the Great Nature to be the grand universe (great heaven and earth; da tian di, 大天地) while a human body is a small universe (small heaven and earth; xiao tian di, 小天地). Since humans are formed in the Great Nature, we copy the same energy pattern and have the same energy similarities. Therefore, a human being incorporates both a physical and a spiritual body.

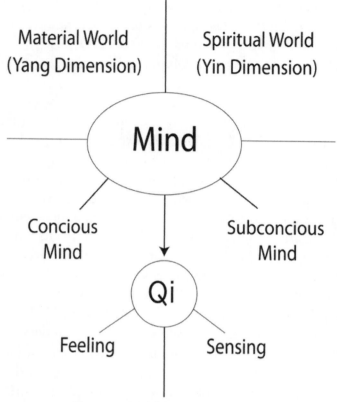

Figure 1-2. Yin/Yang Worlds and Mind

Naturally, the physical body is considered as yang while the spiritual body is considered as yin. Between this yin and yang is the mind. Mind is not the spirit but connects to both the spirit and the physical body (figure 1-2).

Throughout Chinese history the Dao has been called different names depending on the school or society. For example, it is called "taiji" (太極) (grand ultimate) in Confucian scholar society, "Dao" (道) or "tai chu" (太初) (grand initiation) by Daoist society, and "tai xu" (太虛) (great emptiness) by Chinese medical society. In the Daoist book, *Yun Ji Qi Jian* (《云笈七鑒·元氣論》), it is said:

> "*extremely profound and deep, it is tai yi (太易); when the original qi is not yet formed, it is then called tai chu (太初);*

when original Qi just begins to initiate, it is called tai shi (太始); when the shape of qi has begun to formalize, it is called tai su (太素); when the shape of qi has been formed into material, it is called taiji (太極)."[9]

In Chinese society, it is believed that this universe began with some unexplainable and incomprehensible deep and profound force. This force is called "tai yi" (太易) and means "extreme change." Then energy (original qi) was produced, but not formed into shape. This second stage is called "tai chu" (太初) and means "great initiation." After this, the original qi began to be formed and is called "tai shi" (太始), which means "grand commencement." Then, the original qi began to formalize into shape and is called "tai su" (太素), which means "great simplicity." Once the original qi began to formalize into material; it is called "taiji" (太極) which means "great or grand ultimate." Therefore, taiji is the force that formalizes material from the wuji state.

Cheng, Yi and Cheng, Hao (程頤/程顥) said: "What is taiji? It means the 'Dao.'"[10] Then, what is taiji? In order to understand qigong, you must first comprehend the definition of taiji or Dao. Taiji is usually translated as "grand ultimate." However, its meaning is still vague. Let us take a look at a classic written by Wang, Zong-Yue (王宗岳). In it he says: "What is taiji? From it, wuji is born. It is a pivotal function of movement and stillness. It is the mother of yin and yang. When it moves, it divides. At rest it reunites."[11] From this, we can see that taiji is a natural force or Dao that activates movement (actions or variations of nature) and also causes the cessation of the movement. When this happens, wuji (nothingness) can manifest into yin and yang, two poles. Once you are in the yin or yang state, you can resume the wuji state from either. From the influence of taiji, this yin and yang can be further divided into more yin and yang, and so on. Consequently, millions of objects are derived (figure 1-3).

Thus, myriad objects can usually be classified as yin or yang. Yin and yang are relative and not absolute. How you define yin and yang depends on your point of view and where you stand as the reference position. For example, female is yin while male is yang and the moon is yin while the sun is yang. The seed is yin and the plant, the manifes-

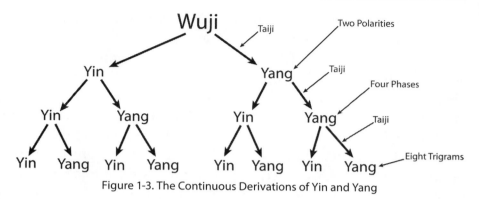

Figure 1-3. The Continuous Derivations of Yin and Yang

tation of the seed, is yang. Sadness is yin while happiness is yang. Naturally, this can change, depending on your reference point.

We can thus see that "nothingness" is the beginning of myriad objects' derivations and "having" (existence) is the manifestation of nothingness. Taiji is the cause of this manifestation, and therefore taiji is the mother of myriad things. When the mind (Dao, 道) is manifested, it is having (De, 德). Having is the manifestation of nothingness (mind). However, this having will eventually return to emptiness, which implies the recycling of manifestations (the material world or actions). Then, what is taiji? It is the Dao of Nature.

From a qigong point of view, when you are in an extremely calm state both physically and mentally, you have returned your being to the wuji state and you do not have any initiation of thought. However, once you have initiated a thought (taiji), movements are also initiated and yin and yang actions are created. When the concept of Dao is applied to a human being, it actually refers to the thought or the mind. It is from this mind that the creation of the human universe or matrix occurs.

Mind or thinking is insubstantial and empty in the material world. However, this mind or thought can be so powerful that it creates things from nothingness. This mind can travel anywhere in the universe without restriction of time or space. Once you can keep this mind open and free, you are able to create myriad things without restrictions. If your mind is restricted in the human matrix, dogmas, or tradition, then your spirit will be in bondage and cannot be developed.

In the grand universe, the taiji or Dao is the natural spirit (God to the Western world) of this universe. However, in a person's small universe, the human spirit is the taiji or the Dao. As is commonly known, we human beings have two coexisting minds—the conscious mind and the subconscious mind. The conscious mind is connected with the matrix we have created in the past and the subconscious mind is more truthful and still connected with our spirit. Our conscious mind has, unfortunately, dominated the body for a long time, and the subconscious mind has been ignored. Consequently, our spirits have been overshadowed and placed behind the human matrix.

However, from a qigong perspective, when you quiet your conscious mind, your subconscious mind will be strengthened. Consequently, the spirit residing at the center of the brain (limbic system) will be awakened and your intuition will be accurate and strong. That is the practice of embryonic breathing.

In embryonic breathing meditation practice, you first bring your mind to the wuji state. When you are in the wuji state, your mind is neutral and without thought. In this state, you will be able to observe and judge things with a neutral mind. From this neutral state, your mind will be clear and able to initiate an idea for further action. Therefore, before making a decision, you should first calm your mind and bring it to the neutral state.

Conclusion

One of the main purposes of practicing qigong is to comprehend the Dao (mind and spirit) in a human body and its relationship with the natural Dao. Daoists are called "xun Dao zhe" (尋道者) which means "Dao searchers." Through qigong practice, they are able to gain health, longevity, and further understand the meaning of life.

The final goal of qigong practice is to reunite your spirit with the natural spirit. This is called "the unification of heaven and human" (tian ren he yi, 天人合一). In order to reach this state, you must first reopen your third eye. The third eye is called "heaven eye" (tian yan, 天眼 or tian mu, 天目) in Chinese qigong society. The crucial key to open the third eye is practicing embryonic breathing meditation in which you must first set your spirit free from the human matrix. That means you have to be truthful. Daoists called themselves "zhen ren" (真人), which means "truthful person." This is because in order to find the truth of the Dao, a Daoist must first be truthful. Only then, will he be able to jump out of the human matrix to experience his true nature. Only when you are truthful will your subconscious mind (the seed of spirit) be awakened. When your subconscious mind is awakened, your spirit will be free and grow.

The mind is the most important and crucial key to qigong practice. This is because this mind (related to spirit) acts just like a god of a human universe.

For any practitioner who wishes to learn qigong at a profound level, he must first understand the meaning and concepts of Dao, taiji, wuji, and yin-yang. The entire qigong theory and practice are built on these basic concepts. Without this foundation, your qigong understanding and practice will be shallow.

Finally, let's summarize the key points of this chapter:

1. This chapter is a summary of the whole book.
2. Recognize and comprehend the root of the Dao—mind and spirit.
3. Recognize the power of the Dao and its possible manifestation (De, 德) and function.
4. Find the correct way of searching the Dao without bias (the neutral mind).
5. Quiet your conscious mind so the subconscious mind can be awakened.
6. When you are in a subconscious state (a semisleeping state), you will be able to reconnect with nature and see the variations (the changes of objects and thoughts) of the universe clearly.

1. 范應元云：“乃入道之門，立德之基，實一經之總也。”
2. 《管子·內業》：“道也者，口之所不能言也，目之所不能視也，耳之所不能聽也。”
3. 《參同契》：“大道無聲無臭，非色非空，有何可言？然無聲無臭中而藏陰陽，非色空裡而含造化。”
4. 《清靜經》曰：“大道無形，生育天地；大道無情，運行日月；大道無名，長養萬物；吾不知其名，強名曰道。”

5. 范應元云：“夫常久自然之道，有而無形，無而有精。其大無外，故大無不包；其小無內，故細無不入，無不通也。”

6. 王安石曰：“道之本出于無，故常無，所以自觀其妙；道之用常歸于有，故常有，得以觀其徼。”

7. 龜井昱曰：“常無者，觀之欲以得其始物之妙也。常有者，觀之欲以得其終物之徼也。”

8. 滕雲山曰：“常無，指道體而言。妙，從無生有。常有，靜極生動。徼者，成物之終，從有還無。”

9. 《云笈七籤·元氣論》：“窈窈冥冥，是為太易；元氣未形，漸謂太初；元氣始萌，次謂太始；形氣始端，又謂太素；形氣有質，復謂太極。”

10. 程頤／程顥說：“何謂太極？道也。”

11. 王宗岳云：“太極者，無極而生，動靜之機，陰陽之母也。動之則分，靜之則合。”

CHAPTER 2
Self-Nourishment—Commonality

第二章
養身—中庸

天下皆知美之為美，
　　　斯惡矣；
皆知善之為善，
　　　斯不善矣。
　　　故
有無相生，難易相成，
長短相形，高下相傾，
音聲相和，前後相隨。
　　　是以
『聖人』處「無為」之事，
　　　行「不言」之教。
萬物作焉而不辭，
　　　生而不有，
　　　為而不恃，
　　　功成而弗居。
夫唯弗居，是以不去。

If (the people in) the world know what beauty is,
  then, there is (an existence of) ugliness;
if (the people) know goodness as goodness,
  then there is (an existence of) non-goodness.
  Therefore,
the having and the nothingness mutually give birth to each other,
  difficulty and easiness are mutually formed,
long and short are mutually shaped (i.e., compared), and high and
  low are mutually quantified,
the sounds mutually harmonized, and the front and the rear are
  mutually following each other.
  Thus,
sages handle matters without doing anything
  and teach without speaking.
(With the Dao), millions of objects are begotten (i.e., created) without being rejected,
  lives are born without being possessed,
  things are done without being proud,
  once accomplished, (they) don't dwell on it.
It is because they don't keep these, thus, (all of) these stay (with
  them).

General Interpretation

Humans have defined what beauty is and what it is not. We also defined what is good and what is bad. In doing this, we set up an emotional matrix and dogma in human society. Once we have these concepts, there exists having or not having, difficulty or ease, and other ideas in comparison to one another. Consequently, competitiveness arises and different classes are discriminated. Du, Guang-Ting (杜光庭) said: "What are beauty and goodness? They are initiated from xin (i.e., emotional mind). From this emotional mind, though ugly, (things) can be beautiful and good. Thus, it is said, those who think beauty is beauty and goodness is goodness, since beauty and goodness cannot be defined, are all absurd."[1] Beauty or ugliness, goodness or evil are all relative and defined by each individual emotional mind. Once we have defined something, we are trapped into the bondage of dogmas.

In the same way, having and not having are relative. Everything was initiated from nothingness and then returns to nothingness. Li, Rong (李榮) said: "All objects under heaven (i.e., the universe) are begotten from the having, and the having is originated from the nothingness. It is from the nothingness that the having is begotten and from the having it returns to the nothingness."[2] This implies all existing objects in this universe were originated from the emptiness. Eventually, all these objects will again return to the emptiness. Lv, Yan (呂岩) said: "It is just like when the heaven and earth began to divide, there were no myriad objects. It was from the qi's (i.e., energy's) existence in the insubstantial nothingness that myriad objects were begotten. This was (a process of) begetting the having from the nothingness. Once there was the birth of myriad objects, then there must be the demise of these myriad objects. The perishing is the returning to the nothingness and is the (process of) begetting the nothingness from the having."[3]

Therefore, it does not matter if it is good or bad, beautiful or ugly; it all originated from our biased mind. Those who have comprehended the Dao understand this and, thus, will do things without doing and will teach without teaching. To them, there is no good or bad, long or short, high or low. All are the same to them. This is the way of the Dao in nature. Consequently, all lives are derived without being distinguished, compared, discriminated, or rejected. Nature gives birth to everything but does not possess them. Nature has accomplished all of the manifestations of the Dao but without feeling proud of it. It is because of all of these that nature owns it and keeps it always.

Qigong Interpretation

In qigong, we should treat all things neutrally. By doing so, we are able to maintain a neutral point of view and be natural. That means we should not be in bondage to the emotions that we have created in this society. In this way, there is no dignity, no glory, no honor, no happiness, and no sadness. Thus, your wisdom and logical mind will be able to govern your emotional mind. You will not be in a state of expectancy at any time during your life. Since there is no expectation, there is no satisfaction or disappointment. Therefore, if we are able to get rid of the emotional desires, we will not be greedy and continuously enslaved by money, glory, dignity, or honor. Our mind will be peaceful and calm. This is the way of following nature. Without this, we will not be able to unite our spirit with the natural spirit.

As mentioned in chapter 1, the conscious mind or thought is part of a human matrix; the mind is not truthful. You must search for the feeling from the subconscious mind that is more truthful and closer to the spirit. In order to reach this subconscious mind, you have to calm down your mind and transcend the bondage that restricts your spirit from growing. If you are able to experience things from a state of neutrality, you will be able to see both the spiritual and material worlds equally. Your judgment will be more accurate.

Furthermore, the yin world is the spiritual world while the yang world is the material world. The yang (De, 德) is the manifestation of yin (Dao, 道). They are two, but one; one, but two. If you see only the material world, you will be attracted by the material enjoyment and ignore your spiritual being. When you apply this concept to your life, the spiritual life is yin while physical life is yang. These two are equally important. When you train qigong, you must train your physical body as well as cultivate your spiritual strength. Without both, you will be weak and sick. The full meaning of life can be clearly comprehended only when these two polarities are treated equally. It is called "dual cultivation of temperament (spirit) and life (physical life)" in Daoist society.[4]

To reach the spiritually peaceful state, you must also have a mind so open there is nothing that can bother or restrict you. In addition, you should also have a huge capacity for forgiveness. Thus, your mind will not be tangled in the biased thoughts that could lead you to an emotional state. In *Yellow Emperor Inner Classic* (《黃帝內經·素問·上古天真論》), it is said:

> *"Then, there are some sages who situate themselves in the harmony of the heaven and the earth, follow the rules of the eight winds (i.e., Nature), wish to stay with laymen society, but without the mind of greediness and desires . . . thus, externally there is no physical fatigue, and internally there is no adversity in thought. Peace and cheer are their main foci. (In this case, the body) achieves its merit (i.e., health) automatically, the shape and body (i.e., physical body) are not awkward and the spirit is not dispersed. One hundred years (of age) can be reached."[5]*

Wang, An-Shi (王安石) said: "The having and the nothingness, high and low, the sound's harmonization, the front and the latter, etc., none can avoid being compared with each other. Only those who are able to forget these six comparisons (i.e., six desires) can enter the spiritual calmness."[6]

Conclusions

This chapter focused on the training of regulating the mind. Only when your mind is regulated can your spirit reach its peaceful and calm state. In order to do this, you must get rid of your seven passions and six desires (qi qing liu yu, 七情六慾). As we have seen, the seven passions are liking (xi, 喜), anger (nu, 怒), sorrow (ai, 哀), joy (le, 樂), love (ai, 愛), hate (hen, 恨), and lust (yu, 慾). The desires are generated from the six roots that are the eyes, ears, nose, tongue, body, and mind (xin, 心). Buddhists also cultivate within themselves a neutral state separated from the four emptinesses of earth, water, fire, and wind (si da jie kong, 四大皆空). That means the emptiness of material desires in the mind.

Once you have reached a state of "regulating without regulating" (tiao er wu tiao, 調而無調) or "doing without doing" (wei er wuwei, 為而無為), your mind will be neutral and peaceful. You will then have reached a stage of "doing nothing, yet nothing is left undone" (wuwei er wu bu wei, 無為而無不為).

1. 杜光庭曰：“美善者，生于欲心，心苟所欲，雖惡而美善矣。故云皆知己之所美為美，所善為善，美善無主，俱是妄情。”

2. 李榮曰：“天下之物生于有，有生于無，從無出有，自有歸無。”

3. 呂岩曰：“如天地之初分，萬物皆無，而虛無之氣，發生萬物，是無中生有也。有萬物之生，必有萬物之死，死者復歸于無，是有中生無也。”

4. “性命雙修。”

5. 《黃帝內經‧素問‧上古天真論》曰：“其次有聖人者，處天地之和，從八風之理，適嗜欲于世俗之間，無恚嗔之心‧‧‧‧，外不勞于事，內無思想之患，以恬愉為務，以自得為功，形體不敝，精神不散，亦可以百數。”

6. 王安石曰：“有之與無，高之與下，音之與聲，前之與后，是皆不免有所對。惟能兼忘此六者，則可以入神。”

CHAPTER 3
Pacifying People—Calming Qi

第三章
安民—平氣

不尚賢，使民不爭；
　　不貴難得之貨，使民不為盜；
　　不見可欲，使民心不亂。
是以『聖人』之治：
　　虛其心，實其腹；
　　弱其志，強其骨。
常使民無知無欲，
　　使夫智者不敢為也。
為「無為」，則無不治。

Not to uphold those achievers, so the people will not compete with each other;
   not to treasure those goods harder to obtain, so the people will not become thieves;
   not to show those desirable things, so the people's mind will not be disordered (i.e., confused).
Therefore, the sages' way of governing
   is to keep their (i.e., people's) hearts (i.e., emotional mind) empty and solidify (i.e., fill) their stomach;
   weaken their will and strengthen their bones.
Always make the people know nothing and desire nothing,
   and make those schemers dare not use their wisdom.
This is the "wuwei"; consequently, there is nothing that cannot be ruled.

General Interpretation

The emotional mind has always been the cause of problems. When we begin to compare one person to the other, there is competition and expectation. When the value of goodness has been set, then there is greediness. When people have been trapped in emotional desires, the society will become disordered. Therefore, if a ruler wishes to govern a country with harmony and peace, he should weaken people's emotional desires and greediness. Instead, he should find the way to let them have plenty of food and other necessities. When material desires are removed and/or sated, then there is harmony in society.

Qigong Interpretation

This chapter talks about the practice of "regulating the emotional mind" (tiao xin, 調心). The king refers to the mind that governs the country. The country implies the physical body. The people imply the qi in the body. The breathing is the policy (strategy) of handling country business.

When the mind does not get trapped in human emotional bondage, the qi can flow smoothly. However, when the mind pays too much attention to emotional disturbance, the qi circulation will be stagnant. Once the qi cannot flow naturally and smoothly, the circulation becomes aberrant. In addition, the mind must be kept calm, neutral, and without emotional disturbance. When this happens, the yi (意) (wisdom mind) will be able to govern the xin (心) (emotional mind).

Du, Guang-Ting (杜光庭) said:

> "Those who cultivate the Dao, when they are at the beginning stage (of cultivation), (the mind) is not complete (i.e., not regulated), (the practice) is not yet mastered, and they are afraid to see temptations and affect their mind by the surrounding environment. They seclude themselves from the public and reside in the mountains and woods

*to avoid noise and influences. When (they) reach the stage
that the mind is calm, the will is steady, and the environ-
mental attractions cannot allure, they are thus able to
control their emotional mind all day long; consequently,
they are peaceful and easy-going (i.e., relaxed). When
their hearts (i.e., emotional mind) are clear and all worries are ceased, the thoughts are real (i.e., firmed) and
righteous, there are no temptations that can lure their
minds externally, and there is a peaceful and harmonious will internally; though managing daily business, the
name (i.e., reputation) and benefit are not related (i.e. in
his concern or intention). Though the mind is busy, it is
not involved in laymen's discord. (In this case,) though
staying in the cities, how can it be harmful to their cultivation of the truth?"[1]*

Therefore, when you practice qigong to a profound stage, you
should have an empty mind (with no desire or emotional disturbance)
and have abundant qi stored. The way to conserve and store qi is to keep
your mind calm and without distraction. When you do this, the qi can
stay at its residence. Ge, Xuan (葛玄) said: "Empty the heart (i.e., emotional mind) means no evil thoughts; solidify the stomach (i.e., fill qi at
lower dan tian) means to close qi (i.e., keep qi at its residence) and cultivate the calmness."[2] Dong, Si-Jing (董思靖) said: "Empty the heart
(i.e., emotional mind) means to forget both objects and I; solidify the
stomach means condense and keep the spirit (at its residence) internally.
When objects and I are all forgotten, then thinking will not be generated and the temptation will be softened automatically; when spirit is
kept internally, then qi will not be weakened; consequently, the bones
are strong automatically."[3]

After you have practiced for a long time and are able to reach the
stage of "regulating of no regulating" (bu tiao er tiao, 不調而調), then
this is the stage of "wuwei" (無為) (not doing) and means "doing of no
doing." Once you have reached this stage, even if you live in an emotional matrix, you will be able to firm your thoughts without being
lured by the temptations.

Conclusions

In order to regulate your emotional mind (xin, 心), you must know how to use your wisdom mind (yi, 意) to analyze and govern the emotional mind. This is the stage of regulating the mind (tiao xin, 調心). Regulating the emotional mind means to free yourself from the bondage of glory, reputation, greed, wealth, and dignity (qu xin yu, 去心慾) to avoid the temptations of material attraction and ownership (qu wu yu, 去物慾) and to eliminate the desires of emotional temptations such as love, hate, sadness, and happiness (qu qing yu, 去情慾). Only when the emotional mind is regulated can the qi be calm, peaceful, and stay at its residence.

To reach this goal, you must also learn how to regulate your breathing and pay attention to your lower real dan tian (zhen xia dan tian, 真下丹田). When this happens, the qi will be conserved and stored at its residence to an abundant level.

1. 杜光庭曰：“修道之士，初階之時，愿行未周，澄練未熟，畏見可欲，為境所牽，乃棲隱山林，以避囂染。及心泰志定，境不能誘，終日指揮，未始不晏如也。”“及其澄心息慮，想念正真，外無撓惑之緣，內保恬和之志，雖營營朝市，名利不關，其心碌碌，世途是非，不介其意，混跡城市，何損于修真乎？”
2. 葛玄曰：“虛其心，無邪思也；實其腹，閉氣養靜也。”
3. 董思靖曰：“虛心者，物我兼忘；實腹者，精神內守。物我兼忘則慮不萌，而志自弱也；精神內守則氣不餒，而骨自強也

CHAPTER 4

Origin of "Nothingness"—Origin of "Thought"

第四章
"無" 源—"思" 源

『道』沖，
　　而用之或不盈。
淵兮，
　　似萬物之宗。
（挫其銳，解其紛，
　　和其光，同其塵；）
湛兮，
　　似或存。
吾不知誰之子？
　　象帝之先。

The Dao is insubstantial (i.e., infinite),
    When used, it cannot be exhausted.
It is so deep,
    as if it is the origin of myriad objects.
Blunt down the sharpness and untie the tangles,
    harmonize the light (with others), and situate with dust.
(It is) so profound,
    it seems to exist.
I don't know whose offspring is it?
    It has existed (even) before the (heaven) emperor.

General Interpretation

The Dao is not a material object. It is some natural force or power that cannot be interpreted by our limited understanding. However, when the Dao manifests its power, myriad objects can be created and this force or power cannot be exhausted.

Though the Dao is so profound and mysterious, it can be so calm, yet so powerful. It is so powerful and flexible that it can be anything and anywhere. Its sharpness can be blunted; all mysteries can be dissolved. It can harmonize and coexist with others or position itself with the dust.

Shi, De-Qing (釋得清) said:

> "This (chapter) is to praise the marvelousness of the Dao that cannot be gauged (measured). 'Chong' (沖) means 'insubstantial'; 'ying' (盈) means 'full'; 'yuan' (淵) means 'calm and deep without movement'; and 'zong' (宗) means 'return and belong to.' It says though the Dao is extremely insubstantial, in fact, it is full (i.e., existing everywhere) in myriad objects (i.e., all objects) in the heaven and the earth (i.e., universe). However, it is shapeless and cannot be seen. Thus, it is said 'when used, it cannot be exhausted' (i.e., cannot be seen). It says, the Dao itself, though deep and profound, yet lonely (i.e., calm and peaceful), can give birth to myriad objects and also accept their returning (i.e., recycling). However, though it gives birth (to myriad objects), it does not govern them. Thus, it is said, 'it seems that it is the origin of myriad objects.'"[1]

The Dao cannot be seen, but it can be felt. It seems it exists but doesn't exist. Nobody can be sure and know how the Dao was originated. It existed before even the universe was created. Wu, Cheng (吳澄) said: "The sentence, 'I don't know whose offspring is it?' is a question and the sentence 'It has existed (even) before the (heaven) emperor' is the answer. Offspring were born by parents. Emperor means the master of the heaven (i.e., Nature). The heaven existed before myriad objects

and the Dao existed before the heaven. That is, the heaven was originated from the Dao. There is nothing else before the Dao."[2]

Qigong Interpretation

If you apply the concept of this chapter to the human body, then
the spirit is an insubstantial being in our body. Spirit (taiji or Dao) cannot be seen, touched, or heard, but it can be felt.

Mind is related and connected to the spirit, but is not the spirit.
Spirit is truthful and natural and, therefore, can reach the natural
spirit. However, the human conscious mind has been contaminated
by humanity's mental constructions established throughout human
history. Therefore, we are living in a mental matrix created by human
dogmas and traditions.

When a person dies, the mind will be gone with the physical body,
but the spirit will be re-united with Nature for a period of time and then
be reincarnated. If you are able to keep your mind simple, pure, honest, neutral, peaceful, calm, harmonious, and without the disturbance
of human emotions and desires, then the spirit will be able to grow and
evolve to a higher level. If your mind is continuously trapped in the
human emotional matrix, your spirit will be confused and disturbed.

When you train embryonic breathing meditation, you are learning
to calm down your conscious mind and allow your subconscious mind
to grow. When this happens, the spirit can be awakened and reconnect
with Nature.

Ni, Yuan-Tan (倪元坦) said: "Sharpness means the qi's strength and
stiffness. Use the softness and weakness (i.e., gentleness) to blunt (i.e.,
subdue) it. Confusion means the chaotic action of qi. Use the tranquil
mind to dissolve (its chaos). Light means the clear observation of wisdom. Use the calm comprehending mind to harmonize it. Dust means
the good and bad conditions of the environment that we should find
the ways to synchronize (i.e., accept and harmonize) with it."[3] This
implies that if you are able to find the Dao (the mind) of your being,
you will be able to soften your over-strong qi, calm down the chaos of
the qi's circulation, use your mind to analyze the situation, and, finally,

find ways to synchronize and dissolve the problem. Fan, Ying-Yuan (范應元) said: "If a person is able to use the Dao to blunt the sharpness of his emotion, dissolve the chaotic condition of events encountered, managing his mind clearly without shining its brightness, situate himself in the dirty laymen's world and not have his truthfulness contaminated, then it seems the Dao will be deeply existing within."[4]

Conclusions

Our conscious mind has been formed by human dogmas and traditions. We all wear masks on our faces in order to survive in this society or matrix. We learn how to lie, to brainwash, and to channel ourselves into false glory and dignity, and to blind our subconscious mind and feeling. This subconscious mind and feeling is the root of our connection to nature.

In order to awaken our subconscious mind, we must calm down our conscious mind. We must learn to take all human emotional disturbances lightly. Only then will our mind be peaceful and profound. When this happens, we will be able to reconnect with Nature (the Dao).

1. 釋得清曰："此贊道體用微妙而不可測也。沖，虛也；盈，充滿也；淵，靜深不動也；宗，依歸也。謂道體至虛，其實充滿天地萬物，但無形而不可見，故曰用之或不盈；謂道體淵深寂寞，其實能發育萬物而為萬物所依歸。但生而不育，為而不宰，故曰似萬物之宗。

2. 吳澄曰："吾不知誰之子，問辭也。象帝之先，答辭也。子，父母所生者。帝，言天之宰也。天，先乎萬物，而道又在天之先，則天亦由道而生，無有在道之先者矣。"

3. 倪元坦曰："銳者，氣之剛強也，以柔弱挫之。紛者，氣之擾動也，以恬淡解之。光者，智之昭察也，以韜晦和之。塵者，境之順逆也，以因任同之。"

4. 范應元曰："人能用道，以挫情欲之銳，解事物之紛，營心鑒而不炫其明，混濁世而不污其真，則道常湛兮似乎或存也。"

CHAPTER 5

Insubstantial Usage—Keeping at the Center

第五章
虛用—守中

天地不仁，
　　　以萬物為芻狗；
『聖人』不仁，
　　　以百姓為芻狗。
天地之間，
　　　其猶橐籥乎？
虛而不屈，
　　　動而愈出。
多言數窮，
　　　不如守中。

The heaven and the earth (i.e., Nature) do not have benevolence,
   thus, they regard all myriad objects as chu gou (i.e., straw dogs).
Those sages do not have benevolence;
   thus, they regard people as chu gou.
Between the heaven and the earth,
   isn't it just like a tuo yue (i.e., wind bellows)?
(Though) insubstantial, yet cannot be exhausted,
   the more it moves, the more it produces.
Too much talking is awkward and deviates from the Dao,
   it is better to keep (ourselves) at the center (i.e., neutral thinking or quiet).

General Interpretation

As explained in chapter 1, Nature (the Dao) does not have emotions such as mercy, love, hate, glory, happiness, or sadness. Even though myriad objects living in this Nature are full of emotions and have limited lives, to Nature, they are just like the sacrificial offering, chu gou (芻狗). Chu gou was a sacrificial dog that was made from straw and used for ceremonies of worship in ancient China. Those sages had cultivated their emotional minds to the neutral state. Therefore, they were not touched by any emotional disturbances from laymen's society. All events are accepted as only part of natural occurrences. Once it is recognized that all lives are in their recycling process, it naturally follows that there is nothing to be emotional about.

The space between the heaven and the earth is just like tuo yue (橐籥). Tuo yue was a wind bellow that was used to assist the air's circulation in ancient times. Lin, Zhao-En (林兆恩) said: "Tuo yue is the bellow used to melt or fuse metals. Tuo is a leather bag made of animal skin and used as a wind bellow. Yue is made of bamboo and is the tube connected to the bellow's entrance."[1] This implies that myriad lives rely on the natural qi (air) circulation to survive. Air is called "space qi" (kong qi, 空氣) and means the energy in space. Though it is insubstantial, the movement of the air can never be exhausted. The more you act, the more the flow of the air will be generated.

All of these principles are the natural rules and the Dao of Nature. The more we talk about it, the farther we are separated from Nature (truth). Therefore, we should comprehend it with our natural instinct. As such, we will be able to feel it and understand it from our heart.

Qigong Interpretation

From a qigong perspective, the head is considered as heaven (qian, 乾) while the abdominal area is considered as earth (kun, 坤). The perineum is the sea bottom (hai di, 海底). The space between the head and abdominal area is where the lungs are located and that corresponds to the space of the natural heaven and earth. In this space, the qi (kong qi, 空氣) (air qi) circulates and keeps millions of cells alive. The lungs are like bellows (tuo yue). The more and the deeper you breathe, the more oxygen you will acquire. From a Western medical science perspective, the body's metabolism heavily relies on the quantity of oxygen. The more oxygen you can provide, the more energy (qi) can be produced. When this happens, cellular replacements will occur smoothly and the immune system may be stronger. Presumably, your life may be healthier and longer.

$$Glucose + 6O_2 \rightarrow 6CO_2 + 6H_2O$$
$$\Delta G^{O'} = -686 \text{ Kcal}$$

The mind (or the spirit, the human Dao) is the motive force that makes the internal qi (bioelectricity) move or stop. The more the mind acts, the more the qi's circulation is excited and out of control. Therefore, in order to calm down the body and keep the qi at its residence, you must keep your mind centered at the neutral state and be undisturbed by emotion.

Taixi Jing Shu (《胎息經疏》) (*The Dredge of Embryonic Breathing*) says: "Valley spirit (gu shen, 谷神) does not die; it is called 'yuan pin' (元牝). 'Yuan pin' is also named 'qi xue' (氣穴) (i.e., qi cavity). Close the eyes and look inward, condense and enter the spirit into it, then spirit and qi will mutually support each other; this is 'shou zhong' (守中) (i.e., keeping at the center)."[2] "Yuan pin" (元牝) means "xuan pin" (玄牝). It is explained in the next chapter that xuan pin is the female animal (mother) that gives birth to new life. It implies the spirit that resides at the center of the brain (shen zhi, 神室) (spirit residence or limbic system). It is believed that when the spirit is able to stay at this center (shou zhong, 守中) the mind will not be wandering and become chaotic. Accordingly, the qi will be gathered in the body and stay at the lower real dan tian (xia zhen dan tian, 下真丹田) instead of being wasted. This is the way of protecting and conserving the qi.

Xiao, Tian-Shi (蕭天石) said:

"If the mouth does not talk much, the heart will be clear and the shape (i.e., physical body) will be peaceful; thus,

the spirit and qi will not disperse. When the eyes do not see much, then the soul will stay at the liver. When the ears do not hear much, then the essence will stay at the kidneys. When the nose does not smell much, then the vital spirit (po, 魄) will remain at the lungs. When the mouth does not talk much, the spirit can be in the heart. When the body does not move much, then the yi (意) (i.e., logical thought) will stay at the spleen. When these five spirits (i.e., the spirit of the five organs) are able to stay, then the organs' five qi will move toward its origin (i.e., normal state). This is the marvelousness of 'keeping at the center.'[3]

This implies that when you don't talk, don't see, don't listen, don't smell, and the body does not move, with the concentration of your mind, you will be able to regulate the five organs' qi to their origins (to their normal and healthy state). This is called "five qi gather toward their centers" (wu qi chao yuan, 五氣朝元). This is the result of "keeping at the center" (shou zhong, 守中).

The qigong practitioner who wishes to reopen the heaven eye (tian yan, 天眼) (the third eye) must learn how to conserve his qi and also know how to build up the qi to an abundant level. Only then, can the third eye be reopened. To keep the spirit and mind inward is the first key of conserving qi. Si, De-Qing (釋得清) said: "When the center is kept, it is the gongfu of entering the Dao."[4]

Conclusion

In order to reopen the third eye, you will need a lot of qi to activate more brain cells so the brain can be charged to a high-energy state. Without this high energy, the third eye cannot be reopened.

Therefore, in order to reach this goal, you must know how to conserve the qi and also know how to generate more qi. The way of conserving the qi is through embryonic breathing meditation (tai xi jing zuo, 胎息靜坐). Furthermore, once you have generated more qi, you still need to store it at the lower real dan tian. The way to store this created qi is also through embryonic breathing.

The key to reaching this goal is cultivation of your emotional mind. Only when your mind is in its calm, peaceful, honest, and harmonious state can the qi be gathered at the center of the brain (the limbic system) or spiritual residence (shen shi, 神室). The way to bring your mind to a regulated state is through deep, soft, and calm breathing.

1. 林兆恩曰：“橐籥鑄冶所用致風之器，橐以皮為之皮囊，以為風袋也。籥以竹為之，袋口之管也。”
2.《胎息經疏》云：“谷神不死，是謂元牝。元牝又名氣穴。閉目反視，凝神入之，則神氣相注，守中也”
3. 蕭天石曰：“口不多言，心清形安而神氣不散。”“眼不多視，其魂在肝。耳不多聽，其精在腎。鼻不多聞，其魄在肺。口不多言，其神在心。身不多動，其意在脾。五神守中，五氣自然朝元。此乃守中之妙。”
4. 釋得清曰：“蓋守中，即進道功夫也。”

CHAPTER 6

Forming Phenomena—Original Spirit

第六章
成象—元神

谷神不死，
　　是謂玄牝。
玄牝之門，
　　是謂天地根。
綿綿若存，
　　用之不勤。

The valley spirit (gu shen) does not die,
    (then) it is called "xuan pin" (i.e., profound female animal).
The door (i.e., key) of reaching this "xuan pin,"
    is the root of the heaven and the earth (i.e., Nature).
It is very soft and continuous as if it exists.
    When utilized, it will never be exhausted.

General and Qigong Interpretation

The spirit (shen, 神) resides at the bottom of the space between the two lobes of the brain at the location of the limbic system. This space is like a valley between two mountains. It is able to trap energy and generate resonant vibrations. These vibrations correspond and resonate with the energy outside the valley. Thus, the shen residing in this valley is called "valley spirit" (gu shen, 谷神) and the valley in which the shen resides is called "spiritual valley" (shen gu, 神谷). It is believed that the shen residing in this valley governs the energy vibration of the entire body and, thus, controls the qi status and its manifestation. When this shen is strong, the qi manifestation in your life will be strong and you will have a long and healthy life (immortality). The *Original Collection of Zi Qing Zhi* (《紫清指元集》) says: "There are nine palaces in the head to correspond with the nine heavens above. There is a palace situated at the center called 'Ni Wan' (泥丸) (Mud Pill), also called 'Huang Ting' (黄庭) (Yellow Yard), again named 'Kun Lun' (崑崙), and again named 'Tian Gu' (天谷) (Heaven Valley). It has many names and is the palace where the original shen (yuan shen, 元神) resides. It is empty as a valley and the shen resides within; thus, it is called 'gu shen' (valley spirit)."[1] It is believed, in Chinese religious society, that there are nine layers of heaven above us. There are also nine layers of energy vibrations in our head that correspond to the nine heavens. However, the one at the center is the most important and is the place where the spirit (shen) resides. Kun Lun (崑崙) is one of the highest mountains in China covering three provinces—Xizang (西藏), Xinjiang (新疆), and Qinghai (青海). The head is called Kun Lun since it is the highest part of the body.

"Xuan" (玄) means "original" (yuan, 元), and "pin" (牝) refers to female animals and means "mothers." Therefore, "yuan pin" means the "origin or root of lives." When the valley spirit is centered (condensed) and functions actively, the life force is strong. Actually, "xuan pin" (玄牝) is what is called "taiji" (太極) (grand ultimate) in the *Yi Jing* (《易經》) (*The Book of Changes*). This taiji is the Dao (道) that produces myriad lives in the natural world. Therefore, we can conclude that "xuan pin" is: "the root of creation, variation, bearing, and raising of myriad objects, and thus is the mother of myriad objects of heaven and earth. It is another name for 'Dao.'"[2]

Achieving xuan pin is the key to connect to the natural shen (spirit). The shen is very soft and continuous as though existing, and yet feels as if it is not existing. The shen cannot be seen but is felt through cultivation. When it is used, it will not be exhausted. Shi, De-Qing (釋得清) said: "Pin means female animals, and is the mother of myriad lives. When used, it is the pivotal function of (spirit's) entering and exiting, thus the Dao is this pivotal function. Therefore, 'The door of profound function' is thus called 'the root of heaven and earth.'"[3] The Dao is taiji and means the spirit residing in the Mud Pill Palace (Ni Wan Gong, 泥丸宮).

According to Daoist and Buddhist societies, in order to reach the natural shen, you must reopen your third eye. The third eye is called "tian mu/tian yan" (天目/天眼) (heaven eye) or "yu men" (玉門) (jade gate) by religious societies, and "yintang" (M-HN-3, 印堂) (seal hall) by Chinese medical society. *Wudang's Illustration of Cultivating Truth* (《武當修真圖》) says: "(the place) under the mingtang (明堂) (ezhong (M-HN-2), 額中) (central area of forehead), above the midpoint of the line connecting two eyebrows, where the spiritual light is emitted, is named 'heaven eye' (tian mu, 天目)."[4] It is also mentioned in *Seventh Bamboo Slips of the Bamboo Bookcase* (《云笈七籤》) that: "The space between the two eyebrows is the 'jade gate' (yu men, 玉門) of ni wan (泥丸)."[5] "Ni wan" (泥丸) is a Daoist term, literally meaning "mud pill" and implies "the brain" or "upper dan tian." The lower center of the spiritual valley (shen gu, 神谷) between the two hemispheres of the brain is called "Ni Wan Gong" (泥丸宮) (the limbic system) and means "Mud Pill Palace."

In order to reach this Mud Pill Palace, one has to learn embryonic breathing (taixi, 胎息) that imitates the soft proto-breathing of an embryo. From embryonic breathing meditation, the spirit can be awakened and kept at its residence. This is the first step to reaching enlightenment. *Four Importances of Nourishing Life* (《養生四要》) states: "Those who wish to nourish life, breathe softly as if they are in an embryonic state. Therefore, it is called 'embryonic breathing.'"[6] If you are interested in embryonic breathing meditation, please refer to the book, *Qigong Meditation—Embryonic Breathing,* by YMAA Publication Center.

Conclusion

The space between the two hemispheres of the brain is called "spiritual valley" (shen gu, 神谷), which echoes and corresponds with Nature. The spirit residing in this valley is known as "valley spirit" (gu shen, 谷神). This spirit is what is called "Dao" or "taiji." When this spirit is strong, you will be able to reach the goal of immortality. If you are able to reopen the third eye, you will be enlightened. Enlightenment precedes Buddhahood.

1. 《紫清指元集》曰：“頭有九宮，上應九天，中間一宮，謂之泥丸，亦曰黃庭，又名崑崙，又名天谷，其名頗多，乃元神所居之宮，其空如谷，而神居之，故謂之谷神。”
2. “指造化生育萬物之根本，亦即天地萬物之母，即道之別稱也。”
3. 釋得清曰：“牝，物之雌者，即所謂萬物之母也。用即出入之樞機，謂道為樞機，皆入于機。故曰『玄機之門，是謂天地根』。”
4. 《武當修真圖》：“明堂下，兩眉連線中點上方。有神光出，而曰天目。”
5. 《云笈七簽》：“兩眉間為泥丸之玉門。”
6. 《養生四要》曰：“養生者，呼吸綿綿，如兒在胎之時，故曰胎息。”

CHAPTER 7
Conceal Radiance—No Selfishness

第七章
韜光—無私

天長地久。
天地所以能長且久者，
　　　以其不自生，
　　　故能長生。
是以『聖人』，
　　　後其身而身先，
　　　外其身而身存。
非以其無私邪？
　　　故能成其私。

The heaven and the earth (i.e., Nature) are everlasting.
The reason they are able to last long
    is because they do not live for themselves;
    thus they are able to live long.
Therefore, those sages
    position themselves last, and thus are in the front,
    less concerned for themselves (i.e., their lives), and thus their
    bodies survive.
Isn't this because (they) don't have selfishness?
    Thus, they are able to achieve fulfillment.

General Interpretation

"The heaven and the earth" refers to Nature (the Dao). The Dao can last forever in comparison to human life. This is because Nature has never been selfish and concerned with its own existence.

Those sages, imitating the Dao, are not selfish and do not have concern for their lives before others. It is because of this that they are always loved and respected. He Shang Gong (河上公) said: "(Those) who are concerned for others first and themselves last, (all the people) under the heaven (i.e., world) respect them and consider them as elders (i.e., leaders)."[1] Si, De-Qing (釋德清) said: "(Those) who are not selfish but concerned with others first are, thus, happily advocated by people without dislike."[2]

Zhang, Qi-Gan (張其淦) said:

> "Only those sages are able to comprehend the Dao so there are not any personal selfish desires. Top and bottom (i.e., mind and body) follow the heaven and the earth (i.e., the Dao). They do not compete with others and are able to consider themselves last, clarify and clean themselves (i.e., mind and body) so they are able to position themselves outside of the circle of desires. It seems there is nothing they are in favor of. However, (because of these) their bodies have always been positioned first and survived. When you see it, it looks like they are able to achieve their personal goals effortlessly. Nevertheless, is this because those sages want to achieve their personal goals? All they do is follow the wuwei (i.e., do nothing) of the Dao, unbiased and with no selfishness."[3]

Qigong Interpretation

When there is no bias in the mind, the mind will be in its neutral state and, thus, the spirit can stay at its residence. When this happens, the spirit can be strong. When the spirit is strong, physical longevity can be reached. Those who are selfishly worrying about their longevity and benefits first and ignore others will be mentally trapped in worries and desires. Thus, the spirit will be weak. Only those who follow the Dao with an opened heart will have spiritual support from others. This is because they are concerned for and love others first before themselves. When this happens, they will gain more respect and love from others. This is the key to spiritual growth. Those who love and respect others will always be loved and respected. In this case, your mind is peaceful and calm. Under this condition, your spirit will be able to grow stronger and stronger. The Chinese have a saying: "Those who respect others will be respected and those who love others will also be loved."[4]

Conclusion

The most challenging cultivation and training in qigong practice is cultivating your temperament. In order for your spirit to grow, you need a peaceful, calm, neutral, and open mind. Without this, you will always be trapped in emotional bondage and desires. Therefore, can you follow the Dao, having no bias, no expectations, no emotional temptations, and no desires? Can you love others more than yourself? If there is something that must be done, can you be the first one to do it? If you have this kind of open heart, you will be respected and loved. Your spirit will grow strong.

1. 河上公曰：“先人而後己者，天下敬之，以為長。”
2. 釋德清曰：“不私其身以先人，故人樂推而不厭。”
3. 張其淦曰：“惟聖人能體道，私慾不存，上下與天地同流。與物無競，能后其身；清淨自身，能外其身；若于此身無所愛者。然而身先身存，人之見之，以為我能成其私也。然聖人豈欲成其私哉？祇法斯道之無為，公而無私而已矣。”
4. “敬人者，人恆敬之。愛人者，人恆愛之。”

CHAPTER 8

Change Temperament—Cultivate Temperament

第八章
易性—養性

上善若水。
水善利萬物而不爭，
　　處眾人之所惡，
　　故幾於『道』。
居善地，
　　心善淵，
　　與善仁，
　　言善信，
　　正善治，
　　事善能，
　　動善時。
夫唯不爭，
　　故無尤。

The top (i.e., Nature or the sage) is as beneficial as water.
The water benefits myriad objects without competing with them.
    It positions itself at the place where others dislike.
    Therefore, it can be near to the "Dao."
Place (yourself) on the good ground
    where the heart is (calm and peaceful) as an abyss,
    give with benevolence,
    speak with trust,
    rule things with righteousness,
    handle matters with good talent,
    and execute action with the right timing.
It is because there is no competition (with others),
    thus, there is no resentment.

General and Qigong Interpretation

When you live in society, can you behave as water, being humble and always positioning yourself at the lowest place? If there is some unpleasant work that has to be done, can you be the one who volunteers to do it? Can you have the humble attitude of water in the way you treat others and practice qigong? If you can do this, you will be as great as water that is favored and accepted by all lives. With this quality of life and attitude, you will be able to govern your qi freely with your generous heart and free mind. If you are able to regulate your mind to this stage, your qi's circulation will be managed smoothly, calmly, peacefully, and harmoniously since qi is led by the mind.

Xun Zi (荀子) said:

> "When Confucius was watching the water flowing eastward, Zi Gong (子貢) (Confucius' student) asked Confucius: 'Those gentlemen (those who are highly educated), whenever seeing the big water, must watch it. Why?' Confucius said: 'This is because water is giving itself to all lives without doing anything (i.e., naturally); this is just like the De (i.e., manifestation of Dao). When it is flowing, it follows the natural rules, always so humble and positioning itself to the lowest place without hesitation; this is just like the yi (義) (i.e., righteousness). It is so abundant without exhaustion, just like the Dao. When there is a rupture (of a dike), it responds with loud sound and without fear, flows thousands of feet to the valley. This is just like bravery. When it is used as a scale, it is always just and balanced. This is just like the law. When it is full, it does not ask more. This is the same as honesty. It can reach even the tiniest place. This is just like investigating a matter carefully. It uses exiting as entering (i.e., to give instead of taking) and keeps objects fresh and clean. This is the same as giving with good deeds. Even if it encounters myriad obstacles, it still flows to the east without changing direction. This is the same as determination.

Therefore, when gentlemen see great water, they must watch it.'"[1]

In the *Yi Jing* (《易·坎》) (*The Book of Changes*), it is said: "When water flows to the dangerous deep abyss, it cannot be filled up. Even in such a dangerous situation, it will still keep its firmness and righteousness without losing its trustworthiness."[2] That means even when water (i.e. the Dao) is situated at the most dangerous position, it can still flow in its righteous way. Thus, it can be trusted.

The Dao is just like water and exists everywhere, gives generously without taking, and treats all lives equally without bias. As a qigong practitioner, you should understand that we are part of the Dao and cannot be separated from it. If we are able to have a heart in accord with the Dao—humble, benevolent, generous, and giving without hesitation—then we are on the correct path of pursuing the Dao. Unfortunately, throughout human history, we have continuously separated ourselves from the Dao, created the illusory matrix of society, and isolated ourselves from Nature.

Therefore, we should always place our position at the goodness of the Dao; the heart (mind) should be calm, deep, and profound. With this goodness and calm mind, we will be able to treat all lives with a benevolent heart, offer our talents to help others without hesitation, handle things with fairness and justice, and act appropriately at the proper moment. In chapter 27, it is said: "Therefore, those sages often help others, so there is no abandoned person, often save things, so there is no abandoned object."[3] That means all of the people exercise their values by offering their talents and all objects have their purpose in serving the world. Sun, Yat-Sen (孫中山) said: "Men are able to contribute their talents, the ground is able to provide its benefits, the objects are able to furnish their usages, and the goods can be circulated smoothly."[4]

Su, Che (蘇轍) said:

> *"Avoid the high and stay toward the low, then there never is adversity. This means (you are) good at choosing the place (i.e., you are able to fit in any environment). Keep*

*the mind empty and calm, and then the depth cannot be
gauged. Then (you are) good at being in a deep abyss (i.e.,
pondering profoundly). To benefit myriad objects, giving
without demanding reward, is a good deed of benevolence. When it is round, it will spin (i.e., flexible) and
when it is square, it will break. When it is blocked, then it
will stop, and once it is ruptured, then it will flow. You
can trust that it will behave with constancy. Knowing
how to cleanse the dirt and to gauge the high and low,
this is being good at ruling. When reflecting the objects
to show their shapes, it can reflect them without changing.
Then it is good in constancy (i.e., talent). When winter
arrives, it is frozen, and when spring comes, it melts, dries
up, or over-flows, not taking precedence; then it is appropriate to the time and season."[5]*

There was no mirror in the past and people used the reflection of the
water to see themselves. The reflection of the water allowed them to
see clearly. That is the talent or constancy of the water.

Chapter 81 of the *Dao De Jing* also says: "The Dao of heaven
benefits (others) without harm; the Dao of sages, does it without contending."[6]

Conclusion

This is the process of regulating the mind. To cultivate the mind, it
must be just like the water's behavior. Water is able to benefit myriad
lives and at the same time does not fight against them. Water is able to
be humble and stay at the lowest place without complaining. It is
because of this that water can be everywhere and anywhere.

It is the same as the mind. If your thinking can be profound, your
manner kind, your talking trustworthy, your behavior righteous, your
handling of things capable, and your action precise, then you will not
be in conflict with others.

1. 荀子曰："孔子觀于東流之水，子貢問孔子曰：「君子之所以見大水必觀焉者，是何？」孔子曰：「夫水遍
   與諸生而無為也，似德；其流也卑下裾拘，必循其理，似義；其洸洸乎不掘盡，似道；若有決行之，其應
   佚若聲響；其赴百仞之谷而不懼，似勇；主量必平，似法；盈不求概，似正；淖約微達，似察；以出為入，
   以就鮮絜，似善化；其萬折也必東，似志。是故君子見大水必觀焉。」"
2. 《易·坎》："水流而不盈，行險而不失其信。"
3. 事善能："『聖人』常善救人，故無棄人；常善救物，故無棄物。"
4. "人能盡其才，地能盡其利，物能盡其用，貨能暢其流。"
5. 蘇轍曰："避高趨下，未嘗有所逆，善地也；空虛靜默，深不可測，善淵也；利澤萬物，施而不求報，善仁
   也；圓必旋，方必折，塞必止，決必流，善信也；洗滌群穢，平准高下，善治也；遇物賦形，而不留于一，善
   能也；冬凝春泮，涸溢不先節，善時也。"
6. 不爭："天之『道』，利而不害；『聖人』之『道』，為而不爭。"

CHAPTER 9

Practicing Placidity—The Deed of the Dao

第九章
運夷—道行

持而盈之，
　　不如其己；
揣而銳之，
　　不可常保。
金玉滿堂，
　　莫之能守；
富貴而驕，
　　自遺其咎。
功成名遂身退，
　　天之『道』。

To take (and keep) until it is overfilling,
    is not as good as stopping (when it is adequate);
To refine and sharpen (a knife),
    may not last for long.
(Having) gold and jade throughout the entire house,
    may not be easy to keep.
(Those who are) rich and hold a high position with pride,
    will (eventually) bring disasters upon themselves.
Withdraw (i.e., retire) as soon as the work is achieved and the name
    is attained,
    this is the Heaven "Dao" (i.e., the Dao of Nature).

General Interpretation

When you take things, you must know when to stop. When pouring water into a cup, you should stop before it overflows. Therefore, you should not be greedy. Greediness has always been one of the human desires. If you have this desire, you will soon be alone by yourself without friendship.

Sharpened knives are usually used first and eventually are damaged and thrown away while dull knives will survive longer since they are not used often. This means you should not keep yourself sharp and get too much attention. Rich people in high positions will not have freedom since they must always be protected. They will always be in an insecure and nervous state. However, if you are at an average or just above average level, you will not attract bad people and will avoid all troubles. Consequently, your mind will be peaceful and calm.

When you have achieved your goal, retreat back and retire. If you glory in your achievment, eventually, you will be envied by others and felt to be threatening to them. Soon, enemies will arise against you.

In the *Han Fei Zi* (《韓非·內儲》) Han Fei said: "Once all sneaky rabbits are hunted, the good hunting dogs will be cooked. Once all the enemies are defeated, all talented planning officers will be killed."[1] This means when you are useful, you will be appreciated. Once the mission is accomplished, often you have no more value and are sacrificed by those who govern you. Therefore, when you have completed your mission, you should retire to a position that is no longer a threat to the rulers.

Qigong Interpretation

This chapter is talking about qigong inner self-cultivation. Your inner feeling and thinking eventually will be manifested externally. If you are able to cultivate your spirit to a neutral and humble level internally, you will be in a neutral state of understanding and practicing qigong. That is the balance of yin (internal cultivation) and yang (external manifestation).

When you have this neutral balance of yin and yang, your heart will be wide open and generous. Even if you have achieved great success, you are not proud, greedy, and ambitious. When the proper time arrives, you simply step aside and offer the opportunity to others. This is the way of the Dao.

From a qigong point of view, if you are able to cultivate your inner spirit to a harmonious and balanced state, your qi circulating in the body can be led smoothly and harmoniously by the mind. The qi can be circulated freely and abundantly only in or with those who have a wide-open and righteous heart. Those who are narrow minded will only restrict their qi from circulating freely. Remember, the mind leads the qi. Only if the mind is open and without emotional bondage can the qi circulate freely.

This chapter has pointed out that the way of attaining this generous and unselfish heart is to take only the right amount. Do not show off how wise you are. Do not be proud about your wealth and glory. If you cannot cultivate these virtues, eventually disaster will befall you. The correct way requires "knowing when to stop and step aside." When you have this attitude, you will not be aggressive and overdo things. Therefore, when you have this wise and neutral judgment, you will be able to use your mind to lead the qi adequately.

Conclusion

When you practice qigong, you should not allow your ego or greediness to control your feelings. Neither excessive qi nor deficient qi is desirable for successful qigong practice. Once you allow your ego or aggressive mind to take over your practice, you will ignore the importance of harmonizing your qi with other parts of the body. For example, you may overemphasize the enhancement of the qi in your liver, and this will trigger your heart to have a problem with excess qi. When you practice qigong, you should keep your emotional mind calm and peaceful. Pay attention to the entire body instead of just a single area. The body is a microcosm of society. If you overdo anything, eventually you may be harmed.

Once your internal emotional mind is regulated, you can then harmonize with others around you. Only when you are able to harmonize with others around you can your mind be peaceful and calm. Without this foundation your mind will be chaotic and disturbed.

1. 《韓非‧內儲》："狡兔盡則良犬烹，敵國滅則謀臣亡。"

CHAPTER 10

Profound De—Embrace Singularity

第十章
玄德—抱一

載營魄抱一，能無離乎？
專氣致柔，能（如）嬰兒乎？
滌除玄覽，能無疵乎？
愛民治國，能無為乎？
天門開闔，能為雌乎？
明白四達，能無知乎？
　　〔生之畜之，
　　　生而不有，
　　　為而不恃，
　　　長而不宰，
　　　是謂玄德。〕

When bearing and managing the po (i.e., vital spirit) and
   embracing singularity (bao yi), can it be not separated (from its
   residence)?
When concentrating the qi to reach its softness, can it be as (soft
   as) a baby?
When cleansing thought to reach its purity, can it be flawless?
When loving the people (i.e., qi) and ruling a country (i.e., body),
   can it be "wuwei?"(i.e., do nothing?)
When opening and closing the Tian Men (Heaven Gate), can it be
   (calm and tender) as a female?
To comprehend (Nature) and reach the four directions (i.e., everywhere), can it be known without knowing?
   [Bearing and raising,
   bearing without possession,
   achieving without arrogance,
   raising without domination,
   this is called "xuan de" (i.e., profound natural virtue)."]

General and Qigong Interpretation

In order to understand this chapter, you must first know a few key Daoist terms. "Po" (魄) is the "vital spirit" that is supported by vital energy (qi) when a person is alive. Often it is called "hun po" (魂魄). "Hun" (魂) means "soul." When a person is dead, then "hun po" is called "gui hun" (鬼魂) or simply "gui" (鬼) (ghost).

In Chinese society, it is believed that when we were born, the spirit incarnated into our physical body. Thus, a human body is constructed of two parts—the physical body (shen, 身) and the spiritual body (shen, 神). This spirit, with qi's nourishment, has become po (魄), enabling us to manage our lives vigorously. When a person is healthy and strong, both the physical body and spiritual body are united tightly and will not be separated. However, when a person is sick or weak, the physical body and spiritual body can be separated. If these two bodies cannot be reunited, then this person will die. Shen, Yi-Guan (沈一貫) said:

> "The Book of Changes said: 'Jing (精) and qi (氣) together become an object. When hun (魂) (i.e., soul) is drifting (i.e., separating), it changes (into ghost).' This means it is normal that all humans have life and death. The spirit of qi (i.e., energy) is 'hun.' The spirit of 'jing' (i.e., essence) is 'po.' When jing and qi are exuberant, the 'hun po' (i.e., living spirit) is exuberant. When jing and qi are weak, the 'hun po' (i.e., living spirit) is weak. When jing and qi have become exhausted, then 'hun' (i.e., soul) is drifting and 'po' (i.e., vital spirit) decreases, consequently separating from the shape (i.e., physical body) and dying."[1]

Therefore, Daoists are always searching for the way to keep the physical body (yang, 陽) and spiritual body (yin, 陰) united as one. This is called "bao yi" (抱一) (embracing singularity) which means the unification of the physical body (physical life) and the spiritual body (spiritual life). He Shang-Gong (河上公) said: "This is talking about when a person is able to embrace singularity and achieve the conditions whereby the (spirit) is not separate from the (physical) body; then they will live long. What is singularity? It is originated from the Dao and the grand harmonization of jing and qi."[2] In order to reach this unification and keep the singularity, through thousands of years of practicing and pondering, Daoists have found out that qigong embryonic breathing (taixi, 胎息) is the key to reaching this goal. The Daoist work, *Ling Jian Zi's Dao Yin Zi-Wu Recording* (《靈劍子導引子午記注》) says: "What is embryonic breathing? It is a method of embracing singularity (bao yi, 抱一) (wuji center) and keeping it in the center."[3]

That is why the first sentence of this chapter asks, ". . . when you are bearing and managing the po . . . can it not be separated (from its residence)?" The way to achieve this goal is to keep the spirit at its residence, ni wan gong (泥丸宮), that is located within the limbic system of the brain (figure 10-1). When the spirit is kept at this center, your mind will be focused, centered, and not entrapped by emotional disturbances. Consequently, the qi will stay in the body and be conserved. If you are interested in this subject, please refer to the book: *Qigong Meditation— Embryonic Breathing*, by YMAA Publication Center.

Qi is the inner energy that supports our physical life and continues to nourish our spirit. Since the air (kong qi, 空氣) (external qi) is related to the inner qi, it is also commonly believed that the qi mentioned in this

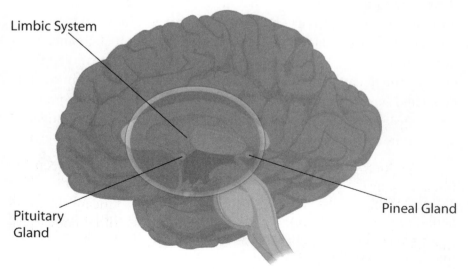

Figure 10-1. Ni Wan Gong (Limbic System)

chapter refers to breathing. We know that the body's inner energy is generated from its metabolism, which converts glucose into bioenergy. During this process, an abundant oxygen supply is necessary. The greater the oxygen supply, the more energy can be produced. That is why when we lift weights or push a car, we must first inhale deeply in order to generate more power.

$$Glucose + 6O_2 \rightarrow 6CO_2 + 6H_2O$$
$$\Delta G^{O'} = -686 \text{ Kcal}$$

The third important point mentioned in this chapter is about the mind. Can we keep our mind simple and pure, so there is no disturbance or confusion about life? In qigong, a common comparison is that the mind is the king of a country, people are qi, and the country is the body. Therefore, the sentence, "When loving the people (i.e., qi) and ruling a country (i.e., body), can it be 'wuwei?'(i.e., do nothing)" This means when you use the mind to love and lead the qi, and use it to nourish the physical body, you can reach the stage of "regulating without regulating" (wuwei, 無為).

Infants' minds are natural, naïve, and innocent so their qi can flow smoothly and softly. In addition, due to an absence of distraction from the surrounding environment, they are able to conserve the qi and keep it in the body. However, when they grow up, their minds can be trapped into emotional bondage making the qi's circulation stagnant, disordered, and wasted. This chapter poses the question, Can you be like a child so the qi can circulate as softly as it does in an infant? In order to do so and have a healthy body, you must first free yourself from emotional enslavement. The way to do so is to cleanse your thoughts and set them free from emotional disturbance. Your mind will become pure and simple. This is the way to attain the softness. Lie Zi (《列子·天瑞》) said: "Talking about an infant, the qi is concentrating (i.e., gathering) and the thought (i.e., mind) is one (i.e., simple). This is the extreme (condition) of harmonization. Consequently, the surrounding objects cannot harm (him) (i.e., distract him and cause harm) and the De (i.e., manifestation of thought) will not fall upon (on him)."[4]

Song, Chang-Xing (宋長星) said:

> *"For those infants not even one year old, the original qi has not been dispersed (i.e., it remains at the center), the born physical body has not been harmed, and they are completely innocent without knowing anything; this is why the marvelous qi can be concentrated (i.e., gathered). (They are) incapable of doing anything, and this is why and how they are able to reach harmonization. It is because (they are able to) gather qi and reach softness, (they have) no desires and know nothing (i.e., they are innocent); (there is) no thought and no thinking; therefore, (they) are able to embrace the singularity of jing and qi."*[5]

In qigong practice, you must see through the attraction of the material world and dissolve your emotional attachment. This is the stage of four emptinesses (si da jie kong, 四大皆空), which all Buddhist and Daoist monks and nuns strive for. The emptinesses of "earth" (di, 地), "water" (shui, 水), "fire" (huo, 火), and "wind" (feng, 風) imply the material world. When you have reached the stage of "regulating of no regulating" (wu tiao er tiao, 無調而調), then you have reached the first step of enlightenment cultivation. This stage is called "wuwei" (無為). When the Fifth Ancestor of Chan (Ren) (禪宗五祖) passed his teaching to his disciples, he asked his disciples about life. One of his top disciples, Shen-Xiu (神秀), said: "The body is like the Bodhi tree (Ficus religiosa) (菩提樹). The mind is like a shining mirror on the table. It should be wiped and cleaned all the time and do not allow any dust on it." Buddha comprehended the Dao and became enlightened when he was meditating under the Bodhi tree. Since then, the Bodhi tree has become a symbol of Buddhahood. After Shen-Xiu finished his statement, another top disciple, Hui-Neng (慧能), responded and said: "Bodhi (Buddhahood) has no tree originally, and the shining mirror and table are not there either. There is no object originally; how can they get dusty?"[6] From this corresponding conversation, you can see Shen-Xiu was still in the stage of regulating his body and mind (cleaning the dust) while Hui-Neng had already passed the stage of cleaning and entered the stage of "regulating of no regulating."

To conclude the last discussion, Cheng, Yi-Ning (程以寧) said:

> "When singularity is embraced, then the jing (i.e., essence) can be converted into qi, qi can be transformed into shen (i.e., spirit), and (finally) the shen can be converted into emptiness. This is the only way to achieve the long lasting Dao of longevity. However, (one) has to begin from embryonic breathing. (When reaching the stage of) seeing (i.e., feeling) the air entering and exiting the nose like smoke (i.e., softly), and this smoke gradually disappears and becomes white (i.e., feels pure). After a long time the breathing becomes so slender, then it is the stage of 'concentrating the qi to reach its softness.' As for pre-heaven (i.e., pre-birth) ancestral qi, only the infant's is complete. For those learners who wish to cultivate qi, can they use the post-heaven body and mind to return to the pre-heaven conditions like infants? What is 'xuan lan' (玄覽)? It means the idea or thought. Whenever there is a slight thought, then the Great Dao will be flawed. Therefore, they must cleanse the thought until it is completely pure white (i.e., pure) and flawless. This is the gongfu of returning the essence to its spirit . . ."[7]

This implies that for you to reach the Dao, you must first regulate your mind until it is without thought, like a baby. Only then can your body and qi be soft and relaxed like a baby. To reach this goal, the first step is through embryonic breathing (taixi, 胎息).

Tian men (天門) (heaven gate) means "the third eye," which allows you to communicate with Nature. There are two locations that are considered tian men (天門) in Daoist society. One is located at the crown (baihui, 百會) where the spirit enters and exits. When a fetus is formed, the spirit enters the physical body through this gate, and when a person dies, the spirit also exits from this gate and the physical body and spiritual body are separated (figure 10-2).

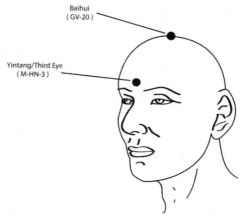

Figure 10-2. Baihui (Gv-20) and Yintang (M-HN-3) (The Third Eye)

The second gate, which Buddhists and Daoists believe is located at the third eye, is also called "heaven eye" (tian yan, 天眼) (tian mu, 天目) (figure 10-2). The third eye is also called "yin tang" (M-HN-3) (印堂) (Seal Hall) in Chinese medicine and qigong society. They believe that if a person is able to train himself to reopen this third eye through meditation, his spirit will be able to exit through this area while the physical body is still alive. Lv Yan (呂岩) said: "When tian men (i.e., heaven gate) is opened, then the spirit has the capability to be steady (i.e., stay in the body) or exit."[8]

To reopen the third eye, you must be soft and tender. Most importantly, you should never forget the spirit valley is the residence of the spirit (shen, 神), the origin of life. Once you have reopened the third eye, you are considered enlightened since you will be able to communicate with Nature and comprehend everything around you. You will also have the capability for telepathy. You will know so many things without any intention of knowing it. Such a person would be considered to be a prophet or a holy man. In Chinese society, this stage is called "De Dao" (得道) that means "has gained the Dao." *The Book of Changes (Yi Jing)* (《易·系辭》) says: "(When one has) changed (to this stage) (i.e., reopened the third eye), there is no thought and there is no action, (and one is) extremely calm without motion. Thus, (one is) able to communicate and sense heaven and earth (i.e., Nature). If he has not reached this extreme (high level of) spiritual (cultivation himself), how can he reach this?"[9]

Song, Chang-Xing (宋常星) said:

"What is ming (明)? It means the inner light of the heart (i.e., mind) is clearly shinning with wisdom. What is bai (白)? It means the original body of the heart (i.e., the origin of mind) exists with purity. Therefore, when (the mind is) insubstantial (i.e., the material world does not exist for it), it is able to shine (i.e., see far) and when (the mind is) calm, it can be white (i.e., pure). (If one's mind can be) insubstantial, calm, shining, and pure, then (he) can reach the four directions (i.e., everywhere) clearly."[10]

Xi, Tong (奚侗) offered this interpretation: "What does it mean by 'insubstantial, calm, shining, and pure, then (he) can reach the four directions (i.e., everywhere) clearly'? It means there is nothing that is not known (i.e., everything is known). Knowing without knowing he is knowing, this is the utmost of the De (i.e., manifestation of mind)."[11] That is why in this chapter it is asked: "To comprehend (nature) and reach the four directions (i.e., everywhere), can it be known without knowing?"

When a person has reached this stage, he will be able to recondition his spirit to be just like a newborn baby. When this spiritual baby is matured, even if the physical body dies, this spirit does not have to reenter the reincarnation process. In this case, this spirit can live forever having reached the stage of Buddhahood. This is also the stage of unification of human and heaven (tian ren he yi, 天人合一). That is why it is asked, 'The opening and closing of the tian men (heaven gate), can it be (calm and tender) as a female?' If you are interested in knowing more about this subject, please refer to the book: *Qigong—Secret of Youth*, by YMAA Publication Center.

Once you have reached the Dao of enlightenment, you must educate others and help them to grow their spirits. You should not control their spirit or abuse them. You should teach them how to be independent spiritually so they will no longer be abused either physically or spiritually. When this happens, everything has become Nature. This is the way of the Dao (道) or "Xuan De" (玄德) (profound natural virtue).

The Complete Book of Principal Contents of Human Life and Temperament (《性命圭旨全書·亨集》) says: "If (you are able to) concentrate the training of qi to reach its softness, the spirit will stay (in its residence) for a long time. To and fro, the real breathing will become natural and smooth. Softly and continuously, lead the qi to its origin. (In this case), the spiritual fountain will always emerge automatically without pumping."[12] This saying implies that in order to keep the spirit at its residence for a long time (longevity), you must first learn how to breathe softly, so you can build up the qi storage to a higher level, and then circulate it in the entire body smoothly and continuously. Through this practice, the original qi (yuan qi, 元氣) can be maintained at its residence. When this original qi is used to nourish the original spirit (yuan shen, 元神), your spirit can be raised up to a high level of longevity and spiritual enlightenment. In qigong breathing practice, "uttering must be slender and receiving must be soft."[13] You must practice regulating the breathing until no regulating is necessary. *Talking Shallow and Near the Dao* (《道言淺近》) says: "Regulating the breathing needs to continue until the real breathing stops." "Condensing the spirit via regulating the breathing can only be reached with a peaceful xin (i.e., emotional mind) and harmonious qi."[14] *The Complete Book of Principal Contents of Human Life and Temperament* (《性命圭旨全書·蟄藏氣穴·眾妙歸根》) says: "When regulating the breathing, the real breathing must be regulated until the regulating has ceased. When you train the spirit, you must train it until no spirit regulating is necessary."[15] This all implies that at the end, the training and cultivation have become natural and no more training is necessary. When this happens, you are training always and everywhere.

Once you have reached this final stage of Buddhahood, can you be like Nature? When you offer, give, or nurture, can you not ask for return or control? It is just like Nature that offers everything without asking for return or control. This is the way of the great, marvelous, and profound De manifested from the Dao (Xuan De, 玄德).

Conclusion

Xuan De (玄德) (the marvelous and profound manifestation of the Dao) is the manifestation of the human and Nature's unification (天人合一). When one has reached this stage, he has reached Buddhahood and become part of Nature. He will have a Buddha heart and embody the saying, "To give birth and raise, to yield without owning, to do without keeping, to raise without controlling" as is natural.

The first step of reaching this Buddhahood is to embrace the singularity (bao yi, 抱一). That means to bring your mind and body to a childlike state so the body and qi can be soft. When this occurs, you will be able to conserve your qi to an abundant level and circulate it smoothly in the body. To have a simple and concentrated mind, you must set yourself free from the bondage of the material and emotional worlds. Only without these distractions can your qi be gathered and strong. You can then lead the qi upward to the third eye (tian yan, 天眼) to reopen it. Once you have opened it, you will comprehend and sense a lot of things other people cannot see or sense (you will be enlightened). Then, you continue your spiritual cultivation until this spirit can be reunited with the natural spirit and become Buddha.

1. 沈一貫曰："《易》曰:「精氣為物,游魂為變」。此言眾人有生死之常也。氣之神為魂,精之神為魄,精氣盛則魂魄盛,精氣衰則魂魄衰,精氣耗竭魂游魄降,與形相離死矣。"
2. 河上公曰:"言人能抱一,使不離於身,則長存。一者,道始所生,太和之精氣也"
3. 靈劍子導引子午記注:"胎息者,抱一守中之法也。"
4. 《列子·天瑞》:"其在嬰孩,氣專志一,和之至也,物不傷焉,德莫加焉。"
5. 宋長星曰:"未歲之赤子,元氣未散,乾體未破,百無一知,正是氣專之妙;百無一能,正是致和之妙。因專氣致柔,所以無欲無知,無思無慮,神氣故能抱一。"
6. 禪宗五祖傳法時,神秀上坐作偈曰:"身為菩提樹,心如明鏡台,時時勤撫拭,勿使惹塵埃。"慧能應曰:"菩提本無樹,明鏡亦非台,本來無一物,何處惹塵埃?"
7. 程以寧曰:"抱一,則精化為氣,氣化為神,神化為虛矣。此不二法門,長生久視之道。然必自調息始,見鼻中氣出入如煙,煙象微消成白,久之而息微,是專氣致柔也。先天祖氣,惟嬰兒完全,學人養氣,能以后天以復先天如嬰兒乎?玄覽者,見解也。稍著見解,即為大道之疵類矣。故必滌除玄覽,渾然純白,能無疵乎?此為練精還神工夫。...."
8. 呂岩曰:"天門開闔是入定出神之能事也。"
9. 《易·繫辭》:"易,無思也,無為也,寂然不動,感而遂通天下之故。非天下之至神,其孰能與于此。"
10. 宋常星曰:"明者,心之內光慧照謂之明。白者,心之本體素存謂之白。蓋以虛能生明,靜能生白。虛靜明白者,方可謂明白四達也。"
11. 奚侗曰:"明白四達,是無所不知也。知而不自以為知,乃德之上也。"
12. 《性命圭旨全書·亨集》:"專氣致柔神久留,往來真息自悠悠。綿綿迤邐歸元氣,不汲靈泉常自流。"
13. "吐唯細細,納唯綿綿。"
14. 《道言淺近》:"調息要調真息息","凝神調息,只要心平氣和。"
15. 《性命圭旨全書·蟄藏氣穴·眾妙歸根》:"調息要調真息息,煉神須煉不神神。"

CHAPTER 11

Usage of Insubstantial—Practical Use

第十一章
虛無—實有

三十幅，共一轂，
　　當其無，
　　　有車之用。
埏埴以為器，
　　當其無，
　　　有器之用。
鑿戶牖以為室，
　　當其無，
　　　有室之用。
故
有之以為利，
　　無之以為用。

Thirty spokes to make a wheel,
    with emptiness (in its axle),
    there is a usage of the wheel.
Using clay to mold a vessel,
    when there is nothing inside,
    then it can be used as a container.
To cut open the door and window to make a room,
    when it is empty,
    there is the usage of the room.
Therefore,
when it is occupied, there is a benefit (of using),
    when it is empty, then it can be useful.

General Interpretation

Thirty spokes made a wheel in ancient China. These spokes were then inserted in the empty space of the axle so the wheel was functional. Without this empty space, the wheel would not be completed. When a vessel is built and empty, the vessel is useful. The same as a house: when it is empty, it can be used. Therefore, once these empty spaces are used, the usages and the benefits of space have been taken. However, when they are still empty, then they can still be used.

Si, De-Qing (釋德清) said:

> "This is talking about people who only know the usage of the usage, but don't know the usage of no usage. It means everyone knows the usage of the spokes, but without knowing the crucial usage of the empty space in the axle. Everyone knows the usage of a vessel but without knowing that it is useful due to the empty space of the vessel. Everyone knows the usage of a room, but without knowing that the usage is due to the empty space of the room. From this, we can compare with the heaven and the earth (i.e., Nature) for their physical appearances. Everyone knows the usage of the heaven and the earth, but not knowing that they are useful due to their insubstantial and invisible divine center. Therefore, it is known that the usage is actually used from nothingness. However, the nothingness cannot be used by itself; it must rely on having for support. Thus, it is said: 'When there is having, it has the benefit of usage, and when there is nothingness, then there is a usage.' Benefit means support. The study of Lao Zi is using the having to observe the nothingness. That means if having is used to observe the nothingness, then it is having, but without having. This is the marvelousness of the Dao and is its major point."[1]

There is a story about a samurai swordsman who was so proud of himself because of his accomplishment. However, he knew there was a very high level master with whom he could continue his advancement. Therefore, he came to see this old master.

"Honorable master, I have reached a high level of samurai skills. But I heard you are very good. Therefore, I come to bow to you and want to learn from you." With his pride, he showed his satisfaction with his accomplishment.

The master did not say a word. He went in the inner room and later came out with a teapot and cups. He put one of the cups in front of this visitor and began to pour the tea. The tea filled up the cup quickly and began to overflow the cup. When this proud visitor saw it, with a little confusion he exclaimed,

"Master, stop. The tea is overflowing the cup."

The master put the teapot down and looked at him with a smile.

"Young man, I am sorry I cannot teach you. Your cup is full. If you wish to learn, you must first empty your cup." After he said this, he went inside.

The Chinese have a proverb: "Satisfaction will incur loss and humility will gain benefit."[2]

Qigong Interpretation

Two parts make up a human body: a visible physical part and an invisible spiritual part. The spiritual part is the origin of physical manifestation. Without this part, the physical shape will not be formalize. However, without physical manifestation, the spirit will not be useful. The spirit (or mind) is the root of physical manifestation. Thus, spirit is yin while the physical body is yang.

From a qigong point of view, we have two minds: a conscious mind and a subconscious mind. It is our subconscious mind, which is more truthful, that connects to our spirit. In order to have a healthy body, we must first have a healthy mind. The root of a healthy mind is a humble mind. Though invisible, its manifestation can be powerfully influential and significant.

When our body is healthy, strong, and long-lived, it is due to our healthy mind's manifestation. Conversely, those who have a strong body initially but are without a healthy mind to govern it may experience bodily harm and damage due to aberrant qi circulation. This makes obvious the value and benefit of the mind's effect. If you keep your mind humble and empty, your heart will be opened and allow for more positive manifestations. Although the spirit is insubstantial, its applications are unlimited.

It is known from Chinese medicine that the status of the qi's circulation in all channels is influenced by the sun and the moon (Nature). It is the up-down sine wave cycle of natural qi that produces the qi potential difference. Consequently, the times for the strongest qi flows for each channel are different. For example, the strongest qi flow of the heart channel is around noon (11 AM–1 PM) while the liver channel is 1–3 AM. Circadian or diurnal processes are evident throughout nature as well as within human biological functions. These rhythms have affected how human beings evolved. One example is that we typically sleep when the sun goes down and are active when the sun rises. Going against these evolved natural rhythms and patterns can ultimately affect our health and well-being negatively.

In addition, it is also known from both Chinese medicine and qigong that the mind (intentions/emotions) can influence the qi's circulation significantly. This is because the mind or emotion will affect the potential difference in the qi and trigger the qi's circulation. For example, lifting our arms to pick up an object is initiated from a thought (intention). From this thought, the qi potential difference is generated. Thus, the qi (bioelectricity) is led to the nerve system of the arms and activates the muscles' function. However, if there is too much mental disturbance (such as emotions), the normal qi's status of each channel can be disrupted. Heightened or chronic anger, for example, may trigger the qi's stagnation in the liver channel. This may cause excitement of the liver, making it too yang and leading to stiffness and tightness in the arm muscles.

It is when the insubstantial mind is empty that it has the potential to be used. Use of the mind occurs once the intentions are initiated and the actions are carried out. That is why regulating the mind is the key to a successful qigong practice. The mind is just like the king of the body's empire. When the mind is calm, peaceful, and empty, there is no thought. Therefore, when we consciously choose to act, our future actions can be under our control. Keeping our mind in a pure state of emptiness provides myriad options of manifestation in the physical world. This is the thought of no thought and the mind of no mind that is the aim of embryonic breathing meditation.

Conclusions

Nature includes two parts: a visible physical part (the material world, or yang space) (yang jian, 陽間) and an invisible spiritual part (the spiritual world) (yin jian, 陰間). The natural spirit is the origin of physical manifestation. A human being is created in this Nature and, thus, also includes two interdependent aspects: a physical life and a spiritual life. While physical life originates from the spiritual world, its function is to express the potential for spiritual manifestation in the material world. Therefore, from a qigong point of view, spiritual cultivation is the key to a healthy body and longevity.

When the conscious mind is empty, you will have a feeling, a connection to the Yin world so it is useful in the Dao (Yin dimension) (i.e., spiritual world). However, if you use the conscious mind, then you are in the De (Yang dimension) and it is useful in the Yang world (material world).

1. 釋德清說：“此言世人但知有用之用，而不知無用之用也。意謂人人皆知車穀有用，而不知用在穀中一竅；人人皆知器之有用，而不知用在器中之虛；人人皆知室之有用，而不知用在室中之空處。以此比喻，譬如天地之有形也。人皆知天地有用，而不知用在虛靈無相之心。是知有雖有用而實在用在無也。然無不能自用，須賴有以濟之。故曰：‘有之以為利，無之以為用’。利猶濟也。老君之學，要即有以觀無。若即有以觀無，則雖有而不有，是謂道妙，此其宗也。”
2. “滿招損，謙受益。”

CHAPTER 12

Repressing Desires—Regulating the Mind

第十二章

檢欲—調心

五色，令人目盲；
五音，令人耳聾；
五味，令人口爽。
馳騁畋獵，
　　　令人心發狂；
難得之貨，
　　　令人行妨。
是以
『聖人』為腹不為目，
　　故
　去彼取此。

Five colors make people blind;
five music tones make people deaf;
five flavors make people lose their sense of taste.
Riding the horse to run in the field for hunting
    makes people's heart (mind) crazy;
Those difficult-to-acquire (precious) goods,
    make people trapped and disabled.
Therefore,
those sages' concern is about their abdomen (i.e., they keep their
    qi full at the abdomen) not their eyes (i.e., material attractions).
    Thus,
repel those (attractions) and take this (i.e., qi cultivations).

General Interpretation

The five colors (wu se, 五色) are: red, yellow, blue, white, and black; from these, all the different colors are constructed. The five music tones (wu yin, 五音) are: gong (宮), shang (商), jiao (角), zheng (徵), and yu (羽), from these all Chinese music is constructed. The five flavors (wu wei, 五味) are: sour (suan, 酸), sweet (tian, 甜), bitter (ku, 苦), pungent (la, 辣), and salty (xian, 鹹). The work, *Huai Na Zi* (《淮南子·精神訓》) says: "Five colors confuse the eyes and prevent the eyes from seeing clearly; five tones clamor in the ears and make sounds inaudible to the ears; and five flavors befog the mouth and dull the tastes."[1]

Most people are looking for beautiful colors, exciting music, and various stimulating tastes. However, they have forgotten that the most important root of color is the colorless. From the colorless, all colors can be derived. The foundation of sound is silence since all sounds are generated from no sound. Furthermore, the tasteless is the origin of all tastes. It is from the tasteless that all tastes are created. Once your mind is attracted by different colors, you are addicted to colorful beauties and forget its root, the colorless. Once your mind is accustomed to your favorite music, you will soon forget the precious value of silence. Furthermore, once you have become habituated to strong tastes, you will forget the feeling of tastelessness. For example, water is tasteless compared with all other tastes. However, it is from water that all juices and other drinks are generated. Once you are accustomed to the special taste, you will soon forget how good "the taste of the tasteless" is. Therefore, you should not forget the root, the origin, and the foundation of everything.

Riding horses and hunting make people excited. This excitement can disturb a peaceful mind. Only when your mind is in a calm and peaceful condition will you be able to think clearly and concentrate.

Precious goods that are difficult to possess can make people's minds unstable and chaotic. Once you own these goods, you will worry about how to protect them and keep them from being taken away.

For these reasons, the sages in the past just worried about keeping their stomach full (that is, keeping qi full in the abdomen) instead of worrying about all emotional desires.

Qigong Interpretation and Conclusions

In Chinese Buddhist and Daoist qigong society, it is understood that in order to have a peaceful and calm mind to cultivate your qi and spirit, you must first regulate the seven passions and six desires (qi qing liu yu, 七情六慾). Recall that the seven passions are joy (xi, 喜), anger (nu, 怒), sorrow (ai, 哀), happiness (le, 樂), love (ai, 愛), hate (hen, 恨), and lust (yu, 慾). The desires are generated from the six roots that are the eyes, ears, nose, tongue, body, and emotional mind (xin, 心). In addition, Buddhists and Daoists are also searching for the way to cultivate within themselves a neutral state separated from the four emptinesses of earth, water, fire, and wind (si da jie kong, 四大皆空). They believe this training enables them to keep their spirits independent so they can reopen the third eye for enlightenment.

Wise qigong practitioners will focus on how to cultivate their qi to an abundant level and store it at the lower dan tian instead of allowing their mind to be in a chaotic condition generated from the emotional mind. As was experienced in the past by accomplished qigong practitioners, in order to reach to a profound level of qigong practice, you must first regulate your mind. This is because the mind is the general that governs your physical and mental bodies.

1.《淮南子·精神訓》："五色亂目，使目不明；五聲譁耳，使耳不聰；五味亂口，使口爽傷。"

CHAPTER 13

Governing the Body—Loathing Shame

第十三章
治身—厭恥

寵辱若驚，
　　貴大患若身。
何謂寵辱若驚？
　　寵為上，辱為下。
得之若驚，失之若驚，
　　是謂寵辱若驚。
何謂貴大患若身？
　　吾所以有大患者，
　　為吾有身。
及吾無身，吾有何患？
故
貴以身為天下，
　　若可寄天下；
愛以身為天下，
　　若可托天下。

Favoritism and disgrace are both frightening,
    so frightening it is as if there is a big disaster coming upon the
    body.
What does "favoritism and disgrace are both frightening" mean?
    Favoritism is for high (i.e., favor) and disgrace is for low (i.e.,
    insulting).
When acquired it, it is fearful and when lost it, it is also fearful.
    Therefore, it is said favoritism and disgrace are both frightening.
What does "as if there is a big disaster coming upon the body"
    mean?
    The reason that there is a big disaster coming upon,
    is because one has concerned (valued) one's body.
If one doesn't have oneself, then what disaster is able to fall upon
    him?
There,
If one values himself as the world,
    then he can be the custodian of the world.
If one loves himself as the world,
    then he can be entrusted with the world.

General Interpretation

Often when we feel unhappy it is because we have thought too much of ourselves. We have taken our own feelings too seriously. If we can treat our feelings and benefits lightly and be concerned with other people's feelings and benefits first, then we will not have emotional bondage or entrap ourselves. For example, if we take our external beauty too seriously and take other people's comments seriously, we will be trapped in emotional turmoil. In time, you will have positioned yourself between favoritism and disgrace. However, once you awaken to realize that real long-lasting beauty is internal instead of external, you will share your valuables and love with others. With this benevolent heart, you will acquire a calm and peaceful life.

In the work *Zhi You Zi* (《至游子·五化》) it is said: "There is no self, does not mean there is no physical body. It is the way to harmonize and match with the Great Dao. Do not pursue glory and wealth selfishly and do not search for advantage. Mind is always peaceful and calm without desires and forgets there is a body (i.e., self)."[1]

Du, Guang-Ting (杜光庭) said:

> "If a ruler really loves himself, he must be humble and frugal. When he is humble, then there is no resented enemy. When he is frugal, then there is no addicted favor. If there is no resented enemy, the country is safe and people are peaceful. If he does not have an addiction, the people will become wealthy. In this case, those who are far appreciate you and those who are near are delighted with you. There is no war with others and no need for guards at borders. The peace and happiness can last and be long. This is the person who can be the custodian of the world."[2]

Dr. Sun, Yat-sen (孫中山) said: "that which is under heaven (i.e., world) belongs to everyone."[3] If you have a wide-open and unselfish heart, value the world as your own self, and love the world as loving yourself, then you can be a good leader.

Qigong Interpretation

The mind is the ruler (the king) of the body and governs the qi (the people). If the mind is selfishly concerned with some special favors and ignores the qi's condition, then the qi's circulation in the body will be imbalanced. For example, if you are addicted to alcohol or some special spicy food and ignore your liver's qi condition, you may soon create a serious liver health problem for yourself. However, if your mind pays attention to the entire body's feelings and treats your entire body as a whole, you will see the harmonization of the body. When this happens, your mind will be peaceful and calm.

It is the same if your mind has been attracted by your own glorification. Eventually, you may bring shame or insult to yourself. That is why it is said: "Do not lose your life due to glory and insult."[4] Wise qigong practitioners take emotional disturbance lightly and are simply humble and frugal. With this attitude, your mind will be peaceful and calm. Naturally, your qigong practice will be able to advance smoothly.

Conclusions

Qigong practice can be compared to a battle against sickness and aging. If you compare your body to a battlefield, then your mind is like the general who generates ideas and controls the situation, and your breathing is his strategy. Your qi is like the soldiers who are led to various places on the battlefield. Your essence is like the quality of the soldiers such as educational background and the skills of combat. Finally, your spirit is the morale of the army.

If your mind is calm and peaceful, you will be able to judge the conditions clearly and set up an effective strategy to govern the soldiers to take care of the situation. However, if your mind is disordered and confused, the battle will be lost for sure. The way of keeping your mind calm and peaceful is to not be distracted by emotional disturbances.

1.《至游子·五化》："無身者，非無此身也。體合大道，不恂乎榮貴，不求乎茍進，恬然無欲，忘此有待之身也。"
2. 杜光庭說："夫人君自愛其身，必歉恭儉約，謙恭則怨敵不起，儉約則嗜好不行；無怨敵則人安，無嗜好則人富，如此則遠懷近悅，外無戰爭，境無勞人，享祚久長，可以永托于天下。"
3. "天下為公。"
4. "不要為榮辱而喪身。"

CHAPTER 14

Praise the Marvelousness—Appearance of the Spirit

第十四章
贊玄─神態

視之不見，名曰『夷』；
聽之不聞，名曰『希』；
搏之不得，名曰『微』。
　　此三者不可致詰，
　　故混而為一。
其上不皦，其下不昧。
　　繩繩不可名，
　　復歸於無物。
是謂無狀之狀，
　　無物之象，
　　是謂惚恍。
迎之不見其首；
　　隨之不見其後。
執古之『道』以御今之有。
　　能知古始，是謂『道』紀。

When looked at, it cannot be seen, named "Yi" (i.e., invisible);
when listened to, it cannot be heard, named "Xi" (i.e., inaudible);
when grasped, it cannot be acquired, named "Wei"(i.e., fine
formless).
These three cannot be completely unraveled;
thus, they are combined into one.
Above it (i.e., in the sky), it is not bright (i.e., clear) and below it
(i.e., on the ground), it is not dim (i.e., concealed).
It is continuous and endless, it cannot be named.
It returns to its state of nothingness.
Thus, it can be called the shape of the shapeless,
with the appearance of nothingness,
and is called "Huang Hu."
When in front of it, its head cannot be seen and,
when following it, its tail cannot be seen.
Use this ancient Dao and apply it to the needs of today.
When able to know the ancient beginning, then it is called
knowing the principles of the Dao.

General Interpretation

He Shang Gong (河上公) called this chapter "Praise the Marvelousness" (Zan Xuan, 贊玄). That means this entire chapter's purpose is to praise the marvelousness of the Dao. "Yi" (夷) means flat or extinguished and implies empty or nothingness. The Dao is so empty that it cannot be seen. "Xi" (希) means sparse or faint. The Dao is also so sparse and cannot be heard. "Wei" (微) means small or weak. It means the Dao is so small and weak that it cannot be felt or sensed. These three things, cannot be seen, cannot be heard, and cannot be felt. Even if we investigate profoundly, we still cannot come to a conclusion about what these three things that cannot be seen, heard, or felt actually are. He Shang Gong (河上公) said: "Colorless means 'Yi', soundless means 'Xi', and shapeless means 'Wei'."[1] He also said: "These three things; called 'yi', 'xi', and 'wei' cannot be unraveled because they are colorless, soundless, and shapeless. It cannot be described orally and cannot be passed down with writing so it can be gained via pondering and profound investigation."[2]

The Dao does not show its shining or dimness either from above or below. Even if we try describing it in numerous ways, it always returns to its origin, nothingness (emptiness). Therefore, it is the shape of no shape and the state of no state. This is called "hu huang" (惚恍). "Hu huang" is the state of existing but not existing and is there but not there. It is the state of semi-existing. When you face it and try to see it and understand it from the beginning, you cannot see it. If you follow and try to see and understand it from the end, you still cannot see it. Chapter 21 of the *Dao De Jing* says: "When describing the Dao as an object, it is ambiguous whether it is there or not. Though it is ambiguous, it seems there is an image; though it is indistinct, it seems there is an object. Though it is so profound and obscure, it seems there is an essence; its essence is so real and truthful, it gives (you) faith."[3]

However, if we are able to grasp the meaning of this ancient Dao and apply its principles and rules to today's world, we can say we have known the ancient beginning. This is the rule of the Dao. He Dao Quan (河道全) said: "If (one is) able to know the theory (or rules) of the ancient beginning, then it can be called 'gaining the principles of the Dao.'"[4]

Qigong Interpretation and Conclusions

The Dao (or taiji or spirit) in the human body is related to the subconscious mind. As known from qigong experience, the subconscious mind connects to the spirit. Both reside at the Mud Pill Palace (Ni Wan Gong, 泥丸宮). Since we don't know what the spirit is yet, we can only feel and sense the spirit through the subconscious mind. The Mud Pill Palace is situated within the limbic system of the head, at the bottom of the narrow space (brain wave resonance chamber) between the two lobes of the brain. This space is called "spiritual valley" (shen gu, 神谷). The spirit that resides in this valley is called "gu shen" (谷神) (chapter 6). The energy is trapped in this valley and resonates with Nature. There is no bondage for this spirit, no restriction of space (dimension) and time. The only way to access this spirit is through a semisleeping state (hu huang, 惚恍) that can be reached by deep meditation. If you are able to use this subconscious mind or spirit to guide you and lead you to the correct path of your life, then you have surely grasped the Dao (Nature) and can apply it in your life.

Du, Guang-Ting (杜光庭) said:

"Applying its (i.e., the Dao's) principle, myriad articles can be expanded (i.e., developed); using its rules, myriad objects can be raised (i.e., created). To regulate the body and govern a country, it is also from this. When governing a country, it should follow the Dao of 'wuwei' (i.e., doing nothing). Thus, people will restore their honesty and return to their simplicity. If regulating the body with the conduct of 'wuwei,' then the spirit will be whole and qi will be abundant. When qi is abundant, the life will be extended and when the spirit is whole, the marvelousness (i.e., spirit) can be raised. This is important in the governing of a country and regulating the body."[5]

1. 河上公說："無色曰夷，無聲曰希，無形曰微。"
2. 河上公說："三者，謂夷、希、微也。不可致詰者，謂無色、無聲、無形；口不能言，書不能傳，當受之以靜，詰問而得之也。"
3. 二十一章："『道』之為物，惟恍惟惚。惚兮恍兮，其中有象；恍兮惚兮，其中有物。窈兮冥兮，其中有精；其精甚真，其中有信。"
4. 河道全說："能知古始之理，是謂得道之綱紀也。"
5. 杜光庭說："引其綱，萬目張；引其紀，萬目起。理身理國，亦猶此歟！理國執無為之道，民復朴而還淳；理身執無為之行，則神全而氣旺。氣旺者延年，神全者升玄，理國修身之要也。"

CHAPTER 15

The Exhibition of Dao's Manifestation—Regulating the Mind

第十五章
顯德—調心

古之善為道者，
　　微妙玄通，深不可識。
夫唯不可識，
　　故強為之容：
豫兮，若冬涉川；
　　猶兮，若畏四鄰；
儼兮，其若客；
　　渙兮，若冰之將釋；
敦兮，其若樸；
　　曠兮，其若谷，
混兮，其若濁：
　　孰能晦以理之徐明？
　　孰能濁以靜之徐清？
　　孰能安以動之徐生？
保此道者不欲盈。
　　夫唯不盈，故能蔽而新成。

Those who were good in following the Dao in ancient times
knew that the Dao was subtle, marvelous and mysterious; its
depth was so deep that it could not be comprehended.
It could not be comprehended,
thus, it could only be described reluctantly with the following
ways:
Cautiously, like crossing a river in winter;
alertly, like fearing problems with the four neighbors.
Solemnly, like a visiting guest;
yieldingly, like ice about to melt.
Genuinely, like a piece of uncarved jade;
openly, like a valley.
When it is muddy like dirty water,
who is able to manage this muddle and make it desist gradually?
Who is able to quiet down this muddiness and make it clear
gradually?
Who is able to activate the calmness and make it alive gradually?
Those who maintain this Dao will not overfill themselves (i.e., they
will be humble).
It is because they do not overfill themselves that they can
preserve the old without creating anew.

General Interpretation

Since ancient times until now, we have known the Dao exists, but we still don't know too much about it. Thus, we cannot use our limited knowledge to interpret the Dao. If we do that, the truth of the Dao will be used to mislead and will be misunderstood. But based on its existence we will be able to describe what it is like and how it feels. Yet, what we can describe is only the part of it that can be detected via a few angles of observation and feelings.

The Dao seems to take care of natural matters cautiously. Everything being taken care of is treated cautiously just like a person crossing a river on thin ice. Not only that, the Dao is always in a state of high alertness so it can sense any disorder in this universe and respond to the changes. Therefore, Nature always corrects itself. The Dao also takes matters seriously. Since the Dao does not have emotion or compassion, it is never compelled to act by emotion. Everything must follow the laws of Nature. It makes you feel like a piece of melting ice: easy, steady, and peaceful. It is natural and genuine just like a piece of raw jade without being decorated or carved. Furthermore, it is generous and open just like a wide valley.

When there is disturbance and disorder in this universe, what is able to make it desist, quiet down, and enable it to regain its order and finally resume its function? There is no question about it; it is the Dao.

From this, you can see that those who have reached the Dao will be able to adjust and correct themselves when they are off the path of the Dao. That is why sages are able to preserve and maintain themselves on the path of the Dao. Not only that, from this path, they are able to consciously create their future.

Qigong Interpretation

As explained in previous chapters, the Dao is what is called taiji. When it is applied to a human body, it is the subconscious mind. Our subconscious mind is mysterious, marvelous, and powerful; it has not yet been fully understood by modern science.

When our subconscious mind is cautious, solemn, calm, alert, loosened, opened, and genuine, we are able to feel or sense the disorder of the qi's circulation or the disturbance in Nature and in our bodies. Not only that, we are able to bring the qi's disorder back to its original healthy path. In order to do this, you must find the center of your subconscious mind (the limbic system) and keep awareness there. As we explained earlier, the subconscious mind is related to your spirit. Therefore, when you keep your subconscious mind at its residence, the spirit will be able to stay there. As long as you are able to maintain your spirit at the center, you will not be disturbed or misled by emotional thinking. Emotional thinking is the main cause of the mind's chaos and disturbances. The way to develop this capability is through embryonic breathing meditation (taixi jing zuo, 胎息靜坐). Once you are able to do this, you can correct the qi to its original path and find other, alternative paths by following the way of the Dao.

For example, if you are able to maintain your mind at a deep subconscious level, whenever there is some qi disorder, such as abnormal qi circulation of the liver (related to anger), you will be able to feel it, sense it, and calm down your emotional mind to relax the liver so the qi can circulate normally again. However, if you find out your liver is qi deficient, you will be able to create the way to nourish and strengthen it.

Zhang, Jin-Gan (張金淦) said: "Peace, is the beginning of calmness. When the peace is able to last long, then the action can be generated gradually. Yi (i.e., *Yi Jing*, 易經) said: 'When the peace is extremely calm to the point of stillness, (i.e., actions of physical and mental bodies), then you will be able to sense and communicate with heaven and earth (i.e., Nature.)' This is what 'activate the calmness' means in this chapter."[1] Communication between Nature and the spirit is called "shen tong" (神通) in Daoist society. This saying implies that in order to be calm, you must first find peace. Only when your mind is peaceful can you then be calm. The way of reaching a peaceful state of mind is by keeping away from emotional disturbance. Once you have reached a high level of calmness, your mind will be clear. With this clear mind, you will be able to sense and communicate with your body and Nature (actions).

It is said in the ancient document, *Yu Ji Qi Jian* (《云笈七鑒·元氣論》): "When the inner mind (i.e., emotional mind) does not arise, the external distractions will not enter. When there is peace and calmness both internally and externally, then the spirit is stable and the qi is harmonious. Consequently, the original qi will arrive automatically."[2] This saying implies that when your inner mind is peaceful and external attractions cannot tempt you, your spirit will be peaceful and qi can be harmonious. When this happens, your original qi (qi from original essence) (yuan jing, 元精) will be produced automatically. It is believed from qigong that there are two kinds of qi circulating in the body: original qi (yuan qi, 元氣) or pre-birth qi (xiantian qi, 先天氣) and post-birth qi (houtian qi, 後天氣). Original qi is converted from the original essence (yuan jing, 元精) that you inherited from your parents while post-birth qi is converted from the food and air after your birth. It is said original qi is pure and when it is circulating abundantly and smoothly in your body, your mind and physical body are calm and healthy. However, when post-birth qi circulates overwhelmingly in your body, your mind is more emotional and scattered, and the physical body may be harmed. Therefore, Daoists would like to enhance the production of original qi and reduce the post-birth qi.

However, it is not easy to reach a peaceful and calm mind. You must be humble and not greedy. You should also prevent the initiation of new desires. Xue, Hui (薛惠) said:

> *"It said that those who wish to protect the Dao will not be overflowing (i.e., with greediness/desires). This is because overflow will not last long and it is what the Dao dislikes. Those who are awkward and lacking are valued by those wise men. But laymen value those who are new and complete (i.e., new accomplishment). Because (those wise men) do not have overflowing desire, thus they are able to keep the lack (i.e., deficiency) and do not wish to pursue the new and complete."[3]*

Cheng, Yi-Ning (程以寧) also said: "With all the objects in this world, when there is something new, then there is something old. When there is something old, then there is something broken. Rarely do things survive without being damaged. When there is no overflow (i.e., desire), then it does not matter if it is new, old, or damaged, nothing can affect the mind. Thus, since ancient times until now, those (sages) that are able to maintain their (humble) incompleteness with Nature, do not even concern the old or broken, how will they see the new and completeness."[4]

Wise men who have attained the Dao have reached the stage of doing without doing (wuwei, 無為). Since these doings are so common for them, they have reached to a level where they don't have to do it and everything will happen automatically. Zhuang Zi (《莊子·刻意》) said: "(Sages) reach the high without intention, cultivate (temperament) without benevolence and righteousness, rule without pursuing merit and reputation, enjoy leisure without rivers and oceans, and live long without Dao-Yin (i.e., qigong). All are forgotten but everything is acquired. They treat things lightly and simply without limitation, yet all the beauties (i.e., good deeds) will follow them. This is the Dao of the heaven and the earth (i.e., Nature) and also the De (virtues) of those sages."[5]

Conclusions

This chapter has made a few points:

1. To have a high level of sensitivity so your spirit and the natural spirit can unite and communicate with each other, you must first keep your mind at its spiritual center (the limbic system). With this method, you will be able to reunite with Nature.

2. To keep the spirit at its residence (spiritual center), you must first get rid of your desire, greediness, and any other emotional allurements. Only then can your mind be peaceful and calm so the spirit stays at its residence.

3. Once you have established this mind, you will be able to do it without even thinking about it. This is the stage of regulating of no regulating and means the stage of "wuwei" (無為).

1. 張金淦說：“安者靜之始也，安而能久，則動徐徐而生矣。《易》曰：‘寂然不動，感而遂通天下之故’。今所謂動者，亦若是耳。”

2. 《云笈七鑒·元氣論》：“內心不起，外境不入；內外安靜，則神定氣和；神定氣和，則元氣自至。”

3. 薛惠說：“此言終身守道之常。保，持守也。言保此道者，不欲盈滿，蓋盈不可久，道所惡也。蔽缺者，至人之所貴；新成者，世俗之所貴。惟不欲盈，故能守其缺，而不願為新成也。”

4. 程以寧說：“天下之物，有新則有蔽，有蔽則有壞，而不蔽則鮮矣。夫惟不盈，則新蔽成壞，無所容心，是以互古互今，能與天壤俱蔽，不見其舊而壞，安見其新而成？”

5. 《莊子·刻意》：“不刻意而高，無仁義而修，無功名而治，無江海而閒，不導引而壽；無不忘也，無不有也，淡然無極，而眾美從之；此天地之道，聖人之德也。”

CHAPTER 16

Return to the Root—Two Polarities

第十六章
歸根—兩儀

致虛極，守靜篤。
　　萬物並作，吾以觀復。
夫物芸芸，各復歸其根。
　　歸根曰「靜」，是謂「復命」。
　　復命曰『常』，知常曰『明』。
　　不知『常』，妄作凶。
知『常』容，容乃公。
　　公乃全，全乃天。
天乃『道』，『道』乃久。
　　歿身不殆。

Attain the ultimate nihility and maintain the serenity sincerely.
   Myriad objects are all in actions; I therefore observe their cyclic
   repetitions.
Though all objects flourish, each individual repeatedly returns to
   its root.
   Returning to its root is called tranquility and means "repeti-
   tion of life."
   Repetition of life is called constancy and knowing constancy
   means clarity.
   Not knowing constancy, recklessness will cause disaster.
Knowing constancy then can be accepted; accepted, then it can be
   impartial.
   Impartial, then it can be completed; completed, then accord
   with heaven.
Heaven is the Dao and following the Dao, is eternal,
   die without perishing.

General Interpretation

All lives originated from nothingness; therefore, in order to see the repetition of lives, we must first attain this nothingness. This nothingness is called the wuji (無極) (no extremity) state. In this state, there is no discrimination of yin (陰) and yang (陽). It is the neutral state of everything. Therefore, nothingness here means the emptiness of the emotional mind and material world. In order to reach this state, the first step is to keep your mind in its extreme insubstantial state and the physical body in its ultimate calmness. The Daoist classic *Xing Ming Gui Zhi* (《性命圭旨》) says: "When there are no objects in the heart (i.e., the mind), it means 'insubstantial,' and when there is no initiation of thought, then the mind is calm."[1] When the mind does not have initiation of thought, the physical body can be quiet and calm. When this happens, you will be able to see the beginning and creation of lives and understand their cyclical nature. Even though there are millions of various living objects, each, at the end, must return to its origin (its root). It is from this origin that the initiation of life begins again. It is said in *Yun Ji Qi Qian* (《云笈七签》): "When returning to its origin and foundation, it is returning to its root to repeat its life."[2] When one has returned to this origin, one is calmed, quiet, and peaceful. When the new life is initiated again, the constant natural routine (chang, 常) will be repeated. If you know this constant natural routine, then there is no doubt about life and you will be enlightened and have understood the way life is. If you do not follow this routine, then you are against Nature and, consequently, various disasters may befall you. If you are able to follow this natural routine and match the way of the natural rules, then you have a better chance to live a long and healthy life. This is what the "Dao" means. He Shang Gong (河上公) said: "If one is able to be impartial, be natural, be communicative with the heaven (i.e., Nature), and be in accord with the Dao; then when all four are acquired, his Dao and De (i.e., mind and its manifestation, meaning morality) will be able to reach wide and far, without disaster and without feelings of self-guilt. Consequently, he is able to live and die with heaven and earth without any danger."[3] The four prerequisites include: be impartial, be natural, be communicative with heaven and earth, and be in accord with the Dao.

Zhang, Qi-Gan (張其淦) said:

"If (the mind) can reach its extreme insubstantial state and (the body) can be maintained to its sincere calmness, and one uses these states to comprehend the Dao, then the state of emptiness is attained. In this case, the variations of myriad objects can be observed. When myriad objects begin their lives, it is the state of moving and action. Those who know the Dao will be able to see 'having' is initiated from 'nothingness.' Knowing there is an action, then the repetition (of lives) can occur. When all various lives return to their roots, then this process is from 'having' to 'nothingness.' When returning to their roots, the calmness will be reached automatically without being pursued. This is the real calmness."[4]

Qigong Interpretation

Actually, this whole chapter is talking about the fundamental concept and practice of embryonic breathing meditation. First, the two polarities in humans is mentioned. One of them is located in the limbic system of the head and is called "Mud Pill Palace" (Ni Wan Gong, 泥丸宮). This center is where the subconscious mind developed. Through the development of the subconscious mind, we will be able to reconnect with the natural spirit. This center is called "spirit residence" (shen shi, 神室) or "upper dan tian" (shang dan tian, 上丹田) in qigong.

When you quiet your conscious mind (which is generated from brain cells) and lead the qi to the limbic system, you are able to awaken your subconscious mind and improve your spiritual feeling. In order to do so, you must first train yourself until your thinking can be in its ultimate empty or insubstantial state.

The second polarity is located at your physical center (the center of gravity) that is known as the second brain in Western science. It is called the "lower real dan tian" (zhen xia dan tian, 真下丹田) in qigong. It is known that this second brain is the human bio-battery that produces and stores the bioelectricity that supplies the entire body's functions. However, in qigong, this center is known as the qi center or qi dwelling (qi she, 氣舍). In order to keep your qi at the center, your physical body must be in a state of extreme calmness and relaxation.

From Chinese qigong, it is understood that the lower qi center provides the quantity of qi to the entire body to nourish the physical life and spiritual life. However, the upper spiritual center governs the quality of the qi's manifestation. Based on qigong theory, you need both pre-birth qi and post-birth qi. One is yin and the other is yang. Both need to balance each other. The quantity of qi includes both. It is understood that these two polarities are connected by the thrusting vessel (chong mai, 衝脈) (spinal cord). Since highly conductive tissues construct the spinal cord, there is no stagnation in this vessel. Therefore, physically, there are two polarities. In function, it is one since these two polarities synchronize with each other.

Once you have cultivated the extreme empty mind and true calmness of the physical body, you will be able to feel the synchronization of the subconscious mind at the upper polarity with the qi in the lower polarity. You can then consciously bring your mind from the upper polarity to the lower one so the spirit and qi can be united at the lower real dan tian. This is called "unification of mother (qi) and son (spirit)," (mu zi xiang he, 母子相合).

According to Chinese qigong, a human life includes two lives in our body: a spiritual life and a physical life. The spiritual life is considered yin, which governs the quality of life (or qi's manifestation) while the physical life is considered yang, which manifests the qi into physical actions. Whenever, your spirit is high and your physical body is strong, you are healthy and will live long. Whenever either is missing, you will be withering and dying.

Once these two polarities have united into one at the lower polarity (real lower dan tian) where the first cell of life was initiated, you will be able to see and feel Nature, the initiation of a life, and how it is repeated. This is the state of embryonic breathing and the state of "embracing singularity" (bao yi, 抱一).

In the book, *Li Ji* (《禮記·大學》), it is said:

> "*The great learning of the Dao is to pursue comprehension of the bright De (i.e., manifestation of Dao) and to influence other people until the ultimate goodness can be reached. Once you know, then your mind is steady without doubt. When the mind is steady, then you can acquire calmness. When you are calm, then you find the peace. When you are in peace, then you are able to ponder. When you are able to ponder, then you gain. All objects have their initiation and termination and all matters have a beginning and an expiration. If one knows the beginning and the end, then one is closer to the Dao.*"[5]

Lu, Yan (呂岩) said:

> "*When this practice is applied to the human body, after the insubstantial mind and physical calmness have been accomplished, the body reaches its extreme yin state, and then yang begins to initiate. When this happens, a regiment of real qi is derived and acts in a profound spiritual space. It cannot be controlled and cannot be relied on; three gates can be clearly opened and the qi can circulate in the entire body. Finally, the qi returns to the dan tian and qihai to complete one cycle. This is the subtlety of returning to the root. Only when returned to the root can there be real calmness. Only when there is real calmness can life then be repeated. When life is repeated, then it is permanent. Through comprehending this constant routine, enlightenment can be reached. When one has reached the real enlightenment, one will not be selfish. When there is no selfishness, then one accords with the heaven's rule. The entire body will follow your order and all qi will gather at its origin. This is the nature of Heaven's Dao.*"[6]

This refers to the profound stage of meditation. When this happens, your body becomes the extreme yin state and the qi will be derived and circulating in your entire body. This qi will eventually open three gates (san guan, 三關). Three gates are the three qi circulation obstacles in small circulation meditation practice named: weilv (尾閭) (tailbone), jiaji (夾脊) (squeeze spine), and yuzhen (玉枕) (jade pillow). Qihai is the medical name of the dan tian's location.

If you are interested in knowing more about embryonic breathing and small circulation meditations, please refer to follow two books: *Qigong Meditation—Embryonic Breathing*, and *Qigong Meditation— Small Circulation*, by YMAA Publication Center.

Conclusions

1. This chapter has pointed out that there are two polarities in our body: a spiritual center and a physical center.
2. In order for us to observe Nature's evolution, we must first bring our mind to its extreme empty state and maintain our physical body to its extreme calm condition. Only then can we feel or sense the two lives residing in our body: the spiritual life and the physical life.
3. The final stage of embryonic breathing is to find the initiation of life that takes place at the center of gravity (real lower dan tian, 真下丹田). This unification of spiritual and physical life is called "unification of mother and son" (mu zi xiang he, 母子相合) in Daoist qigong practice. Spirit is the son while the qi is mother.
4. Once you have reached this stage, you will be able to see the origin of life and how life is repeated.

1.《性命圭旨》: "心中無物為虛,念頭不起為靜。"
2.《云笈七簽》: "還原返本,歸根復命。"
3. 河上公說: "能公能天,通天合道,四者純備,道德弘遠,無殃無咎,乃與天地俱沒,無危殆也。"
4. 張其淦說: "虛能極,靜能篤,然后悟道,即是無,可以觀萬物之變矣。萬物并作之時,即芸芸蠢動之象。知道者觀有于無,知其所以作者,乃其所以復也。芸芸各歸其根,必當自有而無也,歸根則不求靜而自靜,是真靜也。"

5. 《禮記·大學》："大學之道，在明明德，在親民，在止于至善。知止而后有定，定而后能靜，靜而后能安，安而后能慮，慮而后能得。物有本末，事有始終，知所前后，則近道也。"

6. 呂岩說："比之人身，是虛靜之后，陰極陽生，其一圜真氣變動于窅冥之中，而不可御、不可倚，自然三關透徹，遍身周流，以復還于丹田氣海之中，而為一個周天。此所為歸根之奧妙，惟歸根而為真靜，惟真靜而為復命，惟復命而為有恆，為知常而為真明，惟真明而為無私，惟無私而合于天君，百體從命，眾氣朝元，此天道之自然也。"

CHAPTER 17

Genuine Atmosphere—Original Nature

第十七章
淳風—自然

太上，下知有之；
　　其次，親之譽之；
　　其次，畏之；
　　其次，侮之。
信不足焉，
　　有不信焉！
悠兮，其貴言。
功成事遂，
　　百姓皆謂「我自然」。

Regarding the leaders in ancient times, people just knew they exist;
    at the next level, people love them and praise them;
    the next level, people fear them;
    and the next level, people insult (despise) them.
If (the leaders) don't trust enough,
    then people will not trust them.
Those sage rulers manage events calmly and value their words.
When the tasks are accomplished,
    the people all say we did it by ourselves naturally.

General Interpretation

In ancient times, long before history was written, all that people knew was that there was a leader. However, the leader would not interfere with people's activities. Later, when the leader began to establish his power and authority, people tried to honor him and get close to him. Then, when the leader had set up all the rules and laws to restrict people's thinking and freedom, people began to fear the leader. When the leader could not follow the rules and laws he set up by himself, people began to insult him. Since then, the leader who does not trust enough is not trusted. He Shang Gong (河上公) said: "If a sovereign cannot be trusted by heaven and earth (i.e., citizens of a country, then the people will respond with no-trust and deceive their sovereign."[1]

As a leader, he should take it easy and allow the country to be harmonized by itself without a lot of laws and restrictions. When finally the society has reached its final harmonization, people don't even know that it is an achievement led by their leader. Instead, they believe they have accomplished it by themselves.

Song, Chang-Xing (宋長星) said:

> "After the Five Kingdoms, the courtesy and music was formatted, the superiors and inferiors were described, the clothes and hats made for different rankings, the rich and the poor were distinguished. The palace was built to replace the nest and cavern, the bridges were constructed for convenient transportation, the boats and cars were built to transport across the land and water, the contracts were created to replace the rope knots (used for counting in ancient times), the people's mind had gradually opened, and the society had gradually become civilized. Under these circumstances, those with the mind of simplicity and purity could not work (survive). Consequently, the leaders had to teach people what benevolence and righteousness were. Those who had benevolence would be loved and those who were righteous will be praised. This cannot be compared with the habitude of the great ancient period."[2]

This chapter explains that in the beginning, our society was in the wuwei (無為) state. Later, when wisdom was developed, people began to play tricks and lie to each other. Since then, society has had to rely on laws and education to teach people how to obey. The final stage in the evolution of human society is to return to its wuwei state. When this happens, people all know what they should and shouldn't do. In this case, laws and governments are no longer necessary.

Qigong Interpretation

The king or the leader in our body is the mind. At the beginning of our life as a child, we were simple, pure, and innocent. There was not too much contamination in our thoughts. The qi's circulation in our body was smooth and harmonious. Later, we began to learn manners and how to put a mask on and survive in this masked society. We learned how to lie, play tricks, and become sneaky. Our emotional minds have since been allured by greediness, glory, reputation, power, and other emotional desires.

When we grow up, we use our conscious mind to govern our thinking, feelings, diet, and living habits. We ignore the deep feeling in ourselves that is related to the subconscious mind. We often ignore our deepest feelings and listen to other people's opinion instead. This has become the biggest obstacle in qigong practice. We don't trust ourselves and we don't trust our own deep feeling. As a result, our conscious mind has set up many rules and regulations for our body.

In order to have a peaceful and calm mind, we must learn how to return our mind to our infant stage, which is pure and simple. Without this, our qi's circulation will be inharmonious and chaotic. We have to regulate it until no regulating is necessary. Once you have established a good lifestyle through deep feeling, you will believe it has been accomplished without effort. This is the stage of "regulating without regulating" (wuwei, 無為).

To reach this goal, we must slow down the activities of our conscious mind and pay more attention to our subconscious mind. The subconscious mind is related to natural instinctive feeling and is more truthful. The way of reaching this goal is through embryonic breathing meditation.

Conclusions

This chapter emphasizes the importance of the subconscious mind. Trust your deep feeling initiated from this subconscious mind and don't be blinded by your masked conscious mind.

1. 河上公說：“君信不足以天下，下則應之以不信，而欺其君也。”
2. 宋長星說：“次后五帝之時，制禮樂，敘尊卑，造衣冠，分貴賤，作宮室以代巢穴，構橋梁以濟不通，造舟車以行水陸，造書契以代結繩，人心漸漸開明，世道漸漸趨文，渾朴難行，不得不以仁義教化于民，被其仁者故親之，懷其義者故譽之。與太古之風不相比矣。”

CHAPTER 18

Thin (Dao) in Society—The Decline of the Dao

第十八章
俗薄—道微

大『道』廢，
　　有仁義；
智慧出，
　　有大偽；
六親不和，
　　有孝慈；
國家昏亂，
　　有忠臣。

When the Great Dao is abandoned,
    (then) there is benevolence and righteousness.
When cleverness appears,
    (then) there is great hypocrisy.
When the six relatives (i.e., relations) are not harmonious,
    (then) there is filial piety and kindness.
When a country becomes chaotic and disordered,
    (then) there are loyal officials.

General Interpretation

When the Dao is lost, then natural instinctive moralities in society will be neglected. When this happens, then we talk about benevolence and righteousness. If moralities are high in society, then there is no benevolence and righteousness to talk about. Wang, An-Shi (王安石) said: "There is benevolence because there is something to be loved. There is righteousness because there is something to be distinguished. Because there is love and distinction, the Great Dao was abolished."[1]

When the cleverness was developed, people learned how to lie and play tricks. The truth has since been downgraded. People put a fake mask on their face and hide their innocent simplicity and purity. Wang, Bi (王弼) said: "Use brightness (i.e., cleverness) to play tricks and also to examine cunning people and fakes; interested to see the result, knowing how to avoid poor consequence, thus cleverness and wisdom are derived, and the great hypocrisy was developed."[2]

It is the same when there is no harmony among all relatives and friends; then we praise those who have filial piety and kindness. When a country has become disordered and chaotic, then loyal officials can be found and become noticeable. Wang, An-Shi (王安石) said: "Filial piety means to love your parents and kindness is to adore your children. This is why all the six relatives are not harmonious."[3] If there is no special selfish attention to your parents and children and all relatives and friends are treated with the same manners, then there is no problem of harmony. The "six relatives" means: father, mother, elder brothers, younger brothers, wife, and sons (父、母、兄、弟、妻、子).

Li Ji (《禮記·禮運》) said:

> "*Today the Great Dao is concealed and all the people's main concern between heaven and earth (i.e., the world) are their own family; they love their own parents and intimidate their own children, and the goods and efforts are all for themselves. To rank noble and laymen as a way of respect, to build a big city wall and a surrounding river as a method of strength and safety, and to use politeness and righteousness as the laws, so the position of*

*sovereign and officers can be distinguished, the relation-
ship of father and sons can be sincere, the interrelation
among brothers can be amiable, the intimacy between
husband and wife can be harmonious. The system is
established so the rules of the society can be defined.
Those well-known versatile talents and brave warriors
contribute efforts for their own exploits. Thus, schemes
and conspiracies are initiated and wars are launched."[4]*

All of the above are not the way of the Dao. The Dao itself is simple
and pure. It does not have to pretend or be fake. Everything is truthful
without lying. Zhang, Er-Qi (張爾歧) said:

*"When the Great Dao is working, people do not know
there are such things as benevolence and righteousness.
When the Great Dao is abolished, then benevolence and
righteousness can be seen. When people have forgotten
simplicity, then cleverness is developed and its brightness
is demonstrated. Consequently, all the people admire cleverness and the great hypocrisy is derived. When all the six
relatives are harmonious, then filial piety and benevolence
are not noticed. This is because everyone has filial piety
and benevolence. After the harmony has disappeared,
then filial piety and benevolence are noticeable. When a
country is ruled effectively, loyal officers cannot be seen.
This is because all officers are loyal. However, when a
country is disordered and chaotic, then there are loyal
officers."[5]*

Qigong Interpretation

As mentioned before, the Dao or the taiji in our body is our subconscious mind. If we are able to follow the natural subconscious instinct
and accord with the natural way, then the qi will be harmonious. However, if we use our conscious mind to manage our life, then we will be

in the emotional mud of glory, desires, greediness, and selfishness. In this case, the qi in our six yin organs (six relatives)—heart, lungs, pericardium, liver, kidneys, and spleen—will not be harmonious.

When our feelings initiated from our subconscious mind are ignored, then our mind is trapped in emotional thinking and the mask is put on. We begin to compare and forget the truth.

If we are able to be truthful and follow our subconscious feeling, the qi's circulation will be harmonious and a doctor will not be necessary. Those who have followed the Dao will be healthy and will not know what sickness is.

Conclusions

This chapter tells us that we should focus on the development of our subconscious mind and downplay our conscious thinking. When this happens, our mind will not be attracted to the human matrix. Naturally, the qi will be circulating smoothly and healthily.

1. 王安石說：“仁者，有所愛也；義者，有所別也。以其有愛有別，此大道之所以廢也。”
2. 王弼說：“行術用明，以察奸偽；趣睹形見，物知避之。故智慧出，而大偽生也。”
3. 王安石說：“孝者，各親其親；慈者，各子其子：此六親所以不和也。”
4. 《禮記·禮運》：“今大道既隱，天下為家。各親其親，各子其子，貨力為己。大人世及以為禮，城郭溝池以為固，禮義以為紀。以正君臣，以篤父子，以睦兄弟，以和父婦，以設制度，以立田里。以賢勇知，以功為己。故謀用是作，而兵由此起。”
5. 張爾歧說：“大道之行也，民不知有仁義，大道廢而仁義見矣。民相忘于朴，智慧者出而自矜其明，則民各以智相尚，而大偽從此起矣。六親方和，孝慈不著，人皆孝慈也。不和而后，有孝慈矣。國家方治，忠臣不見，人盡忠也。國家昏亂而后，有忠臣矣。”

CHAPTER 19

Returning to Simplicity—Returning to the Foundation

第十九章
還淳—歸本

絕聖棄智，
　　民利百倍；
絕仁棄義，
　　民復孝慈；
絕巧棄利，
　　盜賊無有。
此三者以為文，不足，
　　故令有所屬：
見素抱樸，
　　少私寡欲，
　　絕學無憂。

Abandon wisdom and discard cleverness,
    people will be benefited a hundredfold.
Abandon benevolence and discard righteousness,
    people will recover filial piety and kindness.
Abandon cunning skills and discard profit,
    thieves and robbers will disappear.
Restraining these three things is still not enough,
    thus, set up some rules for people to follow:
Show plainness and embrace simplicity,
    reduce selfishness and decrease desires,
        cease learning and thus there will be no worry.

General Interpretation

In order to make people return to their simplicity so human society can reach the stage of wuwei (無為) again, the leader must teach people not to leverage their wisdom and cleverness. Then there will be no difference among people. Furthermore, if people are taught to ignore benevolence and righteousness, then all the people will regain their benevolence and righteousness. In addition, if all the cunning skills and profiteering are discarded, then thieves and robbers will disappear.

To reach this goal, the people must cultivate their temperament and embrace their simplicity, be less selfish and reduce desires, and stop pursuing more knowledge to increase their cunning. This is the stage of regulating. To reach the goal, the progress will be gradual and slow. Wang, An-Shi (王安石) said: "(This chapter is) not talking about keeping purity, but pursuing purity, not talking about simplicity, but embracing simplicity, not talking about unselfishness, but less selfishness, and not talking about no desire, but less desire. This is because you must first pursue purity. Only then can you keep purity. You must then embrace simplicity and only then can you return to simplicity. You must first reduce your selfishness and only then can you be without selfishness. This is the way of reaching no desires from less desires."[1]

Qigong Interpretation

Since our mind has been contaminated by emotions and desires, it is not easy to return to our original purity and simplicity in a short time. We must first practice regulating our temperament until no regulating is necessary.

In qigong practice, it is recognized that there are four stages of spiritual evolution: self-recognition (zi shi, 自識), self-awareness (zi jue, 自覺), self-awakening (zi wu, 自悟), and finally freedom from spiritual bondage (zi tuo, 自脫). Only when the entire human race has gone through these four required processes will humans reach the final harmony of a wuwei (無為) society.

Conclusions

To reach to a high level of qigong practice, we must return our temperament to our infant stage, pure and simple, and have no desire and emotional bondage. Without these as the foundation, your spiritual cultivation will be shallow. The first step in reaching this goal is dropping your mask and recognizing the real you behind the mask (self-recognition). Only then, can you see the relation between you and nature, you and other humans, and the meaning of your life (self-awareness). Once you have comprehended yourself and what is around you, you then understand what is the aspiration of your life (self-awakening). Finally, you pursue your goal until your spiritual enlightenment has been achieved (spiritual freedom from bondage).

1. 王安石說：「不言守素而言見素，不言返朴而言抱朴，不言無私而言少私，不言無欲而言寡欲。蓋見素然后可以守素，抱朴然后可以返朴，少私然后可以無私，寡欲則致于不見所欲者也。」

CHAPTER 20

Different from Vulgar—Pure and Truthful

第二十章
異俗—純真

唯之與阿，相去幾何？
　　善之與惡，相去若何？
人之所畏，不可不畏。
　　荒兮其未央哉！
眾人熙熙，
　　如享太牢，如春登臺。
我獨泊兮其未兆，
　　如嬰兒之未孩。儽儽兮若無所歸。
眾人皆有餘，而我獨若遺。
　　我愚人之心也哉！沌沌兮。
俗人昭昭，我獨昏昏。
　　俗人察察，我獨悶悶。
澹兮其若海，飂兮若無止。
　　眾人皆有以，而我獨頑且鄙。
　　我獨異於人，而貴食母。

How much difference is there between obsequiousness and flattery?
   How much difference is there between good and evil?
What people are afraid cannot be unafraid!
   Those who are in desolation are far away (from the Dao). How
   limitless it is!
People are gathering and excited,
   as if enjoying a great feast and as if ascending a high terrace in
   spring time.
I am alone quietly without desires, yet not noticeable.
   Just like an infant cannot yet smile, so weary as if there is no
   place to return.
All people have surplus, I alone am still lacking.
   Indeed, I have a heart of a fool; so ignorant!
Most people are bright, I alone am simple and muddled.
   Most people are scrutinizing; I alone am obtuse.
It is tranquil as an ocean; the blowing of high wind seems like it's
   not going to stop.
   People all have purposes; I alone seem stubborn and lowly.
   I am different from others but value the nourishing mother.

General Interpretation

In fact, although there is not much difference between those who are obsequious and those who are flattering, there is a large difference between good and evil. What people say and fear cannot be ignored but instead should make us alert and cautious. People are often confused and use their thinking and emotions to judge everything. Then they talk and spread their thinking to others. However, this is far away from the Dao since the Dao does not see any differences between obsequious and flattering and also good and evil.

There is a story about Confucius' student, Zeng, Shen (曾参). One day, Zeng, Shen's mother was weaving. Someone came to Zeng's home and said: "Zeng, Shen has killed someone." However, his mom was undisturbed and did not believe. She replied: "My son will never kill anyone." Later, someone else came to her and said: "Didn't you know that Zeng, Shen killed some person?" However, his mom still weaved without action. However, a few moments later, when the third person came into her house and told her: "Zeng, Shen killed a person." She disregarded the weaving and ran quickly to see the truth. Naturally, Zeng, Shen did not kill anyone. But due to people's talking, even though it was not real it could still affect her mind. That is why people's talking and doing are reasons to be afraid since these are initiated from people's minds, and that is far away from the Dao.

We all might agree that our entire human society wears a heavy mask that is decorated with glory, dignity, pride, and many other emotional disturbances. Most of these emotions were created during the long history of human conflict. Today, governments still arm themselves with various weapons and prepare to kill each other. Worldwide, almost fifteen thousand nuclear bombs await potential use. This is far away from the Dao.

In order to survive in this masked society, we also carry the mask and talk the way society wants us to talk and do what other people expect us to do. We have hidden our true feelings within. However, subconsciously, we all know that we must lie to avoid being treated as different or unfairly. We often ignore our true feelings and pay more attention to material attractions. Gradually, we have forgotten our human nature. How can we use this misled mind to judge Nature (the

Dao)? As a result, two of our inner minds, the truthful mind and the lying mind, are in conflict with each other. This inner conflict is painful. To ease the pain or numb ourselves, we often indulge in drugs, alcohol, or are addicted to various distractions. We have created a path toward a quick death. Mencius (孟子) said: "Addicted to hunting is called waste and excessive drinking without moderation is called death."[1]

Furthermore, nature has provided us with a comfortable and relaxed living. However, we have kept ourselves busy in pursuing material enjoyment. We have downgraded or ignored our spiritual feelings and development. The book, *Shi Ji* (《史記·貨殖列傳》) says: "All the people in the world are busy coming (i.e., looking) for benefits and rushing here and there for profits."[2]

The attitude we should have is while people are getting excitement and enjoyment from their lives, I, without being noticeable, am alone, quiet like an infant, with no desires and no temptations. I am just like an innocent child, ignorant. I have a simple and tranquil heart. Though people are searching for a better material life, I alone am obtuse. All that I feel is from Nature, such as the oceans, mountains, clouds, winds, and air. Although I am different from others, I don't mind it, since I deeply appreciate what the Dao has provided me, nourishing my life just like a mother.

Huang, Shang (黃裳) said: "It is just like the embryo of a baby that has not been formed yet. A regiment of original qi (yuan qi, 元氣) embraced wholly at the center (womb) is all that exists. This qi can flow up and down freely and ceaselessly, and communicate with the qi of heaven and earth adequately."[3] When you have this feeling, your spiritual and physical bodies are both clean and pure. The book, *Chu Ci* (《楚辭·漁父》) says: "How can I allow my pure and clean bodies to be contaminated with the dirty thinking and objects?"[4]

Qigong Interpretation

In qigong embryonic breathing meditation practice, you are searching for the way to bring your mind to the infant stage. That means you are downplaying the actions of the conscious mind that is full of human dogmas, emotions, and material attractions. Gradually, you want to awaken your subconscious mind that is truthful and is connected to your spirit. To reach this goal, you must think and behave like an infant: pure, simple, and innocent.

Additionally, you would want to lead the qi to its battery located at the center of gravity. This place is called the "real lower dan tian" (真下丹田) or "qi residence" (qi she, 氣舍). When qi can be stored at its residence to an abundant level, you will be able to lead it up to the huang ting (黃庭) (yellow yard) located between the diaphragm and the real lower dan tian. When the fire qi from the middle dan tian (diaphragm) is led down to interact with the water qi from the real dan tian at the huang ting, a spiritual embryo (shen tai, 神胎) can be formed. When this spiritual embryo is matured, you can lead it up to the upper dan tian (brain) to reopen the third eye. The third eye is called "heaven eye" (tian yan, 天眼) because your spirit and the natural spirit can resume their communication through this eye. When this happens, it is called "enlightenment" (shen tong, 神通). The *Huang Ting Classic* (《黃庭經》) says: "All people eat grains and the five spices, but I eat natural great harmonious yin and yang qi." "Hundreds of grains are the fruits of earth essence. The five spices look beautiful (i.e., attracting) but are evil and stink, and can disturb the clarity of my spirit. Consequently, the result of my embryonic qi equals zero. In this case, how can I revert my age and return to babyhood? Why don't we feed ourselves with qi produced by the great harmonious essence? Consequently, we are able to achieve the Dao of huang ting and live with longevity."[5]

Conclusions

To reach the goal of spiritual enlightenment, you must first purify and simplify your mind and bring it to the state of innocence found in childhood. In order to do this, you must downplay your conscious mind and the matrix created by human society. Only then can the subconscious mind be redeveloped and cultivated. The subconscious mind provides you with the path to reestablish the deep feeling and sensing that allows you to reconnect with nature.

In addition, you need to solidify and firm your qi at the lower real dan tian so the qi can be built to an abundant level. Once you have your mind and qi regulated, then you bring your mind to the lower real dan tian. This process is called "unification of mother (qi) and baby (spirit)"[6].

1. 孟子（《梁惠王下》）說：“從獸無厭謂之荒，樂酒無厭謂之亡。”
2. 《史記·貨殖列傳》：“天下熙熙，皆為利來；天下攘攘，皆為利往。”
3. 黃裳說：“如嬰兒之初胎，孩子未成之時，一團元氣，渾然在抱，上下升降，運行不息，適與天地流通。”
4. 《楚辭·漁父》：“安能以身之察察，受物之汶汶者乎？”
5. 《黃庭經》：“人皆食谷與五味，我食太和陰陽氣。”“百谷之實土地精，五味外美邪魔腥臭亂神明，胎氣零，那能反老得還嬰？何不食氣太和精，故能不死入黃寧。”
6. “母子相和。”

CHAPTER 21

Humble Heart—Returning to Its Root

第二十一章

虛心—歸元

孔『德』之容，惟『道』是從。
　　『道』之為物，惟恍惟惚。
惚兮恍兮，其中有象；
　　恍兮惚兮，其中有物。
窈兮冥兮，其中有精；
　　其精甚真，其中有信。
自古至今，
　　其名不去，
　　以閱眾甫。
吾何以知眾甫之狀哉？
　　以此。

The appearance (i.e., action) of the Great De follows only the Dao.
  When describing the Dao as an object, it is ambiguous
  whether it is there or not.
Though it is ambiguous, it seems there is an image;
  though it is indistinct, it seems there is an object.
Though it is so profound and obscure, it seems there is an essence;
  its essence is so real and truthful, it gives (you) faith.
From ancient time till present,
    its name (i.e., the Dao) has never been forgotten,
    so (we are able to) observe the initiation and derivation of all
    objects.
How do I know the nature of all objects?
    Because of this.

General Interpretation

The De (德) is the manifestation of the Dao. The great function of the De is originated from the Great Dao (Da Dao, 大道). Therefore, the De always follows the Dao. Lu, De-Ming (陸德明) said: "The De is the application (i.e., manifestation) of the Dao."[1]

When we talk about the Dao, it is vague, ambiguous, profound, and obscure. It seems it is there, but it is not there; and it seems it is not there, but it is there. Although we cannot see it or hear it, we can feel it. This feeling is real and thus all human races have believed it and trusted it since ancient times. From this belief and also from its manifestation (the De), we are able to trace back the initiation of lives and see their recycling process. If anyone is able to reach this profound comprehension, he will be able to see the natural derivation and changes.

Song, Chang-Xing (宋常星) said:

> "The deep hidden meaning of (comprehending) myriad lives means the real belief (i.e., understanding) of the natural truth (i.e., recycling). Between the beginning and the end, it begins with the initiation (of the Dao); this derives into objects (i.e., lives) and finally ends returning to the Dao again. If we use the Dao to observe the Dao, it is hard to understand the rules or principles of myriad lives. However, if we use the objects (i.e., the De) to observe the Dao, (we will) be able to reach its origin and trace back its root. In this case, the profound natural theory (rules or principles of the Dao) can be understood." "Therefore, those who are good at observing the Dao must always observe the objects (i.e., myriad lives or the De). If separated from the Dao, there are no objects that can be observed; if separated from objects, then the Dao also cannot be observed. When you observe the objects, you are observing how the objects enter their recycling and when you observe the Dao, you are observing how the objects are initiated."[2]

The Dao is the original force or power to initiate all objects. These objects are the manifestation (the De) of the Dao. Therefore, from observing the Dao, you can see how lives are created and derived. From observing the De, you can comprehend the cyle of lives coming into existence, passing away, and then taking birth again.

Qigong Interpretation

One of the main purposes of studying and practicing qigong is to comprehend the meaning of nature and our lives. In order to reach this goal, you must have a neutral and truthful mind to observe the Dao and the De.

In embryonic breathing meditation (胎息靜坐) practice, first you cease the activities of the conscious mind and lead the qi to the limbic system (center of the brain) where the spirit resides. When this happens, the mask on your face will dissolve, and your truthful subconscious mind will be awakened. When you reach this stage, you will feel the truth of nature; it seems it is there but not there; it seems it is not there, but it is there (wei huang wei hu, 惟恍惟惚). It is the stage of the semi-sleeping state. When you are in this state, your thoughts will not be influenced or dominated by the conscious mind that is not truthful and always misleads about the truth of the Dao. When you reach this state, your spirit and the natural spirit can be reunited. This will help you see the initiation of lives.

There is a saying about this state of meditation in taiji Daoist society: "There is no shape and no images, the entire body is transparent and empty. Forget the surrounding objects and be natural, like a stone chime suspended from West Mountain (Xi Shan, 西山)."[3] This means when you reach this state, there is no shape and no image in your mind. All you feel is the energy in you and around you; your physical body is transparent. You are natural and all objects around you are forgotten. Here, the role of your conscious mind is minimized and your subconscious mind has awakened and connected to nature. A stone chime is commonly hung by a thread so it can be moved by the wind to make sound. When the thread is too thick, the mobility of the chime will be restricted and freedom is limited. If the thread is thin, the chime will be able to follow the wind (nature) to move freely. This implies that the thread is the conscious mind while the chime is the subconscious mind. In order to set your subconscious mind free, you must reduce the activities of the conscious mind so the subconscious mind can wake up and be free. When you reach this stage, you will be in a semisleeping state. West Mountain (Xi Shan, 西山) refers to India where the Buddha resides. Reaching Buddhahood or enlightenment is the goal of spiritual cultivation in Buddhist and Daoist society.

Conclusion

To reach the neutral and truthful state, you must cease the activities of the conscious mind and wake up the subconscious mind. The way of reaching this state is through embryonic breathing meditation until you are in semisleeping state. When you are in this state, you are there, but not there; you are not there, but you are there. In this way, you can see and judge things from a neutral state without being misled by the conscious mind.

1. 陸德明說：“德，道之用也。”
2. 宋常星說：“眾甫之密義，即是甚真之真信也。出機入機之間，始則出機，化而為物；終則入機，歸之於道。假使以道觀道，難知眾甫之理。以物觀道，達乎本而窮其元，則眾甫之玄理，始可得而知其然也。”“所以善觀道者，必以物觀之。離道而無以觀物，離物而無以觀道。觀物者，觀物之入機也；觀道者，觀物之出機也。”
3. “無形無象，全身透空。忘物自然，西山懸磬。”

CHAPTER 22

Increasing Humility—Maintaining Neutrality

第二十二章
益謙—持中

曲則全，枉則直；
　　窪則盈，敝則新；
　　少則得，多則惑。
　　是以『聖人』抱一為天下式。
不自見，故明，
　　不自是，故彰，
　　不自伐，故有功，
　　不自矜，故長。
夫惟不爭，
　　故天下莫能與之爭。
古之所謂「曲則全」者，
　　豈虛言哉？
誠全而歸之。

Yield is to maintain wholeness and bend is to become straight;
  to be hollow is to become full and be worn out is for renewal,
  having little can then receive and having much can be confused.
  Thus, those sages embrace one and become the model of the
  world.
Without flaunting themselves, they are therefore illumined,
  without presuming themselves, they are therefore distinguished,
  without praising themselves, they are therefore given credit,
  without boasting about themselves, their achievements are
  therefore lasting.
Because they do not compete,
  thus the world is unable to compete with them.
The ancient saying that 'yield is to maintain wholeness,'
  isn't this saying true?
Become the wholeness and return it (to the one) with sincerity.

General Interpretation

If you are able to yield, you are using soft to overcome the hard. In this case, the wholeness can be maintained. It is harder to be humble and bow to others than stand straight upward and be persistent. That bowing is harder than standing straight implies you are strong and straight inside. When you are able to bow, then things and events can successfully proceed according to the principles of the Dao. You are able to be humble, because you can see far instead of being shortsighted. *Yi Jing* (《易·繫辭下》) (*Book of Changes*) said: "The inchworm bends its body so it can be extended; the dragon and snake hibernate (i.e., calmness) so they can save the body (i.e., life) for action (in spring). When refined essence has entered the spirit, it is for future usage."[1] This saying implies that every action has its reason. Once you are able to see clearly with a deep spiritual feeling, you will be able to see the past and the future and know how to apply it to your life. Once you can see this, you will not mind to bow, act softly, and be humble so the future can be predicted and achieved. He, Shang-Gong (河上公) said: "Bend yourself and yield to others without self-persistence. Then, eventually you are able to complete yourself."[2] From this you can see that if you are able to humble and coordinate with others, eventually, you will be able to accomplish your task. However, if you stubbornly insist upon your opinion, eventually, all cooperation will disperse. Wu, Cheng (吳澄) also said: "Crooked means not straight. The inchworm is able to bend and be crooked; thus, they are able to extend and straighten."[3]

When you position yourself at the low place, eventually, you will acquire more support. Wan, An-Shi (王安石) said: "Oceans, are always positioned at the lowest place and thus become the gathering place of water from hundreds rivers and streams. Thus, the low can be full."[4] When the clothes are old and worn out, it is the time for new ones. If you ask for less, whenever you have more, you appreciate it. However, when you have too much and are greedy, then your mind will become chaotic and confused. This is because of your desires and greediness; your mind has become complicated and is no longer simple.

Therefore, those sages keep their mind simple and in neutral state. This is the way of embracing singularity. Once you have a single and simple mind, then you are able to act freely and fairly. It is just like the power of pure water since from it, all kind of drinks can be produced. It is also like the sound of no sound, the most simple and powerful sound in the universe. Once there is no sound, then you can create any sound. This is why those sages can be used as example for the whole world.

Since they are in a simple neutral state, there is no flaunting, presuming, praising, or boasting. Because their minds are not caught up in such things, they are more powerful and appreciated by others. For this reason, there is nobody and nothing able to compete with them. That is why it is said: '"To yield is to maintain wholeness." In the book, *Shang Shu* (《尚書·大禹謨》), it is said: "Only if you don't boast about your talent will nobody in the world then dare to compete with your talent; only if you don't flaunt yourself, will nobody then dare to compete with your merit and achievement."[5]

Qigong Interpretation

To be enlightened, you must reopen your third eye so your spirit can be reunited with the natural spirit. In order to reopen the third eye, you must have an abundant storage of qi (quantity) and also a focused subconscious mind (quality of manifestation). Therefore, you must know how to condition your bio-battery (real lower dan tian) (zhen xia dan tian, 真下丹田) so the charge of your qi can be raised to a higher level. The stored qi is then led up to the brain to activate more brain cells for functioning. The brain is considered as the upper dan tian (shang dan tian, 上丹田), and the more cells are activated, the more qi the brain can store. Then, you need an undisturbed and calm subconscious mind to focus the qi into a tiny beam like a lens gathers sunbeams to a minutely focused, intense beam of light. With these two conditions met, your third eye may be opened.

To store the built-up qi at the lower real dan tian, you must first regulate your mind and keep it at the center so the qi will not be led outward (embrace singularity). That means the activities of your conscious mind must be minimized and your subconscious mind must be awakened. To minimize your conscious mind, you must cultivate yourself until you are just like a baby, innocent and truthful. This is the cultivation method to bring yourself to the beginning of life. To reach this goal, there are a few requirements.

1. First, you must be humble and know how to yield and be soft. If you cannot, your mind will be hard and thus the emotional mind will be stimulated. Conscious stimulation of the emotional mind will cause your qi to become chaotic and take you further away from calmness and peace. Calmness and peace is the path to reconnect to the spirit.

2. When you downplay your conscious mind (emotional mind) and pay more attention to your limbic system, you will gradually awaken your subconscious mind. It is recognized that the limbic system at the center of your head is the residence of the spirit. There are two glands located in the limbic system, the pineal gland and pituitary gland. This place is called "Mud Pill Palace" (Ni Wan Gong, 泥丸宮) or "spirit residence" (shen shi, 神室) in Chinese qigong. When you are able to use your mind to lead the qi in the brain to the limbic system, you will calm down the conscious mind's activities. Additionally, due to the nourishment of the limbic system with abundant qi, the hormone production from the pineal and pituitary glands can be increased and maintained. This is the key to longevity. Furthermore, when you have reached a certain level, you will be able to sense the spirit is getting stronger and stronger each day. The higher you have reached, the more humble you should be. My White Crane master often said: "The taller the bamboo grows, the lower it bows."[6]

3. Finally, you can bring your subconscious mind to the lower real dan tian located at the center of gravity (the physical center). When this happens, the two polarities have become one, achieving singularity. When your subconscious mind (related to spirit) and qi are united, you begin to return to your embryonic state, innocent,

simple, and pure, with no contamination from brain-washing by dogmas, traditions, material attractions, and emotional disturbances. This is the stage of "embracing singularity" (bao yi, 抱一). When this happens, your spirit is calm, gentle, soft, and innocent like a child's, and your qi can be conserved at an abundant level.

Conclusions

The subconscious mind is more powerful than the conscious mind. The conscious mind is temporary while the subconscious mind is long lasting. Once you have reached to the stage of "regulating of no regulating" (wuwei, 無為), you will be regulating the qi's imbalances automatically.

The way to trace back to the beginning of life is returning yourself to the embryo stage. To do so, first you find your two polarities, the spiritual center and physical center. Once you are able to find and feel these two centers, then bring the spirit down to the physical center where the embryo was formed. When the spirit (related to subconscious mind) and qi both stay at the real lower dan tian, the qi can be conserved, controlled, and built up to an abundant level. It is the final goal of embryonic breathing. When you get deeper, you will be able to sense and observe the initiation of life. This is the state of "embracing singularity" (bao yi, 抱一). Huang, Shang (黃裳) said: "If not by 'embracing singularity,' then how can we acquire the complete return, and go back to the initiation of ultimate beginning?"[7]

1. 《易·繫辭下》："尺蠖之屈，以求信（伸）也；龍蛇之蟄，以存身也；精義入神，以致用也。"
2. 河上公說："曲己從眾不自專，則全其身也。"
3. 吳澄說："枉者，不直也。尺蠖之屈而枉，所以能伸能直。"
4. 王安石說："海者，常處於卑，而為百川之所委，故窪則盈。"
5. 《尚書·大禹謨》："汝惟不矜，天下莫與汝爭能；汝惟不伐，天下莫與汝爭功。"
6. "竹高必躬。"
7. 黃裳說："非抱一者烏能全受全歸，以返其太始之初乎？"

CHAPTER 23

Insubstantial Emptiness—In Accord with the Dao

第二十三章
虛無—循道

希言自然。
　　故
　　飄風不終朝，
　　驟雨不終日。
孰為此者？天地。
　　天地尚不能久，
　　而況於人乎？
故從事於『道』者，同於『道』；
　　『德』者，同於『德』；
　　失者，同於失。
同於『道』者，『道』亦樂得之；
　　同於『德』者，『德』亦樂得之；
　　同於失者，失亦樂得之。
信不足焉，有不信焉！

Nature speaks sparsely.
    Thus,
        a gusting wind does not last the entire morning,
        a rainstorm does not last whole day.
What causes this to be so? Heaven and earth (i.e., Nature).
    Even heaven and earth cannot make it last long,
        how can human beings?
Thus those who follow the Dao will be with the Dao,
    those who follow the De will be with the De,
        (and) those who abandon them will be abandoned.
Those who are with the Dao will be welcome by the Dao,
    those who are with the De will be welcome by the De,
        (and) those are with abandonment will be welcome by aban-
        donment.
Those who cannot be confidently trusted will not be trusted.

General Interpretation

Pursuing the Dao is done through following Nature. There is nothing much to talk about. The Dao is hard to understand but the De (manifestations) is easier to see. For example, the gusting wind and rainstorm are the manifestations of the Dao and can be seen, but do not last long. How do these phenomena occur? They happen because of the Dao (Nature). Even the manifestations of Nature cannot last long, so how can humans? Humans are also the manifestation of the Dao, and thus they will not last long. Confucius (孔子) said: "What does the heaven need to say? The four seasons are carried out and hundreds of objects are growing. What does the heaven need to say?"[1] That means nature does not have to say anything. But from its manifestation, we can see the four seasons change from one to another regularly so all lives can grow accordingly. There is nothing Nature needs to say.

The way of cultivating the Dao is by following it. If we follow the Dao, the Dao will be with us. If we manifest thinking in accord with the Dao, the De (manifestation of Dao) will also be with us. However, if we abandon the Dao, then the Dao will abandon us as well. Xue, Hui (薛惠) said:

> "Nonaction of the mind means the Dao and conducting good deeds means the De. When it is excessive or deficient means fault. The minds of those who follow the Dao are insubstantial and tranquil, quiet without acting. If they follow the Dao, they can last as long as the Dao. This is what 'nature speaks sparsely' means. Those who tirelessly conduct good deeds, even if they are as small as loyalty and trust, are following the De. Those who follow the De will also be treated with good fortune and goodness (or "well-being"). Those who are in contention with the Dao and against the De, will face danger and decease. Those who have abandoned the Dao and the De, will also be abandoned and lost in misfortune."[2]

Du, Guang-Ting (杜光庭) also said: "To those who are in accord with the Dao, the Dao will respond. For those who abandon the Dao, the abandonment by the Dao will come."[3]

Qigong Interpretation

The nature of the Dao is calm, peaceful, and harmonious. Whenever there is an imbalance, it will try to regain its balance; thus, wind must blow and the rain must fall. The formation of a tornado or hurricane is the way that nature tries to regain its balance. However, once it is balanced, the calmness, peace, and harmony will return. In addition, Nature has its routines of energy change. Therefore, repetition or cycling, such as the four seasons or the daily sunrise and sunset, is happening all the time. All lives are developed under this routine cycling and, thus, our body's structure and qi circulation must also adjust and follow the cycle. For example, our body's qi status changes and corresponds to different organs when seasons change. We sleep when the sun goes down and awake and become active when the sun is up. If we understand the natural patterns and follow them, then we are in accord with Nature. If we are against these natural patterns, our qi circulation will become chaotic. When this happens, we will get sick or even die.

Whenever there is qi imbalance in our body, as long as you follow the Dao and the De, your body will regain its balance by itself. However, if you go against it, qi imbalance will continue to worsen and eventually you will become ill and die. For example, smoking causes the lungs' qi circulation to be imbalanced. If you persist with your smoking habit, eventually harm will befall you. However, if you can follow the Dao and the De and resume your healthy lifestyle, the imbalance will be corrected by itself.

From a qigong understanding, there are a few keys to maintain the qi's balance so the body can remain in a healthy state. First, bring your mind to a neutral state. Too much excitement, either happiness or sadness, is harmful, and the qi's normal circulation can be disrupted. For example, too much sorrow and excitement can trigger a heart attack, too much worry can trigger the spleen and stomach's qi imbalance, and too much anger can disrupt the liver's qi balance. Therefore, when you keep your mind in a neutral state, you are in accord with the Dao. Once you follow it, then the manifestation of the Dao, qi's circulation and physical health (the De), can be maintained.

You must maintain a healthy lifestyle that is in accord with the Dao and the De. A regular healthy lifestyle not only makes your body healthy and last long, it can also maintain your mind's healthy functioning. Most of our hormones are produced during the nighttime when we sleep. If we don't have a regular sleeping pattern, the hormone production will be affected and the qi's circulation will become imbalanced.

Then, you must know the concept of yin and yang. Yin and yang is a natural rule or law. When there is a yin, there is a yang, and vice versa. In the Dao, yin and yang are balanced. However, when they are not balanced, Nature will seek the way to regain its balance. For example, your physical body is yang while your qi body is yin. To be healthy, your qi and physical body must be balanced; otherwise, you will be sickened. According to Chinese medicine, each physical part of the body, such as the heart, liver, spleen, or even a tiny cell needs an appropriate amount of qi to maintain their lives and function. Whenever the qi supply is either excessive or deficient, the physical part will be sickened. The treatment strategy of Chinese medicine is to bring the qi supply and circulation back to its normal and balanced level so there is no resulting physical damage.

Finally, other than governing your mind, you also need to know how to control your qi, either its storage or consumption. Naturally, this includes how you use your mind to lead the qi so its manifestation can be the most efficient and effective. This is called "embracing singularity" (bao yi, 抱一). Embryonic breathing is the meditation for this practice.

Du, Guang-Ting (杜光庭) said: "What is qi? It is the reason that lives can exist. Heart (i.e., mind) is used to support the total spirit. However, if (the mind) and qi are fiercely urgent and aggressively require attention, then on the contrary, it will be harmful to the body. Political affairs are used to manage people and the laws are applied to put people in order. If the politics are harsh or practiced aggressively and the laws are stringent and fiercely enforced, the people will disperse and put the country in danger."[4]

Conclusions

To reach the final goal of "embracing singularity," you need to regulate your body, breathing, qi, and mind. Only then will you be able to govern your qi and keep it at its residence. When the spirit and qi are united at the real lower dan tian (the center of gravity), you have reached the stage of embryonic breathing. This means you are in the state of "embracing singularity."

1. 孔子說：「天何言哉？四時行焉，百物生焉，天何言哉！」
2. 薛惠說：「無為之謂道，為善之謂德，過差之謂失。虛無恬淡，寂漠無為，從事于道者也。同于道亦如道之長久矣。所謂希言自然者是也。小題忠信，樂善不倦，從事于德者也。同于德亦如德之吉善矣。反道背德，安于危亡，從事于失者也。同于失亦如失之凶丑矣。」
3. 杜光庭說：「同道者道應，同失者失來。」
4. 杜光庭說：「氣者，所以生身也；心之所以總神也。若其狂疾暴急，反以害身矣。政之所以理民也，令之所以齊民也，若政嚴而狂疾，令峻而暴急，則民散而國危矣。」

CHAPTER 24
Painful Graciousness—Self-Insult

第二十四章
苦恩—自侮

企者不立，
　　跨者不行；
自見者不明，
　　自是者不彰；
自伐者無功，
　　自矜者不長。
其在『道』也，
　　曰：餘食贅形。
物或惡之。
　　故有『道』者不處。

Those who stand on their tiptoes will not be steady;
   those who strain their strides will not be able to walk.
Those who flaunt themselves will not be luminous;
   those who are presumptuous will not be praised;
Those who make claims about their achievements will not receive
   merits,
   those who boast of themselves will not last long.
Those with the Dao
   call these "leftover food or tumors."
Despise them.
   Therefore, those who possess the Dao will not put themselves
   (there).

General Interpretation

Those who stand on their tiptoes to increase their heights will not be steady. Those who strain their strides to step further to increase distance will not be able to walk. Those who like to show off are usually not appreciated. Those who are presumptuous about their capabilities are usually despised. Those who like to boast of themselves usually do not receive credit from others. There is a famous story about Xiang, Yu (項羽) in the Chinese Han Dynasty (漢) (202 BCE–220 CE) history. The book *Shi Ji* (《史記·項羽本紀》) says: "Xiang, Yu (項羽) always boasted his merits in conquering." "He wished to use force to conquer and manage the world. In only five years, he decimated his country and died at Dong'a County (東阿縣). When he died, he still did not wake up and blame himself. Thus, he lost."[1]

In fact, those who are asking for respect are usually those who despise themselves. Those who say they are telling the truth are often untruthful. Those who are dishonest are frequently speaking honestly. Those righteous sages who follow the Dao would despise all of these fake and cunning actions. People who are doing such actions will actually bring more insults upon themselves than if they had taken no action at all.

Those who follow the Dao will be benevolent, unselfish, and concerned with other people's feelings. The book *Shang Shu* (《尚書·大禹謨》) recorded a conversation between Confucius and two of his students:

> "Yan, Yuan (顏淵) and Ji, Lu (季路) are waiting on Confucius. Confucius asked: 'Why don't you talk about your aspiration?' Zi Lu (子路) (Ji, Lu's nickname) said: 'I would like to share my carriage and horse, clothes, and fur coat with my friends. Even if they become worn out, I will not complain or have regrets.' Yan, Yuan said: 'I wish not to flaunt my expertise and not to claim my merit.' Zi Lu then asked Confucius: 'We would like to hear, sir, your aspiration.' Confucius said: 'My wishes are: let the elders have a peaceful living, have my friends trust me, and make sure the youngest are taken care of.'"[2]

When we do things, we should know that everything has its appropriate and adequate level or amount. If it is too little, then it will not work. If it is too much, then it becomes a burden. Su, Che (蘇轍) said: "Use eating as an example. When we have the right amount, stop. If we have excess, then this surplus can make us sick. Use our four bodies (i.e., head, torso, legs, and arms) as another example. When we have all these four, then it is complete. If there are more, such as lumps, then it will become a burden."[3]

Qigong Interpretation

This chapter has pointed out three important things in qigong practice. First, when you practice qigong, do not overdo it. The body has its limitations and tolerances. If you overdo it, it can bring you harm instead of benefit. For example, if you like some special food so you eat a lot of it, eventually this can bring you more harm than benefit.

Second, you should remain humble. When you are humble, you have more friends and support. When you are proud of yourself and boast about it, eventually you will lose all your friends.

Finally, a good heart of benevolence and concern for others can always bring you peace, generous feelings, and righteousness. The reason this feeling exists deeply inside of you is because you have followed the Dao.

Conclusion

Three things may help to build your righteous qi (zheng qi, 正氣) deep inside of you. This righteous qi is usually generated because of your kindness, concern, and righteousness. When you have these virtues within, you will feel peaceful, calm, and harmonious. This will keep your spirit strong and firm. However, if you have committed some bad deeds that make you feel guilty, subconsciously, you feel void spiritually deep inside as well. Remember, the inner righteous feeling is always the major key to balance your qi and spirit.

1.《史記·項羽本紀》：項羽"自矜攻伐""欲以力征經營天下，五年卒亡其國，身死東城（東阿縣），尚不覺悟而不自責，過矣。"

2.《尚書·大禹謨》：顏淵、季路侍。子曰："盍各言爾志？"子路曰："願車、馬、衣、裘與友共敝之而無憾。"顏淵曰："願無伐善，無施勞。"子路曰："願聞子之志。"子曰："老者安之，朋友信之，少者懷之。"

3. 蘇轍說："譬如飲食，適飽則已，有餘則病；譬如四體，適完則已，有贅則累。

Part IV

Representation of Data Mining Knowledge

CHAPTER 25
Representations of the Mystery—Following the Laws
第二十五章
象元—法規

有物混成，先天地生。
　　寂兮寥兮，獨立而不改，
　　周行而不殆，可以為天下母。
吾不知其名，字之曰『道』，
　　強為之名曰『大』。
大曰逝，
　　逝曰遠，
　　遠曰反。
　　故
『道』大，天大，地大，人亦大。
域中有四大，
　　而人居其一焉。
人法地，地法天，天法『道』，『道』法自然。

There is something mysteriously formed before heaven and earth;
    so silent and ethereal, independent and changeless,
        moving with cycle ceaselessly that can be regarded as the
        mother of heaven and earth (i.e., the Nature).
I don't know its name, so word it as "Dao."
    If forced to define it, I call it "great."
Great means to ceaselessly function,
    ceaselessly function means extending far,
    extending far means returning to its beginning.
    Thus,
the Dao is great, the heaven is great, the earth is great, and the
    humans are also great.
There are four greats in this universe,
    and humans are one of them.
The humans follow the laws of the earth, the earth follows the laws
    of heaven, the heaven follows the laws of the Dao, and the Dao
    follows the laws of Nature.

General Interpretation

This chapter describes what the Dao is. Actually, we don't know what the Dao really is. The Dao is invisible, vast, profound, and mysterious. It existed even before the universe was formed (the De). It is quiet and spiritual, yet independent and changeless. This force or energy creates ceaseless cycles of Nature (the De) so it can be regarded as the mother of Nature.

Since there is no definition for the Dao, it is impossible to name it. If we are forced to name it, we may just call it "Great." This greatness covers the ceaseless functionings of the universe that are far beyond what we know. When it reaches to its extremity, it will return to the beginning. This is the cyclic function or pattern of the Great Nature. Wang, Dao (王道) said: "(The universe) has its cyclic energy flow without stagnation. This is a ceaseless phenomenon. (The qi) within is full without limitation. This is a phenomenon of extending far. Observe the phenomena near you to see these cycling patterns, and conceal yourself in seclusion for pondering, so to trace back to these roots."[1] This means that the natural cyclic patterns ceaselessly repeat themselves and the qi existing in this nature is unlimited beyond what we can imagine. The way to see these patterns is to observe these natural patterns near us, such as breathing, on a yearly, monthly, and daily cycling. From observation, if we meditate and ponder quietly, we will be able to find out the roots of this recycling. Xiao, Tian-Shi (蕭天石) said: "The universe has its large and small cyclic patterns, to and fro cycling repeatedly and ceaselessly. This is the Dao of Nature."[2]

There are four recognized great powers in this universe: the Dao, the heaven, the earth, and the human. Human is the last, derived from the cycle of the other three. Thus, humans will copy the laws of the earth. Earth follows the laws of the heaven, and the heaven accords with the laws of the Dao. Wang, An-Shi (王安石) said:

> "Humans follow the quietness of the earth; thus they can achieve their merit without doing (i.e., efforts). The earth copies the heaven's wuwei (i.e., doing nothing); thus, with-

out growing, myriad objects arise. The heaven models the nature of the Dao; thus, myriad objects are derived without bearing (i.e., intention of production). The rule of the Dao has its root by itself; it has existed since ancient times, even before nature was present. That's why there is nothing for the Dao to follow. If there is nothing to follow, then it is just by itself naturally. That's why it is said: 'the Dao follows the laws of the Nature.'"[3]

Qigong Interpretation

The Great Nature has countless cyclic patterns. Some of the patterns are near us and we can see or even experience them; for example, yearly, monthly, and daily cyclic changes due to the positions of the sun, earth, and the moon. All these changes are near us and immediately influence our body's energy and activities. All these are considered as the De, the manifestation of the Dao. Then, what is the Dao? Is the Dao the spirit or God of nature? Since we don't know too much about the Dao, it is still a huge mystery for us.

However, from others' past experience we know that if we meditate correctly, we are able to reconnect our spirits to the natural spirit. But to reach this profound meditative state, we have to minimize our conscious mind (the human matrix) and allow our subconscious mind to grow. Our lives were originated from a single cell. Our spirits were still closely connected with Nature while we were in the embryonic stage. However, after our birth, we began to acquire the usual human dogmas, traditions, and emotional bondage to fit into this society. In this matrix, our spirit gradually parted during our growth and became isolated from the natural spirit. Now, we are separated far from Nature.

As we have seen, Chinese qigong holds that we have two minds coexisting in our body, the conscious mind and the subconscious mind. The conscious mind is where the thought and conscious memory is generated from the brain cells. The conscious mind is also the mind that is related to what we have learned and been taught after birth.

Since we are growing up in a false social construct that exerts a heavy emotional influence, we also become untruthful in order to survive. In this matrix society, we all have a mask on our face.

We have noted that the subconscious mind resides in the limbic system located at the center of the head. The subconscious mind is more truthful and responsive for profound feeling and intuition. This place is called "Mud Pill Palace" (Ni Wan Gong, 泥丸宮) and is the residence of the spirit (shen, 神). Chapter 6 of the *Dao De Jing* states that the spirit that resides at the center is called "valley spirit" (gu shen, 谷神) and the space between the two lobes of the brain is called "Spirit Valley" (shen gu, 神谷).

In the past, many qigong practitioners were able to reconnect to the natural spirit through cultivation of the subconscious mind via embryonic breathing. The way to do this is to bring your mind to the innocent, simple, and pure state of an infant. From this, the subconscious mind will gradually grow stronger. In order to do this, you must be truthful to yourself and others. You have to downplay the role of your conscious mind in this society. However, it is hard to survive if you are truthful in this lying society. Thus, many qigong practitioners, such as Buddhist and Daoist monks, lived in seclusion. This was the reason Daoist monks called themselves a "truthful person" (zhen ren, 真人).

Additionally, to reconnect with the Dao, we have to follow the Dao instead of being against it. The matrix we have created since the beginning of human history has been leading people farther and farther away from the Dao. Now, the entire matrix we have created is often against the Dao (Nature).

Conclusions

The way to find the meaning of life is through meditation and tracing back to the beginning of our lives. From deep meditation, we may reconnect ourselves with the natural spirit. Furthermore, to have a healthy life and live long, we must also follow the Dao. If we continue to live against the Dao, we will never figure out the meaning of the Dao and our lives.

1. 王道說：“自其周流無滯也，有逝之象；自其充周無窮也，有遠之象。近取諸身，而退藏于密，復歸其根也。”

2. 肖天石說：“宇宙有宇宙之大小周天；往復周行，循環不息，此自然之道也。”

3. 王安石說：“人法地之安靜，故無為而天下功；地法天之無為，故不長而萬物育；天法道之自然，故不產而萬物化。道則本自根，未有天地，自古已固存，無所法也。無法者，自然而已。故曰‘道法自然’。”

CHAPTER 26

The Emphasis of the De—Steadiness

第二十六章
重德—穩重

重為輕根，
　　靜為躁君。
　　是以
『聖人』終日行，
　　不離輜重。
雖有榮觀，
　　燕處超然。
奈何萬乘之主，
　　而以身輕天下？
輕則失根，
　　躁則失君。

Heaviness (i.e., steadiness) is the root of lightness (i.e., flightiness),
   calmness is the monarch of restlessness.
   Therefore,
those sages, traveling the whole day,
   will not separate from their heaviness (i.e., steadiness).
Though glory falls upon on them,
   they position themselves lightly.
Nonetheless, how can a lord with ten thousand chariots (i.e., a
   king),
   position himself lightly before the kingdom (i.e., to rule the
   country)?
When frivolous, then the root is lost;
   when restless, then the monarch is lost.

General Interpretation

Heaviness means solemn, steady, and serious. Lightness means careless, frivolous, and irresponsible. As a ruler, if he rules the country solemnly and seriously, he will govern the country effectively and efficiently. However, if the ruler is irresponsible, careless, and frivolous, then the country will become chaotic due to the poor leadership. He, Shang-Gong (河上公) said: "As a ruler, if one is not solemn and serious, then one is not respected by the people. When the mind governs the body without being solemn and serious, then the spirit is lost. The flowers of plants and trees are light; thus, they are withered and fallen. The roots are heavy, thus they last long."[1]

Those sages will be solemn, steady, and treat affairs seriously in the journey of their lives. Even when glory and praise fall upon on them, they will take it lightly. This is because the serious inner self-cultivation and principle are the roots while those glories and praises are just like flowers. The inner temperament lasts long while the glories and praises are temporary.

According to the same principle, if a ruler governs the country without being solemn, steady, confident, and sincere, the country will become disordered and chaotic. Naturally, the safety and stability of the country will not last. On the contrary, if the ruler is solemn and serious, then people will trust him, respect him, and follow his orders; thus the country will be safe and lasting. Du, Guang-Ting (杜光庭) said:

> "When a ruler is steady and calm, then country affairs can be managed effectively and thus are in order. He does not ask much but receives sufficient supports, does not give much but is benevolent, does not speak but is trustworthy, does not ask but still acquires, and does not make an effort but things are accomplished. He simply follows Nature and embraces true simplicity; thus the world (i.e., country) is peaceful and steady. When a person takes things seriously with calmness, the harmonious qi can be cultivated and stored, the mind is peaceful, and the vision and hearing will not be attracted to and confused by the outside

*world. Lust will not be assaulting the mind internally;
thus the life can be extended long."*[2]

There is a story about the kingdom of Yue (越), and its king, Wu Ling (武靈王), in the book, *Han Fei Zi* (《韓非子·喻老》). Han, Fei (韓非) said:

*"The kingdom is the heaviness (zizhong, 輜重) of a king.
When King Wu Ling was still alive, he gave his power to
his son. This is leaving his heaviness. Though he had
acquired the joys at Dai He (代和) and Yun Zhong (雲中),
he had already lost the country, Yue (越), complacently.
King Wu Ling was a lord of myriad chariots (i.e., of a big
country), but decided to position himself lightly and so was
despised by the people. When the power is lost, it is called
'lightness.' When he left his position as a ruler, it is called
'restless.' Finally, he died of starvation while imprisoned.
Therefore, Lao Zi said: 'When frivolous, then the root is
lost; when restless, then the monarch is lost.' This is talking
about the story of King Wu Ling."*[3]

Heaviness (zizhong, 輜重) means the luggage carriage that travels with a traveler. It implies that heaviness is the safeguard of a traveler. Once he lost his luggage carriage, he had lost his safeguard.

Qigong Interpretation

In qigong, the body is like a country or a kingdom, the mind is the king or the ruler, the qi is the people, the breathing is the strategies of governing, and the spirit is the morality or morale of the people. The mind governs the entire body's qi circulation and functions. If the mind is solemn, serious, responsive, calm, and steady, the body's qi can be governed efficiently, the political strategies can be carried out effectively, and the spirit of the country can be high. Cheng, Yi-Ning (程以寧) said:

"When the body is calm, the qi's status (i.e., storage and circulation) will be stable. When the qi is stable, then life can be completely fulfilled.

When the heart (i.e., mind) is calm, the cultivation of the spirit can be completed. When the spirit is completed, then the cultivation of temperament can be achieved. Consequently, when one is completed (i.e., mind), all hundred others can also be completed. Therefore, it is said: 'calmness is the monarch of restlessness.'"[4]

From this, you can see the most important qigong practice is "regulating your mind." This is because the mind is the king who governs the entire body's functions. When the mind is taking care of the body seriously and respectfully, the body will be healthy.

Guan Zi (管子·內業) said:

"A human look for enjoyments in life. If he is worried, he will lose his regular routines and when his is angry, he will forget his discipline. Whenever there is worry, sorrow, joy, or anger, the Dao will not accommodate. When there is lust, then use calmness to stop it. When encountering chaos, then correct it into its right order. You don't need to lead or push; the happiness will fall upon you automatically. When the Dao arrives by itself, you can apply the Dao for your deliberation. When you are calm, you will acquire it, and when you are restless, you will lose it. The spiritual qi resides within your heart (i.e., mind), and comes and goes occasionally. This qi can be small without limitation and can be so large that there is no border. When a human loses his spiritual qi, it is because of the restless' harm (i.e., the harm of being restless). When the heart (i.e., mind) is calm, the Dao (i.e., the body's Dao, the natural behaviors of the body) will become steady and firm by itself."[5]

Confucius (孔子) (《禮記·大學》) also said: "Once you know how to stop (thoughts), then there is a steadiness. When there is a steadiness, then you are able to be calm. When there is calmness, then you are in peace. Once you are in peace, then you are able to ponder (i.e., meditate). Through pondering, you will be able to acquire."[6]

Conclusions

This chapter has pointed out that the crucial key to a successful qigong practice is regulating your mind. When your mind is in a calm and peaceful state, you are able to feel deeply. Remember, feeling is a language that allows your mind and body to communicate. When this feeling is developed to a profound stage subconsciously, you will be able to feel or sense Nature or the Dao. All of these practices are the manifestations (the De) of the Dao.

1. 河上公說："人君不重則不尊，治身不重則失神。草木之華輕，固零落；根重，故長存。"

2. 杜光庭說："人君之重靜也，則事省而理，求寡而贍，不施而仁，不言而信，不求而得，不為而成。懷自然，抱真朴而天下泰矣。人身之重靜也，則和氣積，心慮平，視聽不惑于外，情慾不攖于內而壽命延矣。"

3. 《韓非子·喻老》："邦者，人君之輜重也。主父生傳其邦，此離其輜重者也；故雖有代、雲中之樂，超然已無越矣。主父萬乘之主，而以身輕天下，無勢之謂輕，離位之謂躁，是以生幽而死。故曰'輕則失臣，躁則失君'，主父之謂也。"

4. 程以寧說："身靜則氣定，氣定則了命；心靜則神全，神全則了性；而一了百了矣。故曰靜為躁君。"

5. 管子說："凡人之生也，必以其歡，憂則失紀，怒則失端，憂悲喜怒，道乃無處。愛欲靜之，遇亂正之，勿引勿推，福將自歸。彼道自來，可籍與謀。靜則得之，躁則失之。靈氣在心，一來一逝，其細無內，其大無外。所以失之，以躁為害。心能執靜，道將自定。"《內業》

6. 《禮記·大學》曰："知止而後有定，定而後能靜，靜而後能安，安而後能慮，慮而後能得。"

CHAPTER 27
Use Skillfully—Borrow Examples

第二十七章
巧用—借鑒

善行，無轍跡；
　　善言，無瑕讁，
　　善數，不用籌策，
　　善閉，無關楗而不可開，
　　善結，無繩約而不可解。
是以『聖人』
　　常善救人，故無棄人；
　　常善救物，故無棄物。
　　是謂『襲明』。
故
善人者，不善人之師；
　　不善人者，善人之資。
不貴其師，不愛其資，
　　雖智大迷。
　　是謂『要妙』。

A good traveler leaves no trace,
  a good speaker makes no fault,
  a good accountant uses no devices,
  a good door needs no bolts to remain shut,
  a good fastener needs no rope to hold its bond.
Therefore, those sages
  often help others, so there is no abandoned person,
  often save things, so there is no abandoned object.
  This is called "inheriting bright wisdom."
Thus,
those who are good are the teachers of the bad,
  those who are bad are the admonishment of the good.
Those (who are not good) do not value their teachers and do not
  appreciate their admonishment,
  though intelligent, (they are) actually greatly deluded.
  (Understanding this principle) is called "subtle and
  mysterious."

General Interpretation

This chapter is talking about the applications of the De (the manifestation of the Dao). For those experts in traveling, they will not leave any trace that would let people know where they are heading. For those who are good at speaking, people cannot find fault with what they say. A well-designed door will not require a bolt to keep it shut. Those who know how to fasten do not need rope to keep the bond tight and secure. All of these sayings are talking about those sages who are in accord with the Dao. They will not leave any trace to show what they have done, and they know how to contain their thoughts within themselves and keep their good deeds to themselves. They have reached the stage of "regulating without regulating." Du, Guang-Ting (杜光庭) said: "Those who are good at cultivation of the Dao know how to keep the truth with them and embrace singularity . . . They know how to keep the three gates shut and calm down naturally. They know how to repel all thoughts and be peaceful naturally. The sounds and colors cannot confuse their hearts (i.e., minds); official position and social status cannot tempt their wills. How can these gates be opened for those who are good at shutting them?"[1]

The three gates (三關) means the gates for the life, mind, and spirit. They are the same as what Buddhists have defined: the body, the mind, and the spirit. This implies the connections of the sensing organs with outside world. If you know how to shut them down from external enticements, then you are considered as one who is close to the Dao.

Once you have reached this level, you can say you have established a firm foundation for your spiritual cultivation and rechanneled your spirit into the inherited path as an infant. Du, Guang-Ting (杜光庭) said:

> "What is xi (襲)? It means to inherit and continue. What it says is that the human's spirit at the spiritual residence was originally bright and clean. But it was shaded (i.e., contaminated) by the dusts (i.e., emotional contaminants) so the innocent mind has been enticed. Today, (we) should conduct the five goodness practices to clean the heart (i.e.,

mind) internally so the real (i.e., original) human nature can be returned to its brightness. This intelligent brightness will bring you to your original being. (We) should always conduct our good deeds to save others and stop the initiation of those fantastic emotional thoughts so the intelligent brightness can be resumed and continued. (We) should not allow our mind to be confused, not to linger on the trace (i.e., past), and not to become stagnant from routine. Then, it can be said: 'inheriting bright wisdom.'"[2]

"The five goodness practices" means to be good at speaking (teaching), doing (conducting good deeds), calculating (planning), closing (self-control), and concluding (reach to the end). Stagnant means the stagnation (obstacles) caused by dogmas and traditions. It implies that we should be flexible and dare to evolve from the traditional bondage.

Therefore, you should teach and help others without discriminating against different kinds of people. Wang, An-Shi (王安石) said: "What does it mean to be a good person? It is to teach those who are not good."[3] Ma, Qi-Chang (馬其昶) said: "When you see those who are not good, use them as an admonishment. You still need to teach them to be good. This, then, will make the quantity of my good deeds more sufficient. This is how those who are not good help those who are good."[4] This phrase means that when you help those who are not good, other than the fact that their bad deeds can serve as warnings and examples of how not to conduct yourself, you will also have built up more good deeds. This is how those who are not good help you.

However, even when you have tried hard to help those who are not good, often you will find some who do not welcome your help. Although they are intelligent, they cannot see this fact. Wang, Bi (王弼) said: "Though they have intelligence, they are opinionated with their wisdom, and without seeing obstacles in their way, will be lost. Thus, it is said: 'Thought intelligent, but greatly deluded.'"[5]

Qigong Interpretation

Good qigong practitioners or followers of the Dao, after doing a good deed, will not leave a trace of their actions. Cui, Zi-Yu (崔子玉) (座右銘) said: "After doing a good deed for others, do not keep your mind there. However, if you received the favor from others, you should not forget."[6] Their talking makes perfect sense and there is no fault that can be found. When they practice, since they have reached the stage of regulating of no regulating, no plan or schedule is needed. They know how to keep their essence within and preserve the qi without wasting. They know how to govern their emotions, and nothing—such as glory, dignity, wealth, or lust—is able to influence their minds.

They have a benevolent heart and will share and help others without hesitation. There is no one in the world who will be abandoned by them. They will not waste their gifts but will use and appreciate all of them. These deeds are the performances of the Dao and are the demonstrations of wisdom.

They are humbly teaching others without hesitation or discrimination of good or bad. Even the deeds of bad people can be used as examples for them. Thus, if you wish to become a proficient qigong practitioner, you must share your understanding and help others. The more you teach, the more you understand. Other people's mistakes serve as examples for your learning. The Chinese have a saying: "Teaching and learning mutually help and support each other."[7]

Conclusions

This chapter discusses that, as a follower of the Dao, though you have done and contributed many good deeds to the world, you should not dwell on them. You should treat them lightly. When you have this heart, then you can continue to accumulate your credit in the yin world (spiritual world).

1. 杜光庭說：“善修行之人，守真抱一，無欲無營···，閉三關而自靜，祛眾念而自安，聲色不能惑其心，軒冕不能啟其志，此之善閉，其可開乎？”

2. 杜光庭說：“襲者，承續也。言人靈府之性，本來明淨，為塵所翳，迷惑天真，今以五善之行，內洗其心，真性復明，慧照如本然，當常行善救，無起妄塵，承襲慧明，無使昏翳，不矜于跡，不滯于常，可謂襲明也。”

3. 王安石說：“善人，教不善人者也。”

4. 馬其昶說：“見不善非徒以為戒，又必教之使善，然後吾之善量足，是不善人正善人為善之質。”

5. 王弼說：“雖有其智，自任其智，不因物于道，必失。故曰：‘雖智大迷’。”

6. 座右銘“施人慎勿念，受施慎勿忘。”崔子玉（漢）

7. “教學相長。”

CHAPTER 28

Returning to Simplicity—Returning to the Origin

第二十八章
反樸—還原

知其雄，守其雌，
　　為天下谿；
為天下谿，常『德』不離，
　　復歸於嬰兒。
知其白，（守其黑，
　　為天下式；
為天下式，常『德』不忒，
　　復歸於無極。
知其榮，）守其辱，
　　為天下谷；
為天下谷，常『德』乃足，
　　復歸於樸。
樸散則為器，
　　『聖人』用之，則為官長。
故
　　大制不割。

Know the male and hold to the female,
  become the valley stream of the world.
Becoming the valley stream of the world, the eternal De will not
  depart.
  Return to the innocence of an infant.
Know the white and hold to the black,
  become an example to the world.
Becoming an example to the world, the eternal De will not deviate.
  Return to the wujii (i.e., no extremity, beginning, or nothing-
  ness).
Know the honor and hold to the humility,
  become the valley of the world.
Becoming the valley of the world, the eternal De will be sufficient,
  and return to simplicity (i.e., nature).
When simplicity is disseminated (i.e., manifested or applied), then
  it becomes tools.
  Sages use them, then become leaders.
  Thus, great control is achieved without cutting (i.e., becoming
  damaged).

General Interpretation

The male is aggressive and likes to manifest his power externally; thus, more merits can be achieved. The female is gentle, loving, and humble, and usually humbly stays at home to maintain the home's integrity. This implies that the male is an external manifestation (the De) while the female is the inner thought and feeling (the Dao). A sage will keep his internal thoughts humble even though externally he has done many good deeds. He will then receive great respect and people will gather around him. He, Shang-Gong (河上公) said: "The male means dignity while the female implies humility. Though a person knows how to manifest his dignity, he should also keep himself humble and small, repelling the male's strength and positioning himself in softness and harmony. In this case, the world will come to him like water entering a deep stream."[1]

White implies that what you have done or contributed is obvious. Black means you should keep it quiet and in the darkness as if you don't know it exists. He, Shang-Gong (河上公) also said: "White means visible and black implies silence. Although a person knows his merits are obvious and clear, he should keep himself in silence, as if he sees nothing. He can then be an example or model of the world."[2] Once you have become an example for other people and are followed by them, your external virtue (manifestation of the Dao) will last long and will not deviate.

Therefore, when you know your honor but can keep your humility, the people of the world will come to you and stay around you just like the valley streams collecting the water from all directions. When you have achieved this level of leadership, you have built a sufficient eternal De. Then you should return yourself to simplicity. Applied to the world, this simplicity can be an effective tool. When sages use this tool, they can become the unselfish masters or leaders of myriad objects. Wang, Bi (王弼) said: "Simplicity means truth. When truth is disseminated, then hundreds of variations are merged and a variety of lives are generated. Therefore, they are like tools (i.e., root or origin of variations and applications). Sages, due to the dissemination (i.e., applications) of simplicity, can become leaders. Apply it (application of simplicity) to those who are good and they will become teachers and those who are not good will serve as admonishments. These will, thus, change the (poor) customs and return them to singularity."³ Song, Chang-Xing (宋常星) said: "When one is fair and impartial, one can be called an officer (i.e., leader) and when one is able to master myriad objects, one can be called a magistrate."⁴

When sages apply this simplicity to the world or themselves, there is no damage done or abuse committed. He Shang Gong (河上公) said: "When those sages use it (i.e., simplicity) for the world, then they are able to use the Great Dao to rule and administer the world without damage. When it is used for themselves, then they can use the Heaven Dao to control their lust so their spirit will not be harmed."⁵

Qigong Interpretation

Male implies yang, external manifestations or actions, and activity. Female implies yin, internal mind and qi's cultivation, calm and soft. When we live in this society, we need to manifest our mind and qi in daily activities. We also need to use our qi efficiently to maintain our bodies' health. Therefore, yang (male) is consumption of qi while yin (female) conserves the qi with the mind staying at the center (center of gravity and singularity). Yang is physical actions while yin is conserving and centering. Yin preserves qi and governs it so the qi can be used efficiently.

From this, you can see that yin (mind) should be humble and kept at the center (valley stream) so the qi can flow to this center and be stored. To consume is to lead the qi outward so the guardian qi (wei qi, 衛氣) can be expanded and physical actions can be carried out. To keep our bodies healthy, we must have a strong guardian qi for our immune system and a firm body for physical functions and endurance. However, if you overconsume your qi, your qi will be void internally. Eventually, you will get sick simply because of a shortage of qi. Therefore, you must know how much qi you have, how much physical activity you can do, how to conserve the qi, and how to create more qi and store it at the real lower dan tian (bio-battery) situated at the center of gravity.

From this, you can see that the yin practice is considered as the mother of your body. Yin practice can be done through embryonic breathing meditation (taixi jingzuo, 胎息静坐). From this meditation, you will learn how to bring your mind and qi to the center and keep them there. This is called "embracing singularity" (bao yi, 抱一). It is called "the state of no extremity" (wuji, 無極). In order to reach this state, your mind must be soft, simple, extremely calm, and centered. If you are interested in embryonic breathing meditation, please refer to the book and DVD: *Qigong Meditation—Embryonic Breathing*, by YMAA Publication Center.

Conclusions

To learn how to conserve the qi and store it to an abundant level at the lower real dan tian is the crucial key of qigong training. This is considered as the mother (female) of the entire qigong practice. How healthy your body is and how much you are able to accomplish in small circulation and grand circulation all depend on how much qi you can accumulate at the center.

1. 河上公說："雄以喻尊，雌以喻卑。人雖知自尊顯，當復守之以卑微，去雄之強梁，就雌之柔和，如是則天下歸之，如水之入深谿也。"
2. 河上公說："白以喻昭昭，黑以喻默默。人雖自知昭昭明白，當復守之以默默，如闇昧無所見。如是則可以為天下法式。"
3. 王弼說："朴，真也。真散，則百行出，殊類生，若器也。聖人因其分散，故為之立官長，以善為師、不善為資，移風易俗，復使歸于一也。"
4. 宋常星說："公而無私謂之官，主宰萬物謂之長。"
5. 河上公說："聖人用之，則以大道制御天下，無所傷割；治身則以天道制情欲，不害精神也。"

CHAPTER 29

Doing Nothing—Be Nature

第二十九章
無為—自然

將欲取天下而為之，
　　　吾見其不得已。
天下神器，
　　不可為也，不可執也。
　　為者敗之，執者失之。
故
物，或行或隨，
　　或歔或吹，
　　或強或贏，
　　或載或隳。
是以
　　『聖人』去甚、去奢、去泰。

For those who wish to take over the world and act upon it,
    I can see that they cannot succeed.
The world is a sacred vessel,
    it cannot be acted upon it and cannot be controlled.
    Those who act upon it will fail; and those who control it will
    lose.
Therefore,
all objects either lead or follow,
    either blow hot or blow cold,
    either strong or weak,
    either on it or off it.
Thus,
sages eliminate excess, extravagance, and arrogance.

General Interpretation

This chapter is talking about applying wuwei (無為) (doing nothing) when ruling this world. That means a ruler should govern according to Nature. Too much of acting on the world (using force) will fail. He, Shang-Gong (河上公) said: "(If a ruler) wishes to be the master of the world and intends to act upon the people (i.e., to use force) for it, I can see clearly that he will not acquire the help from the Heaven Dao and the support from the people."[1] In chapter 64 it is also said: "Whoever meddles, will fail; whoever persists will lose. Thus, sages do not meddle, thus they do not fail."[2]

That is the reason those sages know how to maintain balance within themselves: neither too much of anything nor too little. They keep their mind simple, pure, calm, and peaceful without being allured by the outside world. They know if you are happy, eventually you will be sad. If you go up, you have to come down. The emotional life is like roller coasters going up, down, and around ceaselessly. Only if you are able to keep your mind neutral will you be undisturbed by these emotional disturbances. He, Shang-Gong (河上公) said: "Excess means being addicted to the joys of lust, sounds, and colors. Extravagance implies the luxuries of dressing and eating, and arrogance means the exaggeration of the residence and gardens."[3]

Du, Guang-Ting (杜光庭) said:

> *"The way that those sages situated themselves in the world was to observe the trends of the up and down changes and see the opportunity of pushing and moving (i.e., actions). Then when they execute their actions, they will not be excessive. They know that whoever has been too excessive will have their situation reversed. Those who are in luxury will become greedy and those who exaggerate will become too prosperous. When things have reached their extremity, the course will surely be reversed. Those who become greedy will complain and those who are prosperous will become feeble. When there is just one of these excesses committed, failure or death is certain. Thus, they get rid of these."[4]*

The Chinese have a saying: "Greediness is a bottomless hole."[5] This implies that the more you desire something, the more you want it, without ceasing.

Qigong Interpretation

This chapter is talking about regulating the mind (tiao xin, 調心). When you practice qigong, your mind must be in a neutral and calm state. If your mind is disturbed by the continuous ups and downs of the emotions, you will not be able to develop the truthful feeling of the subconscious mind. Most emotional turmoil comes from false feeling and desires. If you can be simple, pure, and neutral in your mind, you will have the correct feeling and judgment for your practice.

As we have noted, water is neutral, but from it various drinks can be made. Thus, water is the most universal drink you can ever find. The most powerful sound is the one without sound. When there is no sound, then you can create all kinds of sounds. Though you keep your mind in a neutral state, you must also be flexible. Otherwise, your mind will become too stubborn. When this happens, your mind will be narrowed and closed. This is not the way of learning. In order to learn, you must be humble, open minded, and flexible. Confucius (孔子) (《論語·子罕》) said: "Do not be prejudiced, do not be expectant, do not be stubborn, and do not be selfish."[6] What this sentence means is that you should have an open mind to accept other people's opinions and advice. You should not expect the result that may not necessarily happen. You should not stubbornly persist in your prejudice. And you should not be selfish and concerned only for yourself. These are a few of the important mental cultivations you need in order to reach a proficient level of qigong learning and practice.

Conclusions

The mind is the general or the king who is governing and in charge of the entire body's qi. As a general, you must keep your mind calm and neutral. You should be opened minded and not stubborn in your think-ing. Those who have reached a high level of qigong practice did so because they were able to jump out of the human matrix so that their mind is free to accept, to change, to listen, and to develop. It is the same for your practice. If you cannot be humble and open minded, then your learning and practice will be limited.

1. 河上公說：“欲為天下主，欲以有為治民，我見其不得天道人心已明矣。”
2. 六十四章說：“為者敗之，執者失之。是以聖人無為，故無敗；無執，故無失。”
3. 河上公說：“甚謂貪淫聲色，奢謂服飾飲食，泰謂宮室台榭。”
4. 杜光庭說：“聖人之于天下也，觀倚伏之勢，見推移之機，于施為之中，不使過分；知甚者必極，奢者必貪，泰者必盛；極則必反，貪則必怨，盛者必衰。有一于此，必為亡敗，故皆去之。”
5. “貪是無底洞。”
6. 孔子說：“毋意，毋必，毋固，毋我。”（《論語·子罕》）

CHAPTER 30

Limiting the Use of War—Ways of Treating People

第三十章
儉武—待人

以道佐人主者，
　　不以兵強天下。
其事好還。
　　師之所處，荊棘生焉；
　　大軍之後，必有凶年。
善者果而已，
　　不敢以取強。
果而勿矜，
　　果而勿伐，
　　果而勿驕，
　　果而不得已，
　　果而勿強。
物壯則老，
　　是謂『不道』。不『道』早已。

Those who use the Dao to advise the ruler,
   do not (advise to) conquer the world with an army.
The use of an army tends to cause retribution.
   Wherever armies stay, thorns and brambles grow;
   after the great armies' (action), there must be an inauspicious
   year.
A skillful leader stops after achieving the goal,
   dares not demonstrate his power (for domination).
Achieves the goal without bragging,
   achieves the goal without flaunting,
   achieves the goal without arrogance,
   achieves the goal out of necessity,
   and achieves the goal but without dominance.
When objects have reached the peak of their strength, and then
   get old,
   this is contrary to the Dao. Without the Dao, things soon perish.

General Interpretation

As a leader, your mind must be confident and firm and your spirit must be strong. However, you must also be humble enough to take counsel from others before your final decision. Advisors around a leader are crucially important. Often a wise leader is successful due to his humility and willingness to listen. A stubborn leader will usually fail. Good and wise advisors would offer suggestions to their leader to follow the Dao. This is because when the leader follows the Dao, the country will be peaceful and harmonious. Mencius (《孟子 · 公孫丑下》) said: "The people cannot be kept within by relying on the border. A country cannot be safe just relying on the mountains and rivers. Showing a country's prestige to the world does not rely on sharp weapons. Those who have acquired the Dao will receive much help while those without the Dao will receive less."[1]

Sometimes, force is necessary. For example, when enemies have invaded your homeland, negotiation has failed, and you need to use force to protect your country. In this case, as a leader, you must firmly lead the troops and work to keep morale high. However, you must recognize that it does not matter if it is offense or defense; war will only bring disaster and misfortune to the country. That is the reason any leader should always avoid war. Wang, Bi (王弼) said: "Talking about deploying troops is a fiercely harmful matter. It does not offer any help but brings harm. It brings injuries and death to the people and barrenness to the fields. Thus, it is said: 'thorns and brambles grow.'"[2]

Even if you have defeated your enemies, you should not brag, flaunt, and be arrogant. You should remain calm and kind to your enemies without dominating them. If possible, you should help your enemies regain their normal lives. If you do so, you will build up friendships instead of eternal enemies. The Chinese have a saying: "What you don't desire, you should not apply to others."[3] How you treat others is how others will treat you. Zeng Zi (曾子) (《孟子 · 梁惠王下》) said: "Be aware! Be aware! How you treat others is how others treat you."[4] Wang, An-Shi (王安石) said: "If you kill someone's father, someone will also kill your father; if you kill someone's brother, someone will also kill your brother."[5] One of Lao Zi's philosophies is "using good deeds to repay the resentment."[6] That means when there is fighting, the losing side will be filled with resentment. However, if you are able to treat them kindly and provide them generous help, then you are using good deeds to repay resentment. In this case, your enemies will become friends. Sun Zi (孫子·謀攻) also said: "Thus, a hundred battles with a hundred victories is not the best (policy) of goodness. To be able to defeat the opponent without battling is the best (policy) of goodness."[7] Wang, Bi (王弼) also said: "This is taking the world without using troops."[8]

From this, you can see the best policy is not using force to solve the problem. However, if it is necessary to deploy force, then even if you win, you should—again—not be proud, brag, flaunt, and be arrogant. You should follow the Dao and treat your enemies as friends and help them. He, Shang-Gong (河上公) said: "Those who do not follow the Dao, die early."[9] Mencius (《孟子·離樓上》) said: "To initiate a battle for taking a land, the deaths of people are full in the field. To fight for a city, the deaths of people are full in the city. This is what is called to consume humans for occupying land. This crime cannot be forgiven even when punished by death. Therefore, those who like war should suffer the most severe punishments."[10]

Qigong Interpretation

Often the way of healing or practicing qigong is through softness, gentleness, and gradual progress, but with consistency instead of aggression. This is simply because the body takes time to heal, adjust, and condition. If the practice or treatment is too aggressive, often the mind becomes chaotic, and the qi flows into the wrong path. This is called "walking into the fire and entering into the devil."[11] Walking into the fire means the qi has entered the wrong place and caused fire. Entering into the devil means the mind has entered the state of fantasy. All of these reversed reactions are the rebound of aggression. For example, use of aggressive surgery, chemotherapy, radiation therapy, and many other methods to treat cancers, may just cause more problems. From past experience, these methods have been proven to not work effectively. Even if there is some small percentage of success, cancer often comes back and kills the sufferer. However, if you improve the qi circulation, provide a healthy lifestyle, have an optimal diet, and get adequate exercises, often the effectiveness of treatment is much higher. Naturally, it takes time, patience, and perseverance to accomplish the treatment with the qigong way. But with the reestablishment of a healthy lifestyle and regular exercise, health can be long lasting.

Emotions are always one of the biggest obstacles of treating cancer effectively. From a qigong understanding, the mind leads the qi. Your body's qi status is closely related to your mind. If your mind is under the conditions of fear, distress, and sadness, your qi status will be suboptimal; thus, cancer cells continue to survive and spread. Studies have shown that a positive outlook is associated with increased levels of healing. Set your mind free from emotional bondage. With your mind free, you can develop a healthy lifestyle and make yourself happy again. This will bring the qi's circulation to its normal healthy state. From a Chinese medical understanding, lumps (cancers) are developed due to the qi's abnormal circulation. The way to remove cancer cells is to resume your healthy and smooth qi circulation. After all, cancers are not problems caused by viruses or germs. It is the cells' restructuring of your body. The physical body is yang while the qi body is yin. One is a mechanical part and the other is the energy part. Both must be in balance. If one of them has a problem (for example, the qi supply is excessive or deficient) the physical part will be changed and possibly sickened.

However, in some cases, you need to treat the problem more aggressively. For example, suppose you have already been attacked by breast cancer. In this case, your enemy has already invaded your homeland. You need to take care of it by focusing on treating the problem. You need to enhance the qi circulation at the breast area and then release it. Through this repeated set of exercises, you will remove the cancer cells gradually. However, once you have recovered from sickness, you should still pay attention to the area and take good care of it. Not only that, you should establish a healthy lifestyle so further problems can be prevented.

Conclusions

Your mind is the leader, the body is the country, and qi is the people. As a leader, you should take care of people with care, softness, and kindness. If you abuse your lifestyle, you will be invaded by the enemies and become sickened. However, when you are sick, you must take care of the problem. After the problem is solved, you should treat it carefully and nicely and continue to take care of it.

1. 《孟子·公孫丑下》: "域民不以封疆之界，固國不以山溪之險，威天下不以兵革之利。得道者多助，失道者寡助。"
2. 王弼說: "言師凶害之物也，無有所濟，必有所傷。賊害人民，殘荒田畝，故曰荊棘生焉。"
3. "己所不欲，勿施於人。"
4. 曾子曰: "戒之戒之！出乎爾者，反乎爾者也。"（《孟子·梁惠王下》）
5. 王安石說: "殺人之父，人亦殺其父；殺人之兄，人亦殺其兄。"
6. "以德報怨。"
7. 《孫子·謀攻》: "是故百戰百勝，非善之善者也；不戰而屈人之兵，善之善者也。"
8. 王弼說: "不以兵力取強于天下也。"
9. 河上公說: "不行道者早死。"
10. 《孟子·離婁上》: "爭地以戰，殺人盈野；爭城以戰，殺人盈城。此所謂率土地而食人肉，罪不容于死。故善戰者服上刑。"
11. "走火入魔。"

CHAPTER 31
Quelling War—Ceasing Aggression
第三十一章
偃武—止犯

夫佳兵者，不祥之器，物或惡之，
　　故有道者不處。
君子居則貴左，
　　用兵則貴右。
兵者不祥之器，非君子之器，
　　不得已而用之，
　　恬淡為上，勝而不美。
而美之者，是樂殺人；
　　夫樂殺人者，
　　則不可得志於天下矣。
吉事尚左，凶事尚右；
　　偏將軍居左，上將軍居右；
　　言以喪禮處之。
殺人之眾，以悲哀莅之，
　　戰勝，以喪禮處之。

Strong armed forces are tools of misfortunate, disliked by the
people.
Thus, those who possess the Dao will not deploy them.
Those noble men, when at home (i.e., during peacetime), value the
left,
and while deploying the armed forces (in wars), value the right.
Armed forces are tools of misfortunate, not noblemen's tools,
used only when necessary.
Tranquility should be the first priority; though victorious, be
without glory.
Those who are glorified are those who like to kill people;
those who like to kill people,
will not achieve their ambitions in this world.
Auspicious matters are appropriate on the left while inauspicious
matters are appropriate on the right.
Lieutenant generals are positioned on the left, while the chief
generals are positioned on the right;
War should be regarded as a funeral.
The many who were killed should be mourned with sadness;
Even in victory, war should be regarded as a funeral.

General Interpretation

Any powerful weapons developed and any powerful army are the tools of the devil and bring the people misfortune. Wang, An-Shi (王安石) said: "Military commanders employ cunning as their foundation, use cheating as their talent, commit killing as their accomplishment, and conquer as their routine event. Thus, (armed forces) are the tools of misfortune."[1]

Those leaders who have followed the Dao will not deploy armed forces unless it is absolutely necessary. Traditionally, the Chinese consider the place on the right as the major position in any arrangement while the left is considered the minor position. War or killing is serious and should be decided by the chief general or the lord who is positioned on the right. Those military advisers or lieutenant generals who offer advice to the leaders are positioned on the left. He Shang Gong (河上公) said: "Those lieutenant generals are humble and position themselves on the yang side (i.e., left side) because they don't have the power of killing. However, those supreme generals are noble and position themselves on the right side because they have authority to kill."[2]

Thus, those leaders who follow the Dao will value the left during peaceful times. However, if there is a necessity to deploy the military, then they will consider the events with grave seriousness. Mencius (《孟子·梁惠王上》) said: "Among the leaders of today's world, there is no one who doesn't favor killing people. If there is one who does not favor killing people, the people of the world will be anxious to follow him. As such, all the people will belong to him. It is just like the water that is flowing downward with such a power and no one is able to stop it."[3] That means those leaders who follow the Dao will be loved and respected by their people.

Culturally the position on the right belongs to the sadness and unfortunate events. It was written in Li Ji (《禮記·檀弓》): "Confucius was standing with his students and politely positioned himself on the right. All his students thus also positioned on the right. Confucius said: 'All of you really love to learn. However, the reason I positioned on the right is because my sister has just passed away.' All students then repositioned themselves on the left."[4] From this, you can see that sadness or any unfortunate events should be treated seriously.

Even when war is necessary, it should not be celebrated if victory comes. It should be treated as a sad thing since so many people have to sacrifice their lives for the war.

Qigong Interpretation

The general on the right is the one who makes decisions. Advisers who offer advice are on the left and cool down aggressive actions. In qigong practice, the general is the emotional mind (xin, 心) while advisers are the wisdom mind (yi, 意). The emotional mind makes your thinking and actions aggressive but often out of focus. With the wisdom mind's assistance, you will be able to keep your momentum, but on the correct path. When you practice qigong, you must have patience, strong will, and perseverance. However, you cannot be emotional. Often the emotional mind is the cause of qigong injury.

When you use the army (aggressive qigong practice), usually you have a problem. If you don't have any problem, you should not have an aggressive attitude in your qigong practice. Aggressive practice is harmful and should not be encouraged. It often brings harm. But when it is necessary, aggressive qigong has to be deployed. For example, if you have already had lung cancer or breast cancer, then your qigong practice would be aggressively targeted on healing. Even after you have resolved the problem, you must remain in a state of high alertness and awareness, deploying the wisdom mind's attitude and treat things like you still have cancer. You will then be able to prevent it from happening again.

Conclusions

The emotional mind is aggressive, but decisive in action. The wisdom mind is calmer and executes the policy more gently and wisely. If you are able to coordinate your emotional mind with the wisdom mind, then you will be on the correct path of qigong practice.

Normally, you practice qigong for sickness prevention (maintaining health). However, if you have a special purpose such as treating illnesses or conditioning your body, then you need to be become more aggressive. Even though this is the case, you must be cautious.

1. 王安石說：“兵家以詭詐為本，欺謫為能，殺獲為功，征伐為事，故曰不祥之器。”
2. 河上公說：“偏將軍卑而居陽者，以其不專殺也。上將軍尊而居右者，言其主殺也。”
3. 《孟子‧梁惠王上》：“今夫天下之人牧，未有不嗜殺人者也。如有不嗜殺人者，則天下之民，皆引領而望之矣。誠如是也，民歸之，由水之就下，沛然誰能御之。”
4. 《禮記‧檀弓》：“孔子與門人立，拱而尚右，二三子亦皆尚右。孔子曰：‘二三子之嗜學也，我則有姐之喪故也。’二三子皆尚左。”

CHAPTER 32
The Holiness of the De—Following the Dao

第三十二章
聖德—從道

『道』常無名，
　　　朴雖小，
　　　天下莫能臣。
侯王若能守之，
　　　萬物將自賓。
天地相合，
　　　以降甘露，
　　　民莫之令而自均。
始制有名，
　　　名亦既有，
　　　夫亦將知止，
　　　知止可以不殆。
譬『道』之在天下，
　　　猶川谷之于江海。

The Dao is always nameless,
  though Pu (i.e., simplicity) is imperceptible,
  no one in the world is able to subjugate it.
If those marquis and kings are able to keep it,
  myriad objects will follow orders automatically.
The heaven and the earth harmonize with each other,
  thus the sweet dew is falling,
  without being asked, all people will accord automatically.
At the beginning, all objects were named and classified,
  once classified,
  then one should know when to stop, or temptations will arise;,
  knowing when to stop will avoid danger.
The Dao in this world,
  is like (the water from) the valleys' streams that flows into rivers
  and oceans.

General Interpretation

Pu (朴) means simpicity, innocence, and purity. It implies the virtue of the Dao. Tian-xia (天下) literally translates as "under heaven." It implies the world. Since we don't know what Nature (the Dao) actually is, any name given such as the Dao or taiji will not be accurate. Therefore, the Dao should not have a name and should not be named. In the first chapter, it is said: "The Dao that can be described is not the eternal Dao. The Name that can be named is not the eternal name." Even though this is true, in order to discuss it, we must give it a name. Without the name, it cannot be identified.

Fan, Ying-Yuan (范應元) said: "The Dao is always nameless. It cannot be described with large or small. Those sages saw it was so large and that there is nothing that cannot be contained by it, thus, (they are) forced to name it 'large'; again, because it is so fine and there is no place that cannot be penetrated by it, therefore, they called it 'small.'"[1]

Cheng, Yi-Ning (程以寧) said: "Because it (i.e., the Dao) has not been engraved and polished (i.e., being still in a natural state), thus it was called 'pu.' Because it is inaudible and so fine, thus it is called 'small.' However, the tian-xia (i.e., the world) dares not subjugate it. Why? Because heaven and earth (i.e., the universe) rely on it so myriad objects can be born and depend on it to survive. Who dares to subjugate it so to affect the growth and lives of itself?"[2] That is why Wu, Cheng (吳澄) said: "The merit of the Dao has reached and spread to the entire tian-xia (i.e., the world). For instance, due to the harmonization of heaven and earth, the sweet dews fall. Though nobody makes it happen, it is able to reach myriad objects uniformly and equally."[3]

He Shang Gong (河上公) said: "If marquis and kings are able to keep the Dao and do nothing (wuwei), then myriad objects will be following orders automatically. This is the way of following the De (i.e., manifestation of the Dao)."[4]

Once all objects were named, then a system and rules were established. When these rules were set up, everything was defined, classified, and compared. When there is classification and comparison, then desire and greediness will develop and dominate human's thinking.

Therefore, we should know how to stop these temptations. If we know how to stop these temptations, we will not endanger our thoughts and bodies. Wang, Bi (王弼) said: "When the rules were set, the roles of all officers had to be established so the seniors and juniors (or superiors and inferiors) could be distinguished. Therefore, all the rules have names."[5]

In human society, once we have defined what is good and bad, rich and poor, superior and inferior, happy and sad, we have placed ourselves in emotional bondage and are mentally disturbed by these emotions.

Qigong Interpretation

As we explained at the beginning of this book, the Dao in a human body is the spirit that is residing in our bodies. This spirit is related to our subconscious mind and resides at the spiritual residence, Ni Wan Gong (泥丸宮) (Mud Pill Palace) or the limbic system located at the center of the head. This spirit is not restricted by time or dimension. The spirit can instantly travel to any place in the universe. This spirit can be infinitely small and can be infinitely large. It cannot be seen and cannot be described. Even though we call it spirit, we still don't have an idea of what it is. However, this spirit can be immeasurably powerful when manifested and can be invisible, yet perceptible when it is calm. This spirit is simple, innocent, and can be equated with "pu" (朴).

Marquis and kings (Hou Wang, 侯王) imply the mind. As explained before, there are two minds in our body: the conscious mind and subconscious mind. The conscious mind is generated from the brain cells. This mind plays tricks, lies, and is trapped in the bondage of human dogma (the human matrix) whereas the subconscious mind that is related to the spirit is more truthful, simple, and innocent. Since the spirit is truthful yet powerful, if a person is able to regulate his mind to a peaceful and calm state through meditation, he will be able to wake up his subconscious mind and keep the spirit peacefully at its residence. The qi of the entire body (myriad objects or cells) ("under heaven") will then be regulated automatically. However, if the conscious mind is emotional, scattered, and confused, then the subconscious mind will be disturbed and chaotic, resulting in the spirit separating from its residence. In this case, the qi circulation of the body will be disorderly.

In qigong, we have to know how to regulate our emotional mind that is generated from our desires and sensing organs—eyes, ears, nose, tongue, and skin. If we don't know how to regulate our emotional mind and stop these temptations, we will harm our body. In addition, the conscious mind will block the subconscious mind from awakening and will slow down spiritual development. Therefore, the first step to reaching enlightenment is to regulate the emotional mind.

Following the Dao or spirit, you are following the natural path of Dao. It is just like all of the water in the rivers entering the ocean. Din, Fu-Bao (丁福保) said: "When water enters the gully, it is called 'valley.' Here, it says though the streams and valleys are many, but (the water) all flows into the rivers and seas. Although the tian-xia (i.e., the world) is large, all follow the long-lasting Dao. This long-lasting Dao is what is called pu. It is also known as the 'valley spirit' (gu shen, 谷神)."[6]

Conclusions

This chapter has pointed out a few things related to qigong:

1. Pu (朴) is equated with the Dao, simple and innocent. When this pu is applied to a human body, it is the spirit that is related to the subconscious mind. If the mind (the king) is able to keep this spirit simple, pure, and innocent, then the entire body (with its myriad cells) will follow Nature automatically. It is said: "When (one) rules a country as (one) rules a body, the people under tian-xia (the world) will return to him with their hearts (mind)."[7]

2. Tian (天) (the heaven) implies yang (陽) while di (地) (the earth) implies yin (陰). In qigong, baihui (Gv-20) (百會) (crown) is yang (the heaven) while huiyin (Co-1) (會陰) (perineum) is yin (the earth). When yin and yang are harmonious with each other in the body, the cells in the

entire body will receive a proper and uniform healthy qi supply. Consequently, health and longevity can be achieved.

3. We should learn how to control our emotional mind so it will not dominate our thinking and behavior. If we don't know how to control our emotional mind eventually it will bring harm to us. This will keep our spirit away from its residence and stop us from searching for the true Dao.

4. If we know how to follow the Dao, it is just like the water in the rivers that flows into the ocean naturally.

1. 范應元說：“道常無名，固不可以大小言之。聖人因見其大而無不包，故強名之曰大；復以其細無不入，故曰小也。”

2. 程以寧說：“以其未雕未琢，固謂之朴；以其日希曰微，故謂之小。而天下不敢臣，夫何故？天地資之以始，萬物持之以生，天下孰敢臣其所自始與所自生哉？”

3. 吳澄說：“道之功普遍于天下，譬天地之相合而降為甘露，雖無人使令之，而自能均及萬物。”

4. 河上公說：“侯王若能守道無為，萬物將自賓服，從于德也。”

5. 王弼說：“始制，官長不可不立名分，以定尊卑，故始制有名也。”

6. 丁福保說：“水注壑曰谷。此言川谷雖眾，莫不朝宗于江海。天下雖大，莫不賓服于長道。常道即朴也，亦即谷神也。”

7. “治國如治身，天下自然歸心。”

CHAPTER 33

Discriminating De—Self-Awakening

第三十三章
辨德—自悟

知人者智，
　　自知者明。
勝人者有力，
　　自勝者強。
知足者富。
　　強行者有志。
不失其所者久，
　　死而不亡者壽。

Those who know others are wise,
    those who know themselves are bright.
Those who defeat others have force,
    those who defeat themselves are strong.
Those who know satisfaction are rich,
    those who know how to force themselves have strong will.
Those who know where they are positioned will last long,
    those who are dead but have not perished have longevity.

General and Qigong Interpretations

Knowing yourself is harder than knowing others. That is why it is said if you know others, you are wise; however, if you know yourself, you are more than wise. In this case, you are bright and the mind is clear without a doubt within yourself. Cheng, Yi-Ning (程以寧) said: "Knowing other people is wise; however, it is looking externally. It is no more than just knowing people's kindness and evil, good or bad. Knowing yourself is bright, since it is looking internally. Without quietly returning to one's self-perception (i.e., internal feeling), one cannot reach this since internal vision does not have a shape."[1] To pay attention to inner feeling is called "internal vision and returning to listening to self."[2] That means to pay attention to the inner feeling and see the problem. In order to do so, you must first not be allured by the outside world. The common way of reaching this goal is through meditation.

In addition, it is easier to conquer or defeat others and much harder to conquer yourself. He Shang Gong (河上公) said: "(If one) is able to defeat others, it is because of his power and force. However, if one is able to conquer one's own emotional desires, then there is no one able to compete with him. Therefore, one is strong."[3] Wu, Cheng (吳澄) also said: "(If one) has power to defeat others, this is relying on external force. However, if one is able to win oneself, then (one) is able to conquer (control) oneself internally. Therefore, one can be called 'strong' internally."[4]

Those people who always appreciate what they have will be satisfied. In this case, they always feel they have everything they want. They are always rich, especially spiritually. On the contrary, those who are always demanding and greedy will never be satisfied with what they already have. They are always poor, especially spiritually. Greediness and desire are bottomless pits. They can never make you happy. Only those who are satisfied are happy.

Learning how to conquer yourself is a self-discipline that can lead you into the way of spiritual development. As we know, it is not easy to conquer yourself. You will need a lot of self-discipline to reach this goal. This self-discipline is the self's inner force, strong will, and commitment that make things happen. That is why those who know how to conquer themselves will have inner strength. Wang, An-Shi (王安石)

said: "Those top cultivated (awakened) people, after they hear the Dao, will force themselves to follow it. Therefore, it is said those who force themselves to follow (the Dao) have a strong will. If those who follow it do so for their reputation or wealth, then they do not have a strong will. Only those who force themselves to follow the Dao are the people who have a strong will."[5] Wang is talking about those who are awakened, but still in the stage of regulating. They need a strong will to keep themselves on the path of the Dao till they have reached to the stage of wuwei. This is what he means by "forcing themselves."

In order to have a strong will, you must first understand why you want to follow the Dao and recognize how difficult the path to reach the goal is. If you are able to clearly comprehend these reasons and difficulties internally, you will be ready to establish a strong will. Li, Jia-Mou (李嘉謀) said:

> "When the spirit is manifested externally, it appears as wisdom and force. When it is shown internally, then it is bright and strong. The reason people cannot enter the Dao is because they cannot see themselves clearly and are defeated by the objects (i.e., the desires of the material world). If it is bright (i.e., understood clearly) internally, then (the mind) will not be running wild outside. When (the mind) is not running wild (i.e., confused), then gradually it is able to defeat (the temptation for) objects. After (one) has accumulated days (of practice) and is getting deeper, (he) will enter the Dao automatically. If (one) knows satisfaction, then one's wisdom will become brighter. When one is able to force oneself to follow (the Dao), one is firmed. When this happens, both cultivation and comprehension can be achieved and the self-being can reverse its path back to its origin. This is the verification of the truth from the insubstantial (i.e., cultivation of spirit). When (one) has acquired one's path (i.e., kept on the path of the Dao) without being removed (through temptation toward objects), this is what 'does not lose its position' refers to. These people treat life and death as morning and

evening (i.e., as a natural routine); there is no past and no present, (the spirit) always exists in this universe. This is called 'longevity.'"[6]

From this, we can see the way of longevity is not via the physical body but the spirit. When this spirit has followed the Dao, it can last forever. It is the final goal of Daoist spiritual cultivation, "The unification of heaven and human."[7] Fan, Yin-Yuan (范應元) said: "When a person has a strong will to follow the Dao without separating from its origin (i.e., keep the spirit at its residence), he will therefore not lose his place. In this case, he can last long. Though his shape (i.e., physical body) is dead, his spirit will not die. This is what longevity is."[8] However, to reach the final stage of "regulating of no regulating" (wuwei), you must first force yourself onto the path of the Dao without being tempted by the material world. Only then will you be able to develop your spirit to an enlightened stage.

Conclusions

The first point this chapter makes is that to comprehend and follow the Dao, you must have wisdom that involves not just knowing others but also yourself. In Buddhist qigong, this is called "wu" (悟), which means self-awakening and comprehending things from deep within the heart (self-enlightenment). When you have this, you will not be confused and will have no doubt about your spiritual cultivation. In qigong practice, this is the most important part of training, conquering your mind. In order to do so, you must know what you are doing and how to do it. Without this mental foundation, your will would not be strong enough to fulfill the goal.

The second point is that even after you have made a strong commitment, you still need a lot of patience and perseverance to make it happen. That means you will need a high level of self-discipline or self-conquering. If you are able to do so, then you are strong mentally.

The third point is that your mind must be free from material bondage and emotional desires. When you don't have these temptations

from or for the material world, your mind will be pure, simple, innocent, and satisfied. When this happens, the spirit will be able to reside
at its residence, the Mud Pill Palace (泥丸宮) (limbic system). Your spirit
will then be able to return to its original state.

The fourth point in this chapter is that longevity is not in a physical
body but a spiritual body. When your spirit has returned to its original
state, your spirit will be able to reunify with the natural spirit (the Dao).
In this case, you will naturally have spiritual longevity. This is the stage
of Buddhahood.

1. 程以寧說："知人者智，見于外也，不過識人之善惡優劣而已。自知者明，見于內也，非返聽無聲，內視無
   形者不能也。"
2. "內視返聽。"
3. 河上公說："能勝人者，不過以威力也。人能勝己情慾，則天下無有能與己爭者，故為強。"
4. 吳澄說："有力能勝人，恃外之力；爾能自勝，則內能克己也，故謂之強。"
5. 王安石說："上士聞道，強而行之，故強行者有志。或志于高名，或志于厚利，非所謂志也。惟強行于道，
   斯可謂有志之士。"
6. 李嘉謀說："精神在外為智力，在內為明強。人所以不能入道者，以自見不明，而為物所勝也。若內明則
   自不驚外，不驚外則漸能勝物，積日既深，自然入道。知足而智益明，強行而力益固，修悟兩全，漸反其
   性，虛中證實，所得不移，是之謂不失其所。等視生死，有如旦暮，無古無今，浩然常在，是之謂壽。"
7. "天人合一。"
8. 范應元說："人能有志于道，不離于初，故不失其所，如此者乃可久也。其形雖死，其神不亡。如此者，方
   為壽也。"

CHAPTER 34

Task of Achievement—The Dao of Spirit

第三十四章
任成—神道

大『道』氾兮，
　　其可左右。
萬物恃之而生而不辭，
　　功成而不有，
　　衣養萬物而不為主。
常無欲，
　　可名於小；
萬物歸焉而不為主，
　　可名為大。
以其終不自為大，
　　故能成其大。

The Great Dao is vast and extensive,
    and is (existing) in left and right (i.e., everywhere).
Myriad objects rely on it to survive and have never been refused,
    when the merit has been accomplished, it (i.e., the Dao) does
    not possess them.
    It feeds and nourishes myriad objects and does not master (i.e.,
    control) them.
It never has desire,
    can be called "Small;"
myriad objects all return to it without being controlled,
    can be called "Large."
Because it does not claim its greatness,
    Thus, it can achieve its greatness.

General Interpretation

The Dao is so great, so vast, and so extensive that it exists everywhere in this universe. All lives existing in this universe rely on the Dao to survive. The Dao generously offers all of the necessities to all lives without demanding a return. This Dao can be small, yet so large. It is because it is so generous and humble, that it can be so big and great.

He Shang Gong (河上公) said: "When talking about the Dao, it is vast and extensive. It is as if it is floating, as if it is sinking. It is as if it is there and yet not there. When seeing it, it cannot be seen (i.e., it is invisible). When you talk about it, it is hard to comprehend and marvelous." "The Dao can be on the left or on the right, there is no place that it cannot exist."[1]

If a ruler is able to follow the Dao, give generously to people without asking for anything in return, govern the people without too much interference and disturbance, then he will be a great leader. Confucius (孔子) (《論語·泰伯》) said: "Great! Yao (堯) was so sublime as a monarch. He believed that only the heaven (i.e., the Dao) was the greatest and he only followed it. How can we find words sufficient to compliment him? His merits and achievements are so great and the etiquette system he had set up was brilliant!"[2]

Qigong Interpretation

The Chinese believe that since humans were developed and formed in the energy field of this universe, we have copied nature's energy structure. The Chinese call the Great Nature "grand heaven and earth" (da tian di, 大天地) (or "grand universe") and the human body a "small heaven and earth" (xiao tian di, 小天地) (small universe). To this grand universe, the Dao or taiji (called God in Western society) is the spirit of Nature and the De is the manifestation of the Dao. In this grand universe, each life within is like a tiny cell of the entire universe: all have its life, but are caught in the cycles of birth, death, and rebirth. To the small universe in the human body, the spirit (related to the mind) is the Dao and the De is the manifestation of the Dao (behavior). Morality in the Chinese language is called "Dao-De" (道德), which means thinking and behavior because morality is the thinking that is manifested in action. Again, a human is constructed by billions of cells. All cells have their lives but are recycling. To this small universe, the mind or spirit is the Dao (or God) and the physical body and its actions are the De.

The spirit (or mind) of the body can be profoundly vast, extensive, and able to travel any place without restrictions of time and space. The entire body's life, which includes millions of cells, is relying on the spirit to survive. Though this spirit influences so many lives in a body, it does not rule them or control them. When this spirit is condensed and stays at its residence, the mind and physical body can be calm and peaceful. However, when this spirit manifests into power, it can be so large that no one is able to understand it clearly.

When we practice qigong, we should model the Dao and keep our spirit pure, simple, innocent, generous, and humble. Only when we have this kind of mind will we be able to achieve a high level of spiritual cultivation. When we achieve this, our mind will not be in the emotional bondage we have created. Only then can we set our spirit free and allow it to develop freely.

Wu, Cheng (吳澄) said:

> "Because those sages' Dao (i.e., spirit) is unified with the tian-di (天地) (i.e., the Nature), when the merit has been accomplished, millions of objects have returned to their origins. Thus, the Dao has reached its greatness. Since the tian-di does not take the credit for its achievement, myriad objects do not know there is a master. That is why the Dao of the universe is so strong and great, yet, it does not treat itself as if it were great. This is what those sages have done; therefore, they are able to achieve their greatness. This is also because their Dao (i.e., spirit) is big, but does not need to be treated as big, thus, they are able to become big (i.e., great)."[3]

Conclusions

This chapter has simply pointed out that cultivating spirit is the most important part of qigong practice, especially for those who are looking for spiritual enlightenment. We still don't wholly understand spirit even though we can feel it. We know our body has two lives within, a physical life and spiritual life. Spiritual life is the Dao and physical life is the manifestation of the Dao. Thus, spirit is the god of the human body. If we are able to use our mind to cultivate our spirits in accord with the Dao, then we will be on the right path to reuniting with the spirit of Nature.

1. 河上公說：“言道汜汜，若浮若沉，若有若無，視之不見，說之難殊。”“道可左右，無所不宜。”
2. 孔子（《論語・泰伯》）說：“大哉！堯之為君也！巍巍乎！唯天為大，唯堯則之（效法）。蕩蕩乎！民無能名焉。”
3. 吳澄說：“蓋聖人與天地一也，歲功成而萬物歸，道之至大也。而天地不居其功，萬物不知所主，是天地之道雖大，而不自以為大，聖人亦若此矣，是以能成其大也。亦以其道大而不自以為大，故能成其大焉爾。”

CHAPTER 35
The Virtue of Benevolence—The Dao's Image
第三十五章
仁德—道象

執大象，
　　天下往。
往而不害，
　　安平太。
樂與餌，
　　過客止。
『道』之出口，
　　淡乎其無味。
視之不足見；
聽之不足聞；
用之不足既。

Hold the great image (i.e., the Dao),
    all (lives) under the heaven (i.e., the world) will follow.
Follow harmlessly,
    with peace, calmness, and harmony.
Music and food,
    induce passing travelers to stay.
When the Dao is spoken through the mouth,
    it is insipid without flavor.
Look at it, it is invisible;
listen to it, it is inaudible;
apply it, it is inexhaustible.

General Interpretation

Since the Dao cannot be described and explained, we can just imagine what the Dao is through our limited understanding. Therefore, 'great image' (da xiang, 大象) implies 'the Dao.'

If one is able to keep oneself on the path of the Dao, then the entire world will come and follow him. He Shang Gong (河上公) said: "Zhi (執) means to keep (to hold). Xiang (象) means the Dao. Those sages are able to hold the Dao; thus, the hearts of myriad objects (i.e., people) under heaven (tian xia, 天下) (i.e., the world) will be moved to them and follow them. (If holding the Dao) to govern the self-body, then, the spiritual divine will be sent from the heaven, (and the spirit can move to and fro freely."[1] He also said: "The myriad objects follow without harm; then the country is harmonious and peaceful. When (using) the Dao to govern the body, the spirit will be bright (i.e., clear) without harm; thus the body is peaceful and great longevity can be reached."[2]

Normally, people are tempted by good music, sweet talk, and delicious food. However, the Dao is invisible, inaudible, and tasteless. It is like pure water, tasteless; and like something soundless, inaudible. It is like truthful talking, honest, pure, and straightforward. Du, Guang-Ting (杜光庭) said: "Sweet talk and beautiful words are what is called 'having taste.' However, the theory of 'wuwei' is about the lesson of tranquil and the talking of the precious Dao that are frank without taste. How can they have flavor?"[3]

Qigong Interpretation

In a human body, the spirit is the Dao (or taiji) of the body. We don't actually know what the spirit is; however, we all realize that spirit can be so marvelous and powerful, neutral and natural. The spirit can reach anywhere in the universe and also can travel without the limitation of time. It can be so big, yet so small.

When tian xia (天下) (the world) is applied to a human, it means the body. When our spirit is following the Dao, then the entire body will be calm, peaceful, and harmonious. The mind is not the spirit, though it is connected to it. When the mind is allured by the seven emotions and six desires (qi qing liu yu, 七情六慾), the spirit will become chaotic and confused. In this case, the mental body will lose its center and sickness can occur.

However, if you are able to calm down your emotional mind and allow the spirit to rise, then your qi will be conserved and abundant. When this happens, you will be able to lead the qi to circulate within the entire body freely and smoothly. This will result in good health and a longer life.

Conclusion

Cultivating the spirit (the human Dao) to a calm, peaceful, neutral, and harmonious state is the key to health and longevity.

1. 河上公說：“執，守也。象，道也。聖人守大道，則天下萬物移心歸往之也。治身則天降神明，往來于己也。”
2. 河上公說：“萬物歸往而不傷害，則國安家寧而致太平矣。治身不害神明，則身安而大壽也。”
3. 杜光庭說：“甘言美詞，所謂有味也。無為之理，清靜之訓，玉道之言，其出淡然。安有滋味乎？”

CHAPTER 36
Subtle Clarity—Yin and Yang

第三十六章
微明—陰陽

將欲歙之，
　　　必固張之。
將欲弱之，
　　　必固強之。
將欲廢之，
　　　必固興之。
將欲取之，
　　　必固與之。
是謂微明。
柔弱勝剛強。
魚不可脫於淵；
　　　國之利器，
　　　不可以示人。

In order to shrink it,
    it must be expanded first.
In order to weaken it,
    it must be strengthened first.
In order to discard it,
    it must be built up first.
In order to seize it,
    it must be given first.
This is called subtle clarity.
The softness and gentleness overcome the toughness and strength.
Fish cannot leave the depths;
    the sharp weapons of the states,
    cannot be displayed to the people.

General Interpretation

It is clear that in order to expand something, it must first shrink. It is the same when you want to weaken it: first you should strengthen it. In order to reduce it, you must first build it up. Also, in order to take it, first you must give. This is the theory of yin and yang, which always balance each other. Fang, Yin-Yuan said (范應元): "The furnace's wind bellows has a piston, so it can be used to forge metal. This is because in order for the the wind bellows to contract, it must first expand. If expansion cannot be executed, then it cannot be shrunk."[1] He also said: "Expanding it, strengthening it, building it, and giving it, there is a hidden intention of contracting it, weakening it, discarding it, and taking it. Although the intention does not appear clearly, the facts are apparent. This is what is meant by 'subtle clarity.'"[2]

Si, De-Qing (釋德清) said:

"This saying (i.e., subtle clarity) means that, although it is the way of nature (i.e., yin-yang balance), often people do not see it. This saying is to teach people to be soft and gentle. Objects under heaven (i.e., the world), when they have reached their extremity, always reverse. For example, when the sun is going to be weakened, it must first reach its maximum strength. When the moon becomes a crescent, it must first be full. When a flame is going to extinguish, it first reaches its brightest. These are all natural. Therefore, expanding is the sign of contracting, strengthening is the emblem of weakening, building up is the symbol of discarding, and giving is the indication of taking. This is the natural tendency and theory. However, people we have encountered do not see this, thus, it is called 'subtle clarity.'"[3]

If you can always position yourself in the soft and gentle position, then there is no threat to others; you will always be in a safe position. The Chinese have a saying: "Sharp knives are always thrown away first." Naturally, dull knives are not paid attention to, and thus they last long.

The law of nature is very clear and straightforward. It is just like the fish. Fish cannot leave the water; otherwise they will die. It is the same for a country. The power of a country cannot be given and controlled by others, and its weapons should also not be revealed or demonstrated to the enemy. There is a story in *Huai Nan Zi* (《淮南子·道應訓》).

"In the city of Si (司城), Zi Han (子罕) was a prime minis-
ter of Song (宋). He said to the lord: 'A country's safety or
peace, and the order or disorder of the people, all depend
on the lord's rewards or punishments. Giving rewards is
what people favor so the lord should take care of this part.
Killing and punishing are what people resent. I can take
care of this.' The Song lord said: 'Good. Gua Ren (寡人)
(i.e., I, being humble) should take the favor part and you
will suffer from resentment. I know that Gua Ren will not
be scoffed at by other lords.' Thus, all people in the entire
country know that the power of killing was in the hands
of Zi Han. All officers tried to get close to him and all
common people were afraid of him. It did not last even
one year; Zi Han got rid of the Song lord and took his
power."[4]

Gua Ren (寡人) means "I, being humble." This was the way an ancient
ruler referred to himself. This story tells you that you should not give
the power to others easily.

Han, Fei (韓非) said:

"Rewards and punishments are sharp weapons. When
the lord owns the power, the lord is able to control offi-
cials. If the officials take the power, officials will be able
to subdue the lord. When the lord likes to give rewards,
officials will deduct part of it as their own reward. When
the lord desires to execute punishments, officials will
enhance the punishments to flaunt their prestige. There-
fore, when the lord likes to give a reward, the officials
would abuse the lord's authority and when the lord want
to give a punishment, the officials will use the opportunity
to demonstrate their prestige. Thus, it is said: 'the sharp
weapons of the state cannot be displayed to the people.'"[5]

Qigong Interpretation

Qigong was developed based on the fundamental laws of nature, the balance of yin and yang. Yin and yang are the results. Kan (坎) and li (離) are the actions that lead to the results of yin and yang. Kan represents water and li represents fire in the Eight Trigrams (Bagua, 八卦). Whenever there is too much of yin, li will step in to readjust the situation and make it more yang to manifest yin-yang balance. Naturally, when there is too much of yang, kan will move in to re-adjust it until yin-yang balance is achieved again. The ultimate law of nature is the balance of yin and yang.

To use this strategy for qigong practice, you must know how to maintain your mind in the neutral state. That means without emotional disturbance. Whenever you have emotional disturbance, the qi circulation in your body will become imbalanced and chaotic.

Building up qi and consuming qi are relative. When there is consumption, there must first be production. When you have built up an abundance of qi, then you will have quantity of qi for consumption. For qi exchange practice with a partner, first you help your partner to strengthen and build up the qi, and only then you can gain benefit by qi exchange with your partner.

Remember that your body includes the physical body and also the qi body. Qi is the energy that powers your thinking and physical action. The body is considered as yang and the qi is considered as yin. In order to have good health, you must first have strong qi circulation. When there is strong qi circulation, your physical body can then be built up to a stronger state. Again, without physical strength, you will be weak, sick and tire easily. In order to maintain a machine at peak performance and efficiency, the machine must be strong and you must have the power to run it. If either is missing, nothing will work.

In order to reach a high level of qigong practice, you will need a high level of self-discipline. The discipline is just like the law of punishments and rewards that make things happen. Discipline is like a whip behind you that helps you accomplish your training. However, the discipline you should have is self-discipline. If you give the power to someone else to discipline you, then your mind will be weak. This external discipline will only lead you to dependence instead of independence.

Conclusions

This chapter has pointed out two things. The first one is that yin and yang are mutually influencing each other and always seeking for the way to balance each other. The second is that in order to govern your body effectively and efficiently, you need self-discipline instead of externally imposed discipline. Remember, you are the one controlling your life, nobody else.

1. 范應元說："爐之有鞴，方可冶煉。夫鞴之將歙也，必固張之；張之不固，則不能歙也。"

2. 范應元說："張之、強之、興之、與之之時，已有歙之、弱之、廢之、取之之機，伏在其中矣。幾雖幽微，而事已顯明，固曰'是謂微明。'"

3. 釋德清說："此言物勢之自然而人不能察，教人當以柔弱自處也。天下之物，勢極則反，譬如日之將昃，必盛赫；月之將缺，必極盈；燈之將滅，比熾明。斯皆物勢之自然也。故固張者歙之象也，固強者弱之萌也，固興者廢之機也，固與者奪之兆也。天時人事，物理自然，第人所遇而不測識，故曰微明。"

4. 《淮南子·道應訓》："司城子罕相宋，謂宋君曰：'夫國家之危安，百姓之治亂，在君行賞罰。夫爵賞賜予，民之所好也，君自行之；殺戮刑罰，民之所怨也，臣請當之。'宋君曰：'善！寡人當其美，子受其怨。寡人自知不為諸侯笑矣。'國人皆知殺戮之專制在子罕，大臣親之，百姓畏之。居不至期年，子罕逐卻宋君而專其政。"

5. 韓非說："賞罰者，邦之利器也。在君則制臣，在臣則勝君。君見賞，臣則損之以為德；君見罰，臣則益之以為威。人君見賞而人臣用其勢，人君見罰而人臣乘其威。故曰：'邦之利器不可以示人'。"

CHAPTER 37
Governing Government—Maintain Dao

第三十七章
為政—守道

『道』常「無為」，
　　　而無不為。
侯王若能守之，
　　　萬物將自化。
化而欲作，
　　　吾將鎮之以無名之樸。
（無名之樸，）夫亦將無欲。
不欲以靜，
　　　天下將自定。

The Dao always does nothing (wuwei),
    but nothing is left undone.
If sovereigns are able to follow it (i.e., the Dao),
    myriad objects will be transformed (i.e., in order) automati-
    cally.
Transforming, but the desires are still initiating,
    I will restrain them by nameless simplicity (i.e., the Dao).
(Nameless simplicity), will lead to the desireless.
Using sereneness to stop desires,
    the world will find its peace with its own accord.

General Interpretation

Wu, Cheng (吳澄) said: "The Dao's wuwei (i.e., does nothing) lasts long without changing; it not just temporary. Therefore, it is said: it 'always does nothing.' However, though it does nothing, for whatever needs to be done, there is nothing that cannot be done."[1] Thus, if rulers are able to follow the Dao, the people in the country will be in order automatically.

Even when the mind is in order, ego, desires, and ambitions will still arise. When they do, use simplicity (pure neutral mind) to stop them from arising. Wei, Yuan (魏源) said:

> "'But the desires are still initiating' means that the mind just begins to have an idea of action (i.e., ego). 'Myriad objects will be transformed automatically' means to let them live and die by themselves. When they live and die automatically, the qi's circulation will gradually become gentle. (However), if there is a desire initiated in the heart and (I) use the nameless (i.e., the Dao) to calm it down, then even after three generations have passed and continuing for the next three generations, who is able to stop (me)? Even if (I) calm it down (with the nameless) and the action is still being initiated, I again cease the action with nameless simplicity. What is nameless simplicity? It means to use the calmness to restrain the action, use the purity to calm down the mild disturbance, and use the simple sincerity to vary furtiveness. This is to stop the heart of desire, which seeks to initiate an action, and make it comfortably reverse its desire into no desire. When there is no desire, then there is calm. When there is a calmness, then it straightens and returns itself to the nameless simplicity. This is exactly what is said: 'If I don't have desires, then the people will be simple automatically. If I am in favor of calmness, then the people will be in order by themselves.'"[2]

Ding, Fu-Bao (丁福保) also said: "A human's heart (i.e., mind) is easily plugged (i.e., filled with desires) and is hard to be emptied; it easily initiates actions and is difficult to be calmed, it easily shifts the mind and is hard to keep steady, and it easily changes the path and is hard to maintain. Although these are to be regulated, still there are some desires possibly initiated from external temptations. I will calm them down with the Dao and won't allow them to dare be initiated."[3]

Qigong Interpretation

To qigong, the Dao in the body is the spirit. Though we know and can feel the existence of the spirit, it cannot be seen, touched, or heard. However, this spirit governs the lives of the all the cells in the body. The spirit does not do anything but at the same time does everything in our bodies.

There are two minds in our body: the conscious mind and subconscious mind. The conscious mind is emotional, lying, and filled with desires. The subconscious mind related to our spirit is more truthful and simple. If you are able to calm down the activities of your conscious mind by centering your subconscious mind at its residence (limbic system), then the qi's circulation in your body will be regulated smoothly and automatically by itself.

Conclusions

In order to have smooth and free qi circulation in your body, you must learn to keep your conscious mind calm. That means to regulate your emotional mind until no regulating is required. The way to do that is through embryonic breathing meditation. In embryonic breathing meditation, you will find both your mental center (the subconscious mind) at the center of your head and the physical center at the center of gravity in the body. Once you find these two human polarities, you move your mind to the physical center (lower real dan tian). When you do this, you will be in an extremely calm state both mentally and physically. This will allow the qi to move freely. Consequently, all the cells will be able to maintain their healthy condition. This is the stage of "wuwei" (doing nothing or regulating without regulating) and what is called "embracing singularity" (bao yi, 抱一).

1. 吳澄說：“道之無為，久而不變，非特暫而已，故曰常無為。雖一無所為，而于所當為之事，無一不
   為也。”
2. 魏源說：“蓋欲作者，欲生萌動也。夫萬物自化，則任其自生自息而已。自生自息，而氣運日趨于文，將夫
   有欲心萌作于其間，苟無名以鎮之，則太古降為三代，三代降為后世，其誰止之？然鎮之亦豈能有所為？
   亦鎮之以無名之樸而已。無名之樸者，以靜制動，以質止文，以淳化巧，使其欲心將作而不得，將釋然
   自反而無欲矣。無欲則靜。靜則正而返于無名之樸矣。正謂‘我無欲而民自樸，我好靜而民自正。’”
3. 丁福保說：“人心易塞而難虛，易動而難靜，易遷而難守，易變而難常。雖以相化。而或有復為外物所動
   欲起妄作者，則吾將鎮之以道，使不敢有所妄作也。”

De Jing (Virtue Classic)—Chapters 38 to 81

CHAPTER 38
Discourse on the De—The Dao's Applications
第三十八章
論德—道用

上『德』不『德』，是以有『德』；
　　下『德』不失『德』，是以無『德』。
上『德』無為而無以為；
　　下『德』無為之而有以為。
上「仁」為之而無以為；
　　上「義」為之而有以為。
上「禮」為之而莫之應，
　　則攘臂而扔之。
故
失『道』而後『德』，
　　失『德』而後「仁」，
　　失「仁」而後「義」，
　　失「義」而後「禮」。
夫「禮」者，
　　忠信之薄，而亂之首。
前識者，
　　『道』之華，
　　而愚之始。
是以大丈夫處其厚，不居其薄；
　　處其實，不居其華。
故去彼取此。

(Those) with high virtues do not conduct the De (i.e., virtues); thus
they have the De (i.e., are virtuous).
(Those) with low virtues are always concerned about their De;
thus they don't have the De.
(Those) with high De do nothing yet accomplish anything.
(Those) with low De do things with an intention of doing.
(Those) with high benevolence conduct their actions without
conducting.
(Those) with high righteousness comport their behaviors with
motive.
(When those) with high etiquette conduct their manners but don't
get the wanted response,
then they bare their arms to force their will on others.
Therefore, when the Dao is lost, then there is the De.
When the De is lost, then there is benevolence.
When benevolence is lost, then there is righteousness.
When righteousness is lost, then there is etiquette.
Those who have etiquette are
thin (i.e., weak) in their loyalty and trust; the leaders of chaos.
What is called 'foreknowledge,'
are the flowers of the Dao,
and the beginning of folly.
Thus, those great men dwell in the thickness (i.e., depths) instead
of in the thin (i.e., shallows),
themselves dwelling in the real instead of the flowering.
Therefore, they discard that and accept this.

General Interpretation

Those who have high virtue (the De) do not have the intention to act with virtue, so they are virtuous. This is because they don't have to do it intentionally since the virtues are carried out automatically. Thus, their virtues are complete. However, for those who have low virtues, since they are afraid to lose their virtues, they try hard to maintain it. Therefore, their virtues are not complete.

Those who have high virtues do things by following the Dao without intention; thus, there is nothing that cannot be accomplished. However, those with little virtues have to accomplish things with intention.

Those with much benevolence are benevolent to others without intention. However, those with high righteousness conduct their behaviors with intention. When those who have high etiquette act but don't get the wanted response, they use force to get people to comply. Wei, Yuan (魏源) said: "When those on the top (i.e., leaders) advocate something and those on the bottom do not respond, those on the top raise arms to force it. When there is no response to force, then punishments are generated and weapons are deployed."[1]

From this, you can see that when the Dao is lost, the virtues are emphasized. When the virtues are lost, then we talk about benevolence. When benevolence is lost, we reinforce righteousness. When righteousness is lost, then etiquette emerges. Those who have etiquette are actually hard to be trust. They cause chaos in society. Du, Guang-Ting (杜光庭) said: "When (people's) simplicity is dispersed (i.e., lost), use virtue to keep it. If virtue is in decline and weakened, follow with benevolence. When benevolence is not enough to remedy it, use righteousness to stop the decline. When righteousness is not working, then use etiquette to save it (i.e., righteousness)."[2] Zhuang Zi (莊子) also said: "The Dao cannot be reached and the De (virtue) cannot be acquired, but benevolence can be achieved. Righteousness can be cast aside and etiquette is used to deceive each other. Thus, it is said: 'When the Dao is lost, then there is virtue. When the virtue is lost, then there is benevolence. When the benevolence is lost, then there is righteousness. When the righteousness is lost, then there is etiquette. What is etiquette? It is the flower (i.e., decoration) of the Dao and the leader of disorder.'"³

Those who claim to be persons of foreknowledge are actually like the flowers on the tree of the Dao. This intitiates the follies of society. Therefore, those who have followed the Dao will situate themselves in sincere and profound honesty instead of flowery talk. They will discard the flowery outside decoration (talking and actions) and accept the profound honesty deep in themselves. Han, Fei (韓非) said:

> *"Etiquette is the external look of emotion; writing and painting are the decorations on quality. Those gentlemen would pay attention to emotion, ignore etiquette, appreciate quality, and detest decoration. Those who express their emotions relying on their external appearance, their emotions may detest. Those who must use decoration to talk about quality, the quality may be poor. Why said so? He's jade (和氏璧) does not need five decorations, the pearls of Sui Lord (隋侯) do not need silver and gold to ornament them; they are already extremely beautiful. There is no object able to beautify them. Those objects that need ornaments to show their beauties are not beautiful. Therefore, the relationship between father and son, though etiquette but is not obvious. Thus, it is said: 'thin etiquette.(i.e., Father and son treat each other in a manner that is natural and without pretense, thus it is called thin etiquette)'"⁴*

He's jade (He shi bi, 和氏璧) is a very famous jade known for its beauty. He Shang Gong (河上公) said: "Those who are polite downgrade the quality (i.e., inner feeling), but emphasize the external decoration. Consequently, righteousness is reduced daily and evil chaos grows daily."⁵

When you follow the Dao, the manifestation of the Dao (the De) will be natural and automatic without the conscious mind. If the conscious mind leads you in your virtuous conduct, it will not be the real virtues that manifest. Du, Guang-Ting (杜光庭) said:

"When moving, it matches the heaven, and when calm, it accords with the earth. It mutually gains (i.e., benefits) with the Dao without doing anything (wuwei). The spirit does not have thought, and the sentiment does not have worry. This is the heart (i.e., mind) of doing nothing. Without showing its achievement, its merit is as great as the heaven and the earth. Without displaying its brilliance, its brightness is as shining as the sun and the moon. This is the trace (i.e., proof) of doing nothing (wuwei). This is because this 'wuwei' is not imitating 'wuwei' and becomes 'wuwei.' It is because nothing needs to be done (i.e., imitated). Those who have low virtues know the beauty (i.e., goodness) of 'wuwei' and the evil of 'youwei' (有為) (i.e., intention of doing), (thus) repelling the evil and following the goodness. This is to admire (the goodness of) 'wuwei,' and therefore there is a reason for doing it."[6]

Those high-level Daoists always follow the Dao and manifest their behaviors (the De) accordingly without having to think about it (wuwei). That is why they always have "the De." However, when those lower-level laymen always worry about their behaviors, it means they still don't have the right De (virtues).

It is the same for benevolence and righteousness. If one has to think about it before acting, then it is not the real benevolence and righteousness. How do we define benevolence and righteousness? Han, Fei (韓非) said:

"What is benevolence? It is to have a cheerful heart to love others, a delightful feeling to see others' good fortune and to feel bad about others' disasters. This is originated from a deep heart that cannot be stopped. This is not because of asking for a reward. Therefore, it is said: '(Those) with high benevolence conduct their actions without conducting.' What is righteousness? It is about the relationship between the lord and officials, the difference of the eminent and the humble, the connection with friends,

and the distinction of relatives and outsiders. When offi-
cials serve the lord, the low (i.e., officials) have a loyalty
and the high (i.e., lord) treat officials appropriately. The
son serves the father (i.e., parents) with love and the father
treats the son properly. Those humble persons treat those
eminent persons with respect while those eminent ones
treat those humble ones with proper manners. When treat-
ing friends, it is appropriate to mutually help each other. It
is also proper to be close to relatives and keep a distance
(i.e., respect) with outsiders. Therefore, what is righ-
teousness? It means appropriateness in handling matters.
Thus, it is said: '(Those) with high righteousness com-
port their behaviors with motive.'"[7]

Qigong Interpretation

In order to reopen our third eye, we must be truthful. As was believed in the past, when the third eye is opened, you will resume your telepathic ability. That means you can read and communicate with people's minds without speaking. However, if, to avoid revealing secrets to others, we continue to lie and hide the truth in our minds, subconsciously we will keep our third eyes closed. Therefore, we all have masks on our faces. The masks show what people want to see and say what people want to hear. We are not truthful to our own deep feeling and truth. Daoists called themselves "truthful persons" (zhen ren, 真人) because they are cultivating themselves so they don't have to lie. Only then can the third eye be opened.

Often, people look beautiful outside because of their clothes and make up. However, only they know their true selves. The Chinese always said, "Internal beauty is more important than external beauty."[8] This is because internal beauty is real and truthful and external beauty is temporary and just a decoration. It is the same for talking. A real friend will speak from honest feelings. However, those wearing masks will tell you only what you want to hear. The Chinese always said, "Good herbs are bitter to the mouth and good, honest advice grates on the ears."[9]

To practice qigong for enlightenment, you must be honest and truthful, not just with yourself, but also with others. Since it is not easy in this masked society, Buddhists and Daoists will live in seclusion so they don't have to lie and wear a mask on their faces all the time.

Conclusions

To become truthful to yourself, you must first regulate the emotions of your conscious mind. Only then will you be able to awaken your truthful subconscious mind and feelings. This step in embryonic breathing meditation is called "self-recognition" (zi shi, 自識). What this actually means is "dropping the mask" from your face. This is the first step to reach the final enlightenment.

1. 魏源說："故在上者為之而下不應，至於攘臂而強之，強之而又不應，將刑罰生而兵甲起。"
2. 杜光庭說："朴既散，全德守之；德既下衰，仁愛繼之；仁愛不足，義以制之；義之不行，禮以救之。"
3. 莊子說："道不可致，德不可至，仁可為也，義可虧也，禮相偽也。故曰：失道而后德，失德而后仁，失仁而后義，失義而后禮。禮者，道之華而亂之首也。"
4. 韓非說："禮為情貌者也，文為質飾者也。夫君子取情而去貌，好質而惡飾。夫恃貌而論情者，其情惡也；須飾而論質者，其質衰也。何以論之？和氏之璧不飾以五采，隋侯之珠不飾以銀黃，其質至美，物不足以飾之。夫物之待飾而后行者，其質不美也。是以父子之間，其禮朴而不明。故曰：禮薄也。"
5. 河上公說："禮者賤質而貴文，故正直日以少，邪亂日以生。
6. 杜光庭說："動合乎天，靜合乎地，與道相得而無所為也。神無思，志無慮者，此心之無為也。不顯其功，而功若天也；不彰其明，而明并日月，此跡之無為也。夫此無為，非效學無為而為于無為，是無以為也。而下德之人，知無為為美，有為為惡，舍惡從善，慕此無為，以分別故，是有所以而為也。"
7. 韓非說："仁者，謂其中心欣然愛人也。其喜人之有福而惡人之有禍也。生心之所不能已也，非求其報也。故曰：上仁為之而無以為。義者，君臣上下之事，夫子貴賤之差也，知交朋友之接也，親疏內外之分也。臣事君宜，下懷上宜，子事父宜，賤敬貴宜，知交朋友之相助也宜，親者內而疏者外宜。義者，謂其宜也，宜而為之，故曰：上義為之而有以為也。"
8. "內在美比外在美重要。"
9. "良藥苦口，忠言逆耳。"

CHAPTER 39

The Root of the Law—Holding the Singularity

第三十九章
法本—執一

昔之得『一』者：
　　天得『一』以清；
　　地得『一』以寧；
　　神得『一』以靈；
　　谷得『一』以盈；
　　萬物得『一』以生；
　　侯王得『一』以為天下貞。
其致之。
　　天無以清，將恐裂；
　　地無以寧，將恐發；
　　神無以靈，將恐歇；
　　谷無以盈，將恐竭；
　　萬物無以生，將恐滅；
　　侯王無以貞，將恐蹶。
故貴以賤為本，高以下為基。
　　是以侯王自謂孤、寡、不穀。
此非以賤為本邪？非乎？
（人之所惡，唯孤、寡、不穀，而王公以為稱。）
　　故至譽無譽，
　　不欲琭琭如玉，珞珞如石。

Since ancient times, those who attained the one (i.e., the Dao):
    the skies attained the one and thus are clear,
    the earth attained the one and thus is tranquil,
    the spirit attained the one and thus is divine,
    the valley attained the one and thus is abundant,
    the myriad objects attained the one and thus live,
    the rulers attained the one and thus became the leaders of the world.
These were all achieved (from the one).
    The skies, without clarity, would break apart,
    the earth, without tranquility, would erupt,
    the spirit, without divinity, would dissipate,
    the valley, without abundance, would be barren,
    the myriad objects, without lives, would perish,
    the rulers, without leadership, would fall.
Thus, those nobles use humility as their root (i.e., basis), those with
    high ranks use the low position as their foundation.
Therefore, those rulers called themselves alone, solitary, and
    unworthy.
Isn't this using the low to build their foundations? Isn't it?
(What laymen despise are those who are alone, solitary, and
    unworthy. But those rulers use these as their titles.)
    Therefore, the ultimate honor is without honor,
    Do not wish to be brilliant like a jade but coarse like a rock.

General Interpretation

What is the one? In the *Collection of Confucius' Teachings* (《孔子集語·易者第一》) it says:

> *"In the change (Yi) (易), there is an ultimate change (太易), there is an ultimate initiation (太初), there is an ultimate beginning (太始), and there is an ultimate simplicity (太素). When it was in ultimate change, there is no qi (energy) visible. When it was in ultimate initiation, the qi was just initiated. When it was in ultimate beginning, the shape began to formalize. When it was in ultimate simplicity, it was the beginning of attribute (i.e., quality). When qi, shape, and attributes were generated and gathered, but not separated, it was thus chaotic and turbid. It was chaotic and turbid because when myriad objects were chaotic and turbid, they could not be seen when looked at, could not be heard when listened to, and could not be felt when touched; thus, it was called 'change.' 'Change' does not have a physical boundary, but changes into 'One.'"[1]*

Here, the One means the Dao.

Cheng, Yi-Ning (程以寧) said: "What was the beginning of ancient time? It was when the heaven and the earth (i.e., Nature) were not yet formed. What is the One? When it was chaotic and turbid, but there was an essence within. When encircling it, it was taiji and when straightening it, it was the One. The One means the Dao."[2] Before creation of the universe (or nature) (the De), the space was filled up with chaos and turbid energy. Later, the material universe was formed and through the functions of taiji, spiral actions were created. From these spiral actions and spinning energy, all objects were derived. These spiral actions are what we have seen from nature, as great as black holes and galaxies or as small as tornadoes, hurricanes, seashells, or even DNA. However, when taiji ceases its functions, all manifestations return to their origin (essence). The Dao is this essence.

In addition, Gao, Heng (高亨) had another explanation. He said: "The One has three meanings: first, it means the body (i.e., essence) [see chapter 10]. Second, it means the taiji [see chapter 42]. Third, it means the Dao."[3]

Huai Nan Zi (《淮南子·原道》) said:

> "What the One means is there is nothing equivalent. It is independent by itself. Above, it reaches the nine heavens; below, it penetrates nine boundaries. It is round, but not regular and it is square, but does not follow patterns. When it gives, it is not exhausted and when it is used, there is no an end. When looking at it, the shape cannot be seen; when hearing it, the sound cannot be heard; when touching it, the body cannot be felt. Without the shape, the shapes were then generated; without the sounds, the five sounds were then sung; without the tastes, the five flavors were tasted; without colors, the five colors were derived. Thus, the principle of the One can be applied to four seas (i.e., everywhere) and its usage reaches the heaven and the earth (i.e., the Universe). It is as if it is not existing, but also existing. Myriad objects are all originated from the same cavity (i.e., same origin) and the root of all hundreds of events (i.e., all events) initiated from the same door (i.e., principle). Its movements do not have shapes and its variations are just like the Divine. Its actions do not have traces, often behind, but becoming first.' This is the One. It is a different name for the Dao."[4]

Since we don't actually know the Dao, various interpretations have been presented from ancient times.

From the above statements, we can see that the One means the Dao. When the skies, the earth, the spirit, the valley, the living objects, and even the rulers follow the Dao, then all is peaceful, prosperous, healthy, and delightful. However, if they are against the Dao, then disasters will fall upon them. Wu, Cheng (吳澄) said:

"The sky, the earth, the valley, and the spirit, these four things, though the names are different, actually are the same. When it revolves and becomes clear, it is the sky; when it condenses and becomes tranquil, it is the earth; and the spirit is the marvelousness of the two sides' qi (i.e., heaven and earth, and two sides of a valley). What Zhang Zi (張子) said about the marvelousness (i.e., nature or spirit) between the two sides is that, although it cannot be measured, it can be used to feel and respond (i.e., resonate) in all directions without limitation. Thus, it is divine. Valley means the empty space between two sides. What Zhang said about insubstantial means qi that fills up the space between and is, thus, abundant. Zhen (貞) (the essence of purity and simplicity) is like the tip of a branch. When a ruler has become zhen of heaven and earth (i.e., the world), it means he is the ultimate leader of the people. When it says that the sky is clear, the earth is tranquil, the spirit is divine, the valley is abundant, myriad lives multiply endlessly, and the ruler positions himself above the world, it is all possible because of this One."[5]

Zhang Zi (張子), named Zhang, Zai (張載) (1020–1077 CE), was a founder of the Guan Xue school (關學派) of scholarship during the Chinese Northern Song dynasty (960–1127 CE) (北宋). This paragraph states that we are able to communicate with the universe when the energy (qi) existing between heaven and earth as well as between the two sides of a valley is used to resonate with Nature. For example, when the spiritual qi in the spiritual valley (神谷) (two lobes of the brain) is resonating with the outside world, we are able to communicate with Nature. This spiritual energy is the root of the spirit; when developed, eternal spiritual life can be achieved (chapter 6).

In order to behave like a valley, those rulers were therefore humble and called themselves alone, solitary, and unworthy. They would prefer to be regular rocks instead of precious jade. When humble, they would earn more respect and love from the people. This is the way of the Dao:

to regulate without regulating (wuwei). Zhuang Zi (《莊子·至樂》) said: "This is the highest honor of no honor." "When the sky is doing nothing, it is clear. When the earth is doing nothing, it is tranquil."[6]

Qigong Interpretation

The One means the spirit of the body. The body is like the universe. The top of the head is called "heavenly divine cover" (tian ling gai, 天靈蓋 or baihui, 百會) and the perineum is called "sea bottom" (hai di, 海底 or huiyin, 會陰). The spirit, mysterious and marvelous, cannot be seen, heard, touched, or tasted, but can be felt. This spirit governs the entire body's energy (qi) and manifests it in actions.

This spirit resides at the limbic system under the space between the two lobes of the brain. This place is called "spiritual valley" (shen gu, 神谷) and the spirit residing in this valley is called "valley spirit" (gu shen, 谷神) (see chapter 6). When the qi is abundant in both lobes of the brain, the energy stored in the valley will be strong. When this energy is strong, the spirit is high. When the spirit is high, all lives in the body (cells) will be healthy and vigorous. Naturally, the actions and movements of its manifestation will be powerful and efficient. In addition, due to the abundance of the qi in this spiritual valley, the spirit will be able to communicate with Nature via resonance.

However, this spirit must follow the Dao. If it is against the Dao, disaster will befall the body and it will become sickened or even die. In order to keep our spirit as close as possible to the Dao, we must ignore the emotional bondage or dogmas (the matrix) created from our conscious mind. Once we calm down or cease the activities of our conscious mind, our subconscious mind will awaken and become sensitive. This will allow us to reconnect ourselves to the Dao and follow it through feeling.

The final goal of qigong practice is "regulating of no regulating" (wu tiao er tiao, 無調而調). That means every regulating has become automatic and you don't have to use your conscious mind to make it happen.

Conclusions

This chapter has pointed out three important things. First, when you practice qigong, the most important and ultimate goal is cultivation of your spirit. This spirit is called "the One" or "the Dao" of your body. If you are able to keep your spirit following the way of the Dao and unify with it, then you will already be on the correct path of qigong practice.

Second, in order to reach this goal, you must be humble. When you are humble, you will position yourself in the low place that allows all knowledge and natural divinity to pour in.

Finally, in order to reach the goal of spiritual cultivation, you must regulate your conscious mind and allow your subconscious mind to be awakened. With this subconscious mind, you will be able to reach the stage of "regulating of no regulating."

1. 《孔子集語·易者第一》："易有太易,有太初,有太始,有太素。太易者未見氣,太初者氣之始,太始者形之始,太素者質之始。氣形質具而未離,故渾淪。渾淪者言萬物渾淪而未相離,視之不見,聽之不聞,循之不得,故曰易也。易無形畔,易變而為一。"

2. 程以寧說:"昔者何時?乃未開闢之時。一是何物?即混混沌沌,其中有精,環之而為太極,直之而為一。一即道也。"

3.

4. 高亨說:"一有三義:一曰一者身也,說見十章。二曰:一者太極也,說見四十二章。三曰一者道也。《淮南子·原道》篇:'所謂一者無匹合于天下者也。卓然獨立,上通九天,下貫九野,圓不中規,方不中矩,佈施而不既,用之而不勤(盡),視之不見其形,聽之不聞其聲,循之不得其身;無形而有形生焉,無聲而五音鳴焉,無味而五味形焉,無色而五色成焉。是故一之理施四海,一之解際天地。若無而有,若亡而存,萬物之總皆閱一孔,百事之根皆出一門。其動無形,變化若神,其行無跡,常后而先。'此所謂一,即道之別名也。"

5. 吳澄說:"天地谷神四者,名異實同。其運轉而清者曰天;凝聚而寧靜者曰地;神者兩間二氣之妙,張子所謂兩在故不測者,其用感應無方故靈;谷則兩間空虛之處,張子所謂空虛即氣者,其氣充塞無間故盈;貞猶木之楨干,為天下貞,猶曰民極也。言天清、地寧、神靈、谷盈,萬物之生生不窮,侯王立乎天下之上,而為民極。其所以致之者,皆由此一也。"

6. 《莊子·至樂》:"至譽無譽。""天無為以之清,地無為以之寧。"

CHAPTER 40

Dispensing Utilization—Returning to the Root

第四十章
去用—返本

反者道之動；
　　弱者道之用。
天下萬物生於『有』，
　　『有』生於『無』。

Returning (to the beginning) is the movement of the Dao.
  The weakness (i.e., the gentleness) is the utilization
  (i.e., function) of the Dao.
Myriad objects (i.e., all objects) under heaven (i.e., in the world)
  are begotten from "having,"
  and "having" is originated from "nothingness."

General Interpretation

"Returning" implies "to return to the beginning," which means cycling. He Shang Gong (河上公) said: "Reverse means (return to) the root (i.e., origin). This (returning to the) root is the reason for the Dao's movement. When there is movement, thousands of objects are created. If they go against this rule, they die."[1] Repetition is the main action or movement of the Dao. Without this movement, the Dao cannot be manifested into the De (德). The De is the manifestation of the Dao. The first sentence of chapter 40 was further interpreted by Shi, De-Qing (釋德清):

> "Returning is the main body (i.e., major content) of the Dao. It is said that the body of the Dao is insubstantial, nothingness, extremely calm, and is the master of all movements. In the world, people only know how the movements move and do not know that where there is a movement, there is a calmness. The Book of Changes (《易經》) says: 'The movement under heaven (i.e., the universe or the world) is purely only one.' This is because the movements of all movements all originated from the insubstantial, nothingness, and extreme calmness. Therefore, it is said 'reverse' is the movement (i.e., action) of the Dao."[2]

When the Dao is manifested, it is through soft (weak) action or movement. Therefore, the softness is the application or utilization of the Dao. Song, Chang-Xing (宋長星) said:

> "The movements of the Dao's function do not disobey timing and do not lose qi (i.e., energy). When it gives, it does not choose objects, but is following myriad objects' needs. It does not oppose the usage of objects; thus it is able to follow the property of the objects, yielding entirely. This can be called: 'weak' (or 'soft'). However, when it is in use, it can enter the water and fire without a gap, penetrate the metal and stone without a trace, and satisfy

myriad objects without a shortage. It does not use hardness, but softness. This is what The Book of Changes *(Yi Jing, 易經) said: 'When seeing a group of dragons without the head (i.e., the leader), it is a good fortune.' Therefore, it is said: 'softness is the usage of the Dao.'"*

Song, Chang-Xing also said: "If a human handles business in this world with peaceful and harmonious talking, then listeners will accept this talking easily without being against it. When managing affairs with an open and forgiving heart, all matters can be accomplished without failure."[3]

When there is a group of powerful dragons, without a leader, they will be soft. Thus, it is good fortune. However, if a group of dragons has a leader, they will become aggressive and invasive. Thus, it is a misfortune.

Nothingness is the origin of having. Nothingness and having are two, but one. They cannot exist without the other. The Dao is the one who initiates myriad objects from nothingness and also the one who returns myriad objects to their root, to nothingness. This repeating process is the way of the Dao (Nature). Du, Guang-Ting (杜光庭) said: "Nothingness is the body (i.e., the root) of the Dao and having is the end of the Dao. Thus, because of the root (i.e., nothingness), the end (i.e., having) is produced. All shapes are formed and (thus) 'the having' is initiated. When investigating the causes and pondering the origins of all of this, we can see all of them are created from the Dao. Therefore, ten thousand objects are originated from marvelous nothingness. Whatever is able to return from 'having' to 'nothingness,' it is close to the Dao."[4]

Qigong Interpretation

In qigong society, spirit is considered as the Dao in your body. Spirit is marvelous and mysterious, yet so powerful. Time does not have meaning for spirit and space does not have restriction for spirit. For example, we can travel with our spirit to yesterday or tomorrow without limitation. We can also travel with our spirit to anywhere in this universe instantly without confinement.

The mind is related to spirit, but is not the spirit itself. As we have seen, according to qigong, the mind can be divided into the conscious mind and subconscious mind. The conscious mind is generated from brain cells that provide your thinking and memory. From the conscious mind, humans create the human matrix and dogma. In this matrix, everyone has a mask and lies to each other in order to survive in this masked society. However, the subconscious mind that resides in your limbic system has memory and feeling, but is without thinking. This subconscious mind is more truthful and is the fundamental body of your spirit.

Usually, our spirit has been suppressed due to the active functioning of the conscious mind. Once you learn how to calm down your conscious mind, your subconscious mind will be able to wake up. The first crucial key of calming down the conscious mind is setting you free from emotional bondage.

In order to reach this goal, you must bring yourself to a semisleeping state. When you reach this state, you feel you are there but not there. From this state, you gradually learn how to reconnect your spirit with the natural spirit.

In this condition, you will be in an extremely calm and peaceful state. Not only that, you will be in the state of "regulating of no regulating" (wuwei, 無為). This will allow the qi to circulate anywhere in your body. In your body, qi is the softest and is able to reach every corner of your body. Wang, Bi (王弼) said: "There is no place where the qi cannot enter." "Qi is insubstantial, soft, and weak (i.e., gentle), but there is no place that it cannot be transported, there is nowhere that cannot be reached. It is extremely soft and cannot be bent and broken. From this, the benefits of 'wuwei' are known."[5]

Conclusions

Understanding the natural course is the first step to being in accord with the Dao. First, we should recognize that myriad objects, at the end, all return to their root, nothingness. Second, we must follow the Dao and apply it with softness so the spirit can become evolved. Having and nothingness are only the two faces of Nature. Between these two, the spirit within is the most important and connected with Nature.

1. 河上公說：“反，本也；本者道之所以動，動生萬物，背之則亡也。”
2. 釋德清說：“反者道之體也。謂道體虛無至靜，為群動之主。世人只知動之為動，不知動處即靜。《易》云天下之動，貞夫一者也。以其群動之動，皆自虛無至靜而發，故云反者道之動也。”
3. 宋長星說：“道機之動，不違于時，不失于氣。不擇物而施，能順萬物之情；不逆物而用，能從萬物之性。委曲周遍，可謂弱矣。然其用則入水火而無間，透金石而無痕，體萬物而不匱。不以剛為用，而以柔為用。即《易》曰見群龍無首，吉。故曰弱者道之用。他還說：人之處世，語言平和，則聽者易于受而不違；行事寬恕，則事必易于成而不敗。”
4. 杜光庭說：“無者道之體，有者道之末。因本而生末焉。形而相生，是生于有矣。考其所以，察其所由，皆資道而生，是萬物生于妙無矣。能自有而復無者幾于道矣。”
5. 王弼說：“氣無所不入，虛無柔弱，無所不通，無有不可窮，至柔不可折，以此推云，故知無為之有益也。”

CHAPTER 41

Sameness and Difference—To Awaken to the Dao

第四十一章
同異—悟道

上士聞『道』，勤而行之；
　　中士聞『道』，若存若亡；
　　下士聞『道』，大笑之。
　　不笑不足以為『道』。
故建言有之：
　　「明『道』若昧；
　　進『道』若退；
　　夷『道』若纇；
　　上『德』若谷；
　　大白若辱；
　　廣『德』若不足；
　　建『德』若偷；
　　質真若渝；
　　大方無隅；
　　大器晚成；
　　大音希聲；
　　大象無形；
『道』隱無名。」
　　夫唯『道』，
　　善貸且成。

Those high-level people, after hearing the Dao, practice it diligently;
those middle-class people, after hearing the Dao, seem to
understand, but don't understand;
those low-class people, after hearing to the Dao, (they) laugh
loudly!
If they don't laugh, then it would not be considered the (real)
Dao.
Therefore, there was a saying that:
Understanding the Dao as if it is still in the darkness,
advancing the Dao as if it is retreating,
walking smoothly on the path of the Dao as if on the bumpy
path,
high virtue looks like a valley,
great integrity appears tarnished,
broadening virtue yet seems insufficient,
establishing virtue appears to be weak,
true substance appears contaminated,
a great square has no corners,
a great task (or accomplishment) is often completed late,
the most powerful sound is without a sound,
the greatest form is shapeless.
The Dao is hidden and nameless.
Still, only the Dao is great at beginning and also in final
completeness.

General Interpretation

Those highly educated seekers of the Dao (xun Dao zhe, 尋道者), when they hear of the Dao, will practice it diligently. Those who have only some education, when they hear of the Dao, are confused and wonder about its truth. However, when those uneducated people hear of the Dao, they don't understand it so they laugh about it loudly. Since the Dao is so profound, mysterious, and hard to understand, if those uneducated people do not laugh about it, then it is not the real Dao.

It is said in *Lun Yu* (《論語·里仁》): "If I hear of the Dao in the morning, even if I die in the evening, it is fine."[1] The Chinese have a proverb: "Live to an old age, continue learning until an old age."[2] That means no matter what, there is always something for you to learn since the Dao is so great and profound. Cheng, Yi-Ning (程以寧) said: "High-class means those who have the root (i.e., understood at a deep level) of an education. Hearing does not mean listening with the ears, but hearing with the heart (i.e., feeling)."[3] He Shang Gong (河上公) said: "Those low-class people are greedy and have many desires; when they see the Dao is soft and weak, they believe the Dao is afraid. When they see the Dao is simple and pure, they think it is shallow and awkward; thus, they laugh loudly."[4]

Those who are continuously searching for the truth of the Dao will be deeply humble and believe they are still in darkness. The more they comprehend the Dao, the less they feel they know. Even knowing that the Dao is simple and straightforward, they feel they are walking on a bumpy path and have to be cautious.

Those Dao-seekers' virtues are profound and deep like a valley. They have great integrity but appeared tarnished. They have propagated the truth of the Dao, but still feel insufficient. They have conducted their deeds (the De, manifestation of the Dao) by following the Dao, but still believe they are not strong enough. They are pure, but act as if they are still contaminated.

When the square (the domain or knowledge of the Dao) is large, you cannot even see the corners. To understand it will take time and patience. A great task or accomplishment takes time to complete. The most powerful sound is without sound. Without sound all the many sounds can be created. The soundless is the root of all sounds. All shapes are originated from the shapeless. Thus, the shapeless is also the foundation of all shapes.

The Dao is mysterious, invisible, nameless. Nevertheless, it is only the Dao that is able to initiate and produce everything until their completeness.

Qigong Interpretation

One of the main goals of practicing qigong is to understand the Dao (Nature). As mentioned, those people who are searching for the Dao are called "xun Dao zhe" (尋道者) ("Dao searchers"). Qigong practitioners are Dao searchers who are seeking to understand the Dao and apply it to their lives. Through this practice they are looking for the way to coordinate and harmonize their spirit and physical bodies with the Great Nature, finally reaching the goal of "unification of Nature and humans" (tian ren he yi, 天人合一).

This chapter has pointed out first that, in order to reach a profound level of qigong, you must diligently study, ponder, and practice. Usually, normal laymen cannot comprehend this Dao easily. Only those who are sincere and serious will be willing and be able to put all the effort into pursuing the truth of the Dao.

The second point this chapter has made is, in order to understand the Dao, you must be humble. You must always keep your cup empty so there is space to pour more in. If you are satisfied with your understanding, you have not really comprehended the Dao. Therefore, even though you have reached a profound level of understanding, it seems your understanding is still empty. There is a Chinese proverb: "Satisfaction causes loss and humility receives gains."[5]

In addition, to reach a deeper level of understanding, you must be generous and kind. The more you share what you have with others, the more you gain. It is the way of the Dao; it always gives and never asks for anything in return.

Conclusions

The manner of searching and pursuing the Dao is through intelligent pondering, humble learning, and sharing with an open heart.

1.《論語·里仁》：“朝聞道，夕死可矣。”
2. “活到老，學到老。”
3. 程以寧說：“上士即上根之士。聞非耳聞，乃心聞也。”
4. 河上公說：“下士貪婪多欲，見道柔弱，謂之恐懼；見道質樸，謂之鄙陋，故大笑之。”
5. “滿招損，謙受益。”

CHAPTER 42
Variations of the Dao—Derivation
第四十二章
道化—衍生

『道』生一，
　　一生二，
　　二生三，
　　三生萬物。
萬物負陰而抱陽，
　　沖氣以為和。
（人之所惡，
　　唯孤、寡、不穀，
　　而王公以為稱。）
故
物，或損之而益，
　　或益之而損。
人之所教，
　　我亦教之。
"強梁者不得其死。"
吾將以為教父。

The Dao gives birth to one,
    one produces two,
    two bears three,
    three yields myriad objects.
Myriad objects bear yin and embrace yang.
    through their qi's (energy's) integration, harmony is achieved.
(What people dislike being,
    alone, solitary, and unworthy,
    yet kings and nobles refer to themselves with these terms.)
Thus, things can benefit from a loss,
    and lose as a result of a benefit.
What others teach,
    I also teach.
"Those violent ones will not die peacefully."
I will use this as the principle of my teaching.

General Interpretation

This chapter talks about four important concepts. First, all objects are the manifestations (De) of the Dao (taiji). From taiji, all objects were derived. As explained earlier, the Dao is some power, energy, or force existing in space. From the Dao, things are created and developed into myriad objects in this universe (or universes) and these creations and derivations are called the De. Since our understanding of Nature is so limited, we cannot use our limited knowledge to interpret the Dao. If we do that, we will just mislead ourselves about the truth of Nature. In *The Book of Changes* (*Yi Jing*, 易經) (《易·系辭》), it is said: "There is a taiji (太極) in the 'change' (yi, 易); thus, two polarities (i.e., poles) (liangyi, 兩儀)." "Taiji means before the existence of heaven and earth (i.e., universe), all original qis were mixed into one; this is the singularity of taiji."[1] Taiji is when the Dao is manifested into De at the very beginning. There is no discrimination of two polarities. The space was a mixture of all energies. This is the beginning of the Dao's manifestation that we can see. Since this beginning is so close to the Dao, the Chinese often considered taiji as the Dao. It is said: "What is taiji? It's the Dao."[2] That means taiji was the very beginning manifestation of the Dao.

From taiji, two polarities were generated, then two polarities were derived into four phases, and then continued into eight trigrams, and so on till all objects were created. Si, Ma-Guang (司馬光) said: "The Dao bears one (i.e., singularity), thus creates having (i.e., things) from nothingness. This singularity then bears two so the yin and yang are discriminated. Two is then derived into three due to yin and yang's interaction, and the harmony is then generated. From three, myriad objects are developed. When qi is united harmoniously, objects are produced."[3] The *Yi Jing* (《易·系辭》) says: "The yin and yang qis of heaven and earth (i.e., Nature) interact with each other densely and harmoniously; thus myriad objects are varied and refined diversely. Through male and female's intercourse, myriad objects are generated."[4] In the book *Zhuang Zi* (《莊子·田子方》), Lao Zi's conversation with Confucius is recorded: "The extreme yin is so chilly cold and the extreme yang is so scorching hot. The chilly cold is originated from heaven and the scorching hot is originated from earth. When these two qis interact with each other harmoniously, then myriad objects are derived."[5] Si, Ma-Guang (司馬光) said: "Myriad objects, all carry yin and yang as their bodies, and apply them harmoniously as applications."[6]

Second, this chapter talks about how we should follow the Dao and be humble and flexible. The Dao produces yin and yang from singularity so it can be flexible. From flexibility, Nature is able to balance itself. Since we are created within these yin and yang fields, we should follow the Dao and be flexible. All we need is to be humble and avoid stubbornness. When we allow ourselves to be humble and open-minded, we will have flexibility and, thus, yin and yang can be balanced in our mind and actions. *The Yi Jing* (《易‧謙》) also says: "Those humble and more humble gentlemen always use humility to discipline themselves." "The righteousness of gentlemen is maintaining humility so the deeds (i.e., the De) can be cultivated."[7] In this case, you know how to bow and to bend. The Chinese always say: "Humility is difficult; pride is easy."[8] *The Book* (《書‧大禹謨》) say: "Those who are full (i.e., satisfied) lose while those who are humble gain. This is the Dao of heaven."[9]

Due to humility being the key to ruling a country and harmoniously keeping people together, so those wise rulers were always humble and called themselves alone, solitary, and unworthy. Si, De-Qing (釋德清) said:

"What the laymen dislike is (being) alone, solitary, and unworthy, but those kings and lords commonly used these terms to describe themselves. Is it a fact they were using the softness as the sharp weapon in ruling the country? These words, alone, solitary, and unworthy, are the words of humility. This is because if those kings and lords are not humble, the people of the country will not follow them. Therefore, Yao (堯) and Shun (舜), even though they owned the country, they did not to keep it for themselves. Thus, we have ceaselessly praised them since ancient times until now. This is what it means that when you are self-humble, you gain. However, the lords such as Jie (桀)

and Zhou (紂), who abused the people and asked them to worship them, tyrannous and behaving recklessly, just had regard for themselves without any concern for others. Consequently, when they encountered difficulties, the people rebelled against them. This is what it means that when you are selfishly concerned for your gains, actually you lose."[10]

Yao and Sun were two of the most well-known rulers in ancient China. When they died, they gave the monarchy to the most wise and humble men of the country instead of their own sons. Jie and Zhou were two tyrant rulers in ancient China who eventually died when the people rebelled.

Third, this chapter states that, although the future is unpredictable, you will be able to avoid many possible misfortunes or disasters if you are wise, calm, and have foresight. There is a story about Sun, Shu-Ao (孫叔敖) in *Huai Nan Zi* (《淮南子·人間訓》):

"In the past, the King of Chu (楚莊王), who after his victory had acquired the land between He (河) and Yong (雍), wanted to give a manor to minister Sun, Shu-Ao (孫叔敖) when they returned to the country. Sun declined the offer. When he was dying, he told his son: 'I am going to die soon. After my death, the king will offer you the manor for my loyalty. However, you must decline those fertile lands and accept the land of Qinqiu (寢丘) that is filled with sand and rocks. This place earned its bad reputation due to its rocky surface. Jing people (荊人) treat it as a ghost territory and Yue people (越人) believe this place brings you misfortune. This is the land that nobody desires to have.' Later, Sun, Shu-Ao died, and as predicted, the king wanted to give a manor with fertile land to his son but his son declined. Instead he asked for the land of Qinqiu. According to Chu's custom, those merited officials, after they hold manors for two generations, must return the lands to the king. However, because the manor of Sun,

Shu-Ao was so poor, his land was the only one that remains in his family. This is what is called 'a beneficial loss.'"[11]

The Chinese always say: "Disadvantage is a blessing."[12]

Fourth, this chapter emphasizes the Dao of softness. When you are soft, you will be humble, calm, and peaceful. When you are humble, calm, and peaceful, you will gain harmony. Du, Guang-Ting (杜光庭) said: "When people talk about the lord, it means the chief of politics and education. All countries are transformed due to this person. Thus, Lao Zi said: 'If a lord wishes to use actions and speaking to teach and transform his people, he should teach them the morality of tranquility, calmness, softness, and weakness (i.e., yielding)."[13] Huang, Shang (黃裳) said: "The Great Supreme (Tai Shang, 太上) (i.e., Lao Zi) said: 'What others teach, I also teach.' But what does he teach? There is nothing but softness. If not using softness but using hardness, like those gangsters and robbers,(who) rob as (they) wished; there is no one, at the end, who is able to escape from justice and have a good ending. Thus, we know that those who are violent will encounter death while those who are soft and yielding will survive. This is an important element for cultivating the Dao with sincerity. That is why I teach people to be soft as the first priority."[14] Du, Guang-Ting (杜光庭) also said: "What Lao Zi admonishes is: softness will defeat hardness, and weakness (i.e., yielding) will win against strength. Therefore, the tongue is soft and thus survives, and the teeth are strong and thus decay. From this, it can be seen that violence is not the Dao of protecting the body but the cause of losing life. Hardness and violence are not the ways of advancing the Dao and protecting longevity."[15]

Qigong Interpretation

This chapter describes how myriad objects were derived through the Dao. It does not matter how and what the Dao has created; there are always two polarities, yin and yang. When the yin and yang lose balance, they will interact with each other until they reach harmonization and balance again. When you apply this concept to a human body, a human body also has two polarities. The *Dao De Jing* describes these two polarities as the Mud Pill Palace (Ni Wan Gong, 泥丸宮) located at the central bottom of the spiritual valley (shen gu, 神谷) (the limbic system of brain) and the qi cavity (qi xue, 氣穴) or yellow yard (huang ting, 黃庭) located at the center of gravity (the physical center). The top polarity is the residence of the spirit (shen shi, 神室) that governs the quality of qi's manifestation while the bottom polarity is the storage place of qi (qi residence) (qi she, 氣舍) that stores the quantity of qi to its abundant level. From these two polarities, the entire body's yin (spiritual life) and yang (physical life) can function. When the yin and yang have lost their balance, health will be affected. When yin and yang harmonize and balance each other, health and longevity can be achieved. This is the crucial requirement of reaching ultimate spiritual enlightenment. This is called "dual cultivation of temperament and physical life."[16]

This chapter again points out how important humility and generosity are in qigong practice. Those who give will benefit, and those who take advantage will eventually lose. Those who are aggressive and take advantage of others will earn their retribution (karma) (bao ying, 報應) sooner or later. We don't know the future and it is hard to predict. However, one thing is always true and sure—what seeds you put in the ground is what fruits you will harvest. The Chinese called this "the retribution of the cause and the consequence."[17]

According to Chinese culture, which is heavily influenced by *The Book of Changes* (《*Yi Jing,* 易經》), there are two worlds or dimensions coexisting in this universe: the yang world (yangjian, 陽間) and yin world (yinjian, 陰間). The yang world is the material world while the yin world is the spiritual world. Though there are two worlds, actually, there is only one since both are related and cannot be separated from each other. That is why our bodies, developed in this two-dimensional space, have two aspects, physical life and spiritual life.

Our spiritual life that is connected to the natural spirit is associated with our subconscious mind, and our subconscious mind can be influenced by the repetitive focus of the conscious mind. Therefore, whatever we think or do will influence our subconscious mind and this mind will trigger the qi's redistribution of the yin space (the spiritual world). If we have accumulated good deeds and our subconscious mind is righteous, then the qi accumulated in the yin space will eventually be manifested in the yang space.

From past experience, Daoists realize that those who are calm, peaceful, compassionate, benevolent, and help others will accumulate good deeds and spiritual energy in the yin world.

You should be truthful with yourself and others. Treat affairs with softness, benevolence, calmness, and yielding; consequently, you will acquire a peaceful mind and harmonious qi circulation. Without these, your qigong practice will be shallow.

To regulate the mind is to regulate your thinking and actions. From one thought (wuji state), matter can be moved into myriad actions. For example, one thought of inventing an airplane has manifested in myriad events and consequences. One thought of initiating wars can develop into myriad disasters for the living.

To practice qigong, you should not be allured or influenced by the emotional world. You should keep your mind neutral and stay at its singularity and simplicity. This is the crucial key in following the Dao.

Conclusions

To achieve a high level of qigong practice, you must first regulate your mind. This is because your mind is the governor of your body's qi and actions. If your thinking is righteous and you have accumulated good deeds, your mind will be in a neutral, calm, and peaceful state. In order to reach this state, you must be soft, humble, and yielding. Hard and aggressive minds will trigger emotional imbalance and lead your mind into a chaotic situation. When you have lived righteously, you will accumulate good credit in the yin space that eventually will be redeemed in the yang space.

1. 《易·系辭》："易有太極，是生兩儀。""太極謂天地未分之前，元氣混而為一，即太極初一也。"
2. "何謂太極？道也。"
3. 司馬光說："道生一，自無而有；一生二，分陰分陽；二生三，陰陽交而生和；三生萬物，和氣既合而生物。"

4. 《易·系辭》:"天地絪縕,萬物化醇,男女媾精,萬物化生。"

5. 《莊子·田子方》:"至陰肅肅,至陽赫赫,肅肅出乎天,赫赫出於地,兩者交通成和而萬物生焉。"

6. 司馬光說:"萬物莫不以陰陽為體,以沖和為用。"

7. 《易·謙》:"謙謙君子,卑以自牧。""君子之義,恆已謙卑自養其德也。"

8. "謙難,驕易。"

9. 《書·大禹謨》:"滿招損,謙受益,時乃天道。"

10. 釋德清說:"即如世人之所惡者,惟孤、寡,不穀,王公反以此為稱者,豈不以柔弱為天下之利器耶?且孤、寡、不穀,皆自損之辭也。然而王侯不自損,則天下不歸。故堯舜有天下而不與,至今稱之,澤流無窮。此自損而人益之,故曰或損之而益。若夫桀、紂以天下奉一己,暴戾恣睢,但知有己而不知有人,故難有天下,而天下叛。此自益而人損之,故曰或益之而損。"

11. 《淮南子·人間訓》:"昔者楚莊王既勝晉于河、雍之間,歸而封孫叔敖,辭而不受。病疽將死,謂其子曰:'吾則死矣,王必封女,女必讓肥饒之地,而受沙石之間有寢丘者,其地确石而名丑,荊人鬼,越人橫,人莫之利也。'孫叔敖死,王果封其子以肥饒之地,其子辭而不受,請有寢之丘。楚國之俗,功臣二世而爵祿,惟孫叔敖獨存。此所謂損之而益也。"

12. "吃虧是福。"

13. 杜光庭說:"人謂人君也,人君為政教之首,系乎一人而化。故老君昌言之曰:'人君欲行言教以化人,當須用我沖虛柔弱之義以教之也。'"

14. 黃裳說:"太上所以云:'人之所教,我亦教之也。'所教唯何?至柔已耳。若不用柔而用剛,必如世上強梁之徒,橫行劫奪,終無一人不羅法網而得以善終。是知橫豪者死之機,柔弱者生之路。此誠修道要術,吾之教人以柔弱為先也。"

15. 杜光庭說:"老君所戒,柔必勝剛,弱必勝強。故舌柔則存,齒堅則亡。是則強梁非全身之道。為失生之基耳。剛暴非進道之階,殊保壽之旨矣。'"

16. "性命雙修。"

17. "因果報應。"

CHAPTER 43
The Universal Usage—Without Regulating

第四十三章
偏用—無調

天下之至柔，
　　馳騁天下之至堅，
　　　無有入無間。
吾是以知「無為」之有益。
「不言」之教，
　　「無為」之益，
　　　天下希及之。

The softest things in the world
    are able to override the hardest things in the world,
    the insubstantial is able to penetrate even where there is no opening.
Thus I know the benefits of wuwei (i.e., doing nothing).
The teaching without words,
    and the benefits of wuwei,
    are rarely matched in the world.

General Interpretation

The softest things, like water and air, are able to penetrate the hardest stone or steel. Even if there is no gap, they are able to get through with time; this is the power of nature. Water and air do not have to do anything to accomplish this. This ability is wuwei (doing nothing). Wu, Cheng (吳澄) said: "Though water is extremely soft it is able to penetrate the hardest rock; air is insubstantial but able to permeate the metal or rock without an opening. Thus, though they have the disadvantages of being soft and insubstantial, they also have the advantage of penetrating hardness and even permeating matter without an opening. This is what it is called 'a beneficial loss.' Softness is able to defeat hardness and the insubstantial is able to enter without an opening; all of these are happening naturally without actions. Thus, it is said: 'doing nothing is beneficial.'"[1]

When you are in a wuwei state, you are relaxed, soft, calm, peaceful, and neutral. When you teach people, you don't have to lecture them. All you need is just to be yourself and do nothing. From observing and imitating your thoughts and actions, they are influenced without even knowing it. This is the power of the subconscious mind—teaching without teaching and doing without doing. The Chinese have a saying: "Teaching with talking is not as good as teaching with examples."[2] The reason those sages are able to do so is because they have followed the Dao for a long time to a stage of "regulating of no regulating." That means they don't have to think or make things happen since they have followed the Dao and reached a stage of thinking and doing with their subconscious minds. That means the stage of "regulating of no regulating." Du, Guang-Ting (杜光庭) said: "The ultimate Dao is speechless, but all objects were created. Those sages do nothing, but all people are transformed into purity and clearness. They need not be taught by speaking, but education is done. Out of all the people, there are very few who have reached this state."[3] The book Zhuang Zi (《莊子 · 天道》) says: "Thus, those ancient sage kings, though their wisdom included the whole world, they would not ponder. Though their speaking was able to reach all myriad objects, they would not speak. Though their talent and actions can extend to the four seas (i.e., entire world), they would not act on it. The heaven gives birth to myriad objects without intention and the earth raises myriad objects without doing anything, and the sage kings conduct nothing but all the affairs in the country are accomplished by themselves."[4]

Qigong Interpretation

"Wuwei" means, "doing nothing." In order to reach this stage, you must first learn to do it until it has become natural and you don't have to exert your mind and any effort to do it. However, in order to be extremely natural and soft, you must first establish the discipline for it.

This chapter emphasizes the strength and power of softness. In qigong practice, to reach a high level of physical and spiritual strength, you must first learn to be soft. When the qi can be led softly and smoothly, then you can manifest it powerfully. If your mind and body are not soft and the qi cannot be led smoothly and softly, the qi will become stagnant. This is the cause of stiffness and sickness. Once you have reached to a profound level of softness, then your mind does not have to be there to maintain it since it has already reached the level of "doing without doing" (wei er bu wei, 為而無為) (wuwei, 無為) or "regulating without regulating" (tiao er wu tiao, 調而無調). The most powerful and effective qigong practice is practicing qigong subconsciously. This means that you have built up a natural healthy habit in your lifestyle. For example, one of the most important qigong practices is to, without holding it, regulate the breath until it is soft, slender and long. Once you have practiced to a stage that you have established this breathing habit, you will carry it to your daily life without having to regulate it. This is the stage of wuwei.

It is just like when you are learning to drive. Your mind and body are tensed since you are regulating your driving. However, after you have regulated your driving skill to a profound level, you are relaxed, soft, and easy both mentally and physically. Your conscious mind does not have to be there. This is the stage of "driving without driving." When you practice qigong to cultivate your mind and physical body, you must also be pursuing and aiming for the goal of extreme softness. In order to reach this stage, you must regulate them with a great deal of effort and time. That is the reason that there are not too many people who have reached the profound level of qigong practice.

Conclusions

In conclusion, this chapter focuses on two important qigong points: softness and regulating without regulating. In order to reach the level of "doing nothing" (wuwei, 無為), you must first regulate your body, breathing, qi, and the mind until they have reached the stage of regulating without regulating (調而無調). However, in order to reach this stage, you must be soft, calm, and peaceful. Only through continuous and repeated practice of attaining these states will you be able to establish a subconscious mind to do it without conscious intention. To train qigong with the subconscious mind is the most powerful practice you can achieve since you have already built up the constant habit in your daily life.

1. "言教不如身教。"
2. 吳澄說："水至柔，能攻穿至堅之石；氣無有，能透入無罅隙之金石牆壁。以至柔無有之損，而有馳騁至堅入無間之益，所謂損之而益者，柔能勝剛，無能入有，皆非有所為而自然。故曰無為之有益。"
3. 杜光庭說："至道無言，物以之生；聖人無為，化之以清，即不待立言，然后成教。天下希及之者，言九流百氏，希有能及無為之教者。"
4. 《莊子・天道》："故古之王者，知（智）雖落（包羅）天地，不自慮也；辯雖雕萬物，不自說也；能雖窮四海，不自為也。天不產而萬物化，地不長而萬物育，帝王無為而天下功。"

CHAPTER 44

Set Up Precepts—Knowing Contentment

第四十四章
立戒—知足

名與身孰親？
　　身與貨孰多？
　　得與亡孰病？
是故
　　甚愛必大費，
　　多藏必厚亡。
知足不辱，
　　知止不殆，
　　可以長久。

Fame and life, which one is dearer?
    Life and goods (i.e., material wealth), which one is more valuable?
    Gain and loss, which one is more harmful?
Thus,
    excessive love (i.e., desire) must cause great spending,
    excessive hoarding must lead to a heavy loss.
Knowing contentment prevents disgrace,
    knowing when to stop can prevent danger,
        thus, it can last long.

General Interpretation

Which one is more important to you, your fame or your life? Again, which one is more important to you, your wealth or your life? Have you ever thought about which is more harmful, excess or deficiency?

Anything, when overdone, results in a reduction in or even a reversal of the benefits. He Shang Gong (河上公) said: "Too much lust, then essence and spirit (i.e., the spirit of vitality) will be wasted. Too much love of wealth, then disaster will be provoked." "When alive, the excess wealth is hidden in treasuries and when dead, the excess treasures are hidden in the graves of the hills. When alive, there is a worry of being robbed and when dead, there is worry that the grave will be excavated."[1]

Human beings have created an emotional matrix filled with glory, dignity, wealth, power, and lust. We have been caught up in all these conscious desires and trapped in their bondage. Because of these emotions, we have lied, killed, enslaved, and abused each other. We have become greedy in our desires and hidden and suppressed our true human nature deeply inside of our subconscious awareness. For these reasons, we have been enslaved by these forms of emotional bondage and these material desires. Not only that, we will find any way possible to fulfill our selfish greediness and desires. Su, Che (蘇轍) said: "When there is too much lust after material things, then as long as they can be acquired, they will be pursued through all possible means. In this case, how can there be no waste? When the wealth hidden is too much, then the attackers will be many. In this case, how can there be no death?"[2]

Those who are always greedy and full of desires will be unhappy while those who are satisfied with and appreciate what they have received will be happy.

Qigong Interpretation

One of the most difficult qigong practices is regulating the emotional mind (tiao xin, 調心). We humans have created a society that is filled with human emotions and desires. Then, we have placed ourselves inside this matrix and suffer and fight with each other. This society (matrix) is called "square" (fang, 方) by the Daoists since there are so many square rules and dogmas to retrain human's emotions. These emotions have hindered our spiritual growth. Those who are able to jump out of this matrix are called "persons outside the square" (fang wai zhi ren, 方外之人).

Among the emotions created, just to name a few, are reputation, wealth, and greediness. However, if you compare all of these emotional gains with your health and life, then you must realize that all these emotional gains are worse than nothing. If you are able to stop your desires of pursuing all of these emotional gains, appreciate and be satisfied with what you have already gained without further greediness, then you have regulated your emotional mind. Consequently, your health and longevity can be secured.

If we look at our past, we can see that two parts, the good and the bad, have shaped human history. The good part includes love, compassion, righteousness, benevolence, and justice, and the bad part comprises greediness, selfishness, glory, dignity, and various desires such as power, gold and lust. All of these have become part of our genetic memory. Repetitive thinking and actions that are recorded in our subconscious mind create genetic memory. Behind our masks and due to negative genetic memories, we still hide dark and evil thoughts such as conquering, killing, enslaving, torturing, and raping. In qigong practice, regulating the mind means to regulate the mind of this life as well as previous lives. In order to evolve our spirit, we must continue to fortify our good genetic memory and gradually eliminate bad parts through self-recognition, awareness, awakening, and, finally, through setting our spirit free from the bondage of the past.

Conclusions

The most important thing needed to regulate our mind is seeing through our emotional bondage caused by our desires. If you are able to see through it, your mind will be calm, peaceful, and not trapped in the matrix. Jumping out of this human matrix and facing the true you is the first step to spiritual enlightenment. In order to reopen the third eye, we must first be truthful to others and ourselves. Otherwise, the third eye will remain closed.

1. 河上公說：“甚愛色，費精神；甚愛財，遇禍患”“生多藏于府庫，死多藏于丘墓，生有攻劫之懼，死有掘冢探柩之患。”
2. 蘇轍說：“愛之甚，則凡可以求之者，無所不為，能無費乎？藏之多，則攻之者必眾，能無亡乎？”

CHAPTER 45

Immense De—Modest Manner

第四十五章
洪德—謙虛

大成若缺，
　　其用不弊。
大盈若沖，
　　其用不窮。
大直若屈。
　　　大巧若拙。
　　　大辯若訥。
躁勝寒，
　　靜勝熱。
清靜以為天下正。

Great perfection seems flawed,
    but its function is never impaired.
Great fullness seems void,
    but its usage cannot be exhausted.
Great straightness seems to bend,
    Great skill seems awkward.
    Great eloquence seems inarticulate.
Active movements overcome cold,
    stillness overcomes heat.
Serenity and calmness are the guides of the world.

General Interpretation

Even those who have achieved a high level of success in their cultivations find they are still searching for any remaining flaw. Since their
minds remain humble and stay in high awareness, the search for truth
will not be exhausted. Those who have already acquired abundant
knowledge or experience still believe there are some voids in their learning. Therefore, their learning will never be exhausted. If anyone has
this kind of attitude of learning or doing, then sooner or later he will
reach the stage of wuwei. In order to reach the wuwei state, you must
remain humble and keep your bowl empty. If your bowl is full, then
there is no space for you to learn more. Recall the well-known samurai
story from chapter 11. The young samurai begged the the renown
master to train him, all the while bragging about his level of attainment
in the arts of the samurai. The master did not say a word and went into
the kitchen and came out with a teapot and bowl. He quietly put a bowl
in front of the young samurai and began to pour the tea. Soon, the bowl
filled up and overflowed. The young samurai was confused and said:
"Stop, master. The tea is overflowing." The master put the teapot down,
looked at him with a smile and said, "This is you, young samurai. Your
bowl is full. In order to learn, you must empty your bowl first."

Therefore, if you are satisfied, your regulating process and achievement will be shallow. Zhuang Zi (莊子) said:

> "Yao (堯) wanted to give his ruling power of the country
> to Xu, You (許由). He said: 'The sun and the moon are
> already out but still the torch fire is not extinguished and
> wants to compete with the brightness of the sun and
> moon. Isn't this very difficult? The raining season has
> come and it has rained, but I still water the garden without
> stop. Isn't this effort of irrigation in vain and a waste? If
> sir, you are able to take the ruling power of the country, the
> country will be in great order. But I am still holding the
> position with my limited capability. Please allow me to
> hand the country to you.'"[1]

If anyone can be so humble and always search for ways to improve, soon he will be perfect without even knowing it. Zhang, Er-Qi (張爾歧) said: "Those who have reached a great achievement of the Dao and De do not know their achievement. They always look at themselves as if there are still some flaws. Thus, their functions are not exhausted (i.e., Their work is never at an end.)."[2] Du, Guang-Ting (杜光庭) said:

> *"Those who do not feel proud about what they own, even though there is a surplus it is as if it's empty. Because they do not depend on their surplus, thus when using it, it is not exhausted. When a lord has a surplus of the De (i.e., good deeds), the people have surplus wealth (i.e., qi), which circulates in all directions and reaches far and wide to the four corners. When applying this to rule a country, people will be wealthy by themselves. When applying this to regulate the body, the good deeds will be achieved automatically. There is no limitation for its applications. In this case, how can it be exhausted?"[3]*

Those who are wise and humble know how to keep their knowledge and skills within themselves without showing off. They look as if they are bendable, awkward, and inarticulate. There is a story about Confucius and his student (《論語·為政》). Confucius said: "I talked to Hui (回) the whole day. He listened without disobedience as if he was a fool. After retreating, he would introspect privately and then applied it to his actions clearly. Hui is not stupid."[4] Su, Che (蘇轍) said:

"For those who are straight and not bendable, when they bend they will be broken. However, if they follow the principles and rules, though they are bending, they are still straight. For those who have high skills but do not show awkwardness, their skills must be laborious. Those who take care of the objects (i.e., tasks) naturally, though awkward, are still skillful. Those who are good at eloquence but are not inarticulate, their eloquence must have limitations. However, if they speak according to the rules of logic, though inarticulate they are still eloquent."[5]

Everything and all learning have different levels. Those who think they already know everything and are skillful, due to their satisfaction, will not reach a higher level of understanding and skills. Only those who are humble and continue pursuing the higher level, though they look stupid, are actually the wise ones. Smart people learn things fast. But without humility, they will be satisfied easily and, thus, will not advance to a more profound level. However, those who are not smart but remain humble and continue to learn and improve will one day become the best of experts. These are the wise. Wise persons learn from mistakes and do not repeat their mistakes. This is because they have the right attitude about learning. They know everything has different levels of understanding, feeling, and skills. If they stop learning, their progress will be limited.

The last part of this chapter talks about people who can see winter time is cold, and use movements to keep warm, and summer time is hot and use the stillness to keep cool. However, how can all these efforts compare with the method to just keep yourself calm and quiet internally and allow the imbalance to give way to balance? This is the way of doing nothing and while still doing. Ye, Meng-De (葉夢得) said:

> *"The existence of winter and summer is due to the qi's variations of heaven and earth. Some people recognize this and believe that active movement is able to overcome coldness and stillness is able to subdue summer heat. However, how can all of these be better than doing nothing but maintaining internal quietness and calmness? Won't this be enough to subdue the actions of heaven and earth as a chaste (i.e., pure and simple) person? Thus, it is known that a flaw is better than perfection, a void is better than fullness, bends are better than straightness, and inarticulateness is better than eloquence. However, those laymen in the world do not see these, and the more they have tried to win the more they lost. The internal quietness and calmness are able to put the world into the right order. This is the way of using 'not wining' to win."[6]*

Qigong Interpretation

This chapter has pointed out three important things in qigong practice. First, you must be humble. When you are humble, you will not be satisfied with what you know and how high you have reached. You will continue to search for deeper feeling and knowledge. The more you have, the more you feel you don't have. Confucius (孔子) (《論語·為政》) said: "If you know what you know and what you don't know, this is wisdom."[7] Humble persons will continue to pay attention to what they don't have instead of what they already have. That is how they are able to keep themselves learning and pursuing deeper feeling and understanding.

Second, since your qigong practice is for you and not others, there is no reason to show off or to be proud and self-satisfied. My White Crane master, Zeng, Jin-Zao (曾金灶) always said: "Learning is like plowing."[8] He explained that when you plow, keep your head down and plow. Don't look around and compare with others. If you look around and see you are ahead of others, you feel proud and self-satisfied; then you slow down or stop. If you see you are behind, you feel sad and depressed, and you quit. Why do you look around? Just bow your head and keep plowing. One day, when you are tired, take a break and look around. You will see no one is in sight since you have left them far behind. This has always been my proverb since I was fifteen years old. From his saying I was able to plow my life and follow my dream without being disturbed emotionally.

Third, the best way of correcting qi's unhealthy conditions is to follow the natural way and let the body take care of itself. Often when people's bodies are too yin, they try to use the yang method to correct the problem, and when the body is too yang, again, they will use the yin method. However, since humans are part of nature, we should follow the natural way. Just keep the body and mind calm, quiet, and relaxed and allow the imbalanced body to readjust itself and reach the final yin-and-yang balance again. The crucial key to practice and healing is following the Dao and letting the Dao take care of the problem. The way to reach this goal is to first keep your mind from emotional disturbance.

Conclusions

When you are learning and practicing qigong, you should be humble and natural.

1. 莊子說：“堯讓天下于許由曰：‘日月出矣，而爝火不息，其于光也，不亦難乎？時雨降矣，而猶浸灌，其于澤也，不亦勞乎？夫子立而天下治，而我猶尸之，吾自視缺然，請致天下。’”
2. 張爾歧說：“道德之大成者，不自知其成也，自視常若缺，故其用不敝。”
3. 杜光庭說：“不矜其有，故盈而若虛；不恃其盈，故用之不乏。主有餘德，民有餘財，周流六虛，放曠四極。為國則民自富，理身則德自充。其用無涯，何窮匱之有也。”
4. 《論語·為政》：“子曰：‘吾與回言終日，不違如愚。退而省其私，亦足以發，回也不愚。”
5. 蘇轍說：“直而不屈，其屈必折；循理而行，雖屈亦直。巧而不拙，其巧必勞；待物自然，雖拙而巧。辯而不納，其辯必窮；因理而言，雖納而辯。”
6. 葉夢得說：“寒暑天地之氣也，有人于此，躁猶可以勝寒，靜猶可以勝熱，而況自然無為之清靜，其尚不足以制天下之動而貞夫一者乎？則缺勝成，沖勝盈，屈勝直，拙納勝巧辯，從可知矣。世人不察此，力求勝物而愈莫能勝，清靜正天下，以不勝勝之也。”
7. 《論語·為政》：“知之為知之，不知為不知，是知也。”
8. 曾金灶說：“學如耕耘。”

CHAPTER 46
Moderating Desire—Self-Satisfaction
第四十六章
儉欲—知足

天下有道，
　　卻走馬以糞；
天下無道，
　　戎馬生於郊。
罪莫大於可欲，
　　禍莫大於不知足，
　　咎莫大於欲得。
故
知足之足，
　　常足矣。

When the world is in accord with the Dao,
    fast-running horses are used to carry manure.
When the world is not (in) accord with the Dao,
    battle horses give birth on the (battle) field.
There is no crime greater than greediness,
    there is no disaster greater than discontentment,
    and there is no fault greater than avarice.
Thus,
whoever is content with contentment,
    is always content.

General Interpretation

When the world is ruled according to the Dao, then there is peace, calmness, and harmony. Then even the best horses are useless for battle and instead are used for carrying the dirt and manure on the farms. However, if the ruling of the world does not follow the Dao, even pregnant horses have to give birth on the battlefield.

Han, Fei (韓非) said: "Today, those rulers who have followed the Dao will seldom use troops for wars and will prohibit excessive luxury internally. Thus, the rulers do not use horses to fight and chase enemies, and people do not use horses to carry luxurious objects. All of the efforts are engaged in farming. When they engage in farming, they will need to fertilize and water the plants. Thus, Lao Zi said: 'When the world is in accord with the Dao, fast running horses are used to carry manure.'"[1]

Han, Fei (韓非) also said:

> "When the rulers are not following the Dao, they will violently oppress the people internally and invade neighboring countries externally. When oppressing the people with violence internally, the farming will be interrupted. When invading other countries externally, numerous wars will occur. When there are numerous wars, then soldiers will die and troops will be depleted. The animals will be reduced and the horse will be deficient. If soldiers are exhausted, then the troop will be in danger and those high-ranking officers who are close to the ruler will be drafted for the wars. Due to lack of battle horses, even those pregnant horses have to be used for war. Horses are used greatly in war, and 'on the field' means near the battlefield. Now, what can be offered for battle are those high-ranking officers who are close to the ruler and pregnant horses. Thus Lao Zi said: 'When the world isn't in accord with the Dao, battle horses give birth on the (battle) field.'"[2]

All social disorders like war are caused by human's greed for power, wealth, lust, and luxurious material enjoyment. Greediness is just like a bottomless hole that cannot be filled. The more you have, the more you want. This is the cause of human's unhappiness and disasters. Han Fei (韓非) said: "When a person has a desire, then his thinking will be chaotic. When thinking becomes chaotic, the more desire he will have. When there is a desire, the evil mind will take over. When the evil mind is in charge, the rules for conduct will disappear. When the rules for conduct disappear, then disaster will occur."[3] When you are content, then you are satisfied and appreciate everything you have received. Wang, An-Shi (王安石) said: "All creatures stop taking when they have enough. Contentment exists because there is no mind of (i.e., desire for) contentment."[4] This is the cause of greediness. Du, Guang-Ting (杜光庭) said: "Greediness and contentment are all originated from the heart (i.e., mind). When the mind is content, then there is always a surplus. If the mind is greedy, then there is always discontentment. Those who are greedy, even if they own a huge country with ten thousand horse carriages, are still greedy and demanding of others. Those who are content, even with a single bamboo bowl and simple crude residence, will not forget their happiness."[5]

Thus, those sages will not be allured by these external temptations. They are satisfied, content, and appreciative of what they have already had. When you have such an outlook, your mind will be calm and peaceful. Li, Jia-Mou (李嘉謀) said: "Those rulers who follow the Dao are able to transform soldiers into common people and those who do not follow the Dao can transform common people into soldiers. People have desires because of their love to own (things). Those who are not content will take from others. Thus those who wish to have must have what they wish for. From loving to taking and from taking to owning, transgressions become unlimited. We see those who are not content, though having enough. From this, we know that those who know contentment will always be content."[6]

Qigong Interpretation

Humans have created a matrix that is dominated mainly by emotions and desires. In this matrix, we all carry a mask so we are able to survive in this untruthful human society. Thus, since we were born, we learned how to lie, play tricks, and take advantage whenever possible. In this matrix, we have been brainwashed with glory, false dignity, pride, and blind loyalty. Under these influences, we have become the victims or tools of dictators, kings, or emperors, so their dreams can be fulfilled. We have been separating from the Great Nature and isolating ourselves from the natural spirit. We also learn how to deny our genuine feelings and instincts in our subconscious mind we were born with. We are afraid to face and reveal the dark side of us that is hidden in our genetic memory. We have downgraded the pure feeling of benevolence, love, and compassion. Since then, we have carried weapons and killed each other.

Among these emotions we have created, greediness is one of the major causes driving our behaviors. From this greediness, desires are initiated. Once we have the power to realize the desires, selfishly, without concern for other people, we find the way to fulfill it. You should know all achievement in qigong practice heavily depends on your mind since your mind is the general or king who governs your entire body's qi and functions. If your mind is chaotic and confused, your qi circulation will be imbalanced and your actions will be irrational. From this, you can see how important it is to regulate your mind in qigong practice. Will you be able to face what may be an ugly past and jump out of the human emotional matrix? If you are trapped in your desires, how can you find the true original feelings you were born with?

Therefore, for Buddhists and Daoists, the first task of practicing qigong for their spiritual enlightenment is regulating their emotional mind and desires as well as seeing through material attractions. In order to reach the simplicity and purity of their original spirit, they learn how to repel the seven emotions and six desires (qi qing liu yu, 七情六慾) that we have considered in previous chapters. The seven emotions are happiness (xi, 喜), anger (nu, 怒), sorrow (ai, 哀), joy (le, 樂), love (ai, 愛), hate (hen, 恨), and lust (yu, 慾). The desires are generated from the six roots that are the eyes, ears, nose, tongue, body, and mind (xin, 心). Not only that, they also train themselves so they are able reach the stage of "four emptinesses" (si da jie kong, 四大皆空), the emptiness of earth, water, fire, and wind.

When you are happy and content with what you have instead of being tempted by desires. There is a short story that illustrates this.

A person complained to his friend that he is so poor and unhappy. But his friend looked at him, and said: "How can you be so poor? You already have a few million dollars in your body!"

The person asked, "What do you mean? I don't have any money in my body."

The friend said, "Will you sell me your arms for half a million dollars?"

The person said: "No, of course not."

"Will you sell me your legs for another two million dollars?" the friend asked.

"That's ridiculous, of course not. I will not sell you my legs."

"How about your head? Will you sell it for five million dollars?" the friend asked.

"No! No! Definitely no!"

"Then, you already have a few million dollars in your body. Why did you complain that you are poor? If your body is so valuable to you, why don't you appreciate it and take care of it? Your health is all-important, so you should take care of it and treat it as a body worth a few million dollars."

Conclusions

Regulating your mind is the first important key of qigong practice. Keep your mind content and appreciate everything you have acquired. If you do, you will minimize your greediness and desires. Then you will be able to gain peace, calmness, and harmony.

---

1. 韓非說："今有道之君，外希用甲兵，而內禁淫奢。上不得事馬于戰斗逐北，而民不以馬遠通淫物，所積力唯田疇。積力田疇，必且糞灌，故曰：'天下有道，卻走馬以糞' 也。"（《解老》）

2. 韓非說："人君者無道，則內暴虐其民而外侵欺其鄰國。內暴虐則民產絕，外侵欺則兵數起。民產絕則畜生少，兵數起則士卒盡。畜生少則戎馬乏，士卒盡則軍危殆。戎馬乏則牸馬出，軍危殆則近臣役。馬者，軍之大用；郊者，言其近也。今所以給軍之具于將馬近臣，故曰：'天下無道，戎馬生于郊'。"（《解老》）

3. 韓非說：“人有欲則計會亂，計會亂而有欲甚，有欲甚則邪心勝，邪心勝則事輕絕，事輕絕則禍難生。”
   （《解老》）

4. 王安石說：“萬物常至於足，而有所謂不足者，以其無足心也。”

5. 杜光庭說：“貪之與足，皆出于心。心足則物常有餘，心貪則物常不足。貪者雖四海萬乘之廣，尚欲旁
   求；足者雖一簞環堵之質，不忘其樂。”

6. 李嘉謀說：“有道則能使兵為民，無道則能使民為兵。可欲者愛也。不知足者取也。欲得者有也。由愛生
   取，由取生有，遂為無窮之答。觀不知足者雖足而不足，則知足之足常足可知矣。”

CHAPTER 47
Viewing the Distant—Seeing Clarity

第四十七章
鑒遠—鑒明

不出戶，
　　知天下；
不窺牖，
　　見天『道』。
其出彌遠，
　　其知彌少。
是以『聖人』，
　　不行而知，
　　不見而明，
　　不為而成。

Without going out the door,
    know the world.
Without peering through a window,
    see the the Dao of Heaven.
The further one goes,
    the less one knows.
Thus, those sages,
    know without going out,
    understand clearly without seeing,
    and accomplish without striving.

General Interpretation

The basic foundation or root of the Dao is very simple, yet very difficult to comprehend. Once you are able to understand this basic foundation, you will have seen all possible developments of the Dao. If you look too much for detail and neglect the most basic concept of the Dao, you are paying attention to the branches and flowers and ignoring the root of the Dao. Then, what you have seen is only a tiny portion of the Dao's manifestation. In this case, what you know is very little compared with all other millions of manifestations. However, if you are able to comprehend the root of the Dao and know the basic rules of the Dao's manifestation, even before manifestation happens, you have already seen its coming. This is because the Dao, from its foundation, always follows the same rules to manifest its actions (the De, 德).

Those sages, since they have comprehended the theory of the Dao at a profound level and know the rules or cycles of the Dao's manifestation, can always see and predict what is going to happen since these natural rules or cycles are the foundation of the Dao's manifestations. Confucius said, "I use one (i.e., the same basic foundation) to thread through (i.e., comprehend) my Dao."[1] This means once you have comprehended the basic rules and routines, you will be able to see how the De manifests from the Dao. Thus, you can foresee what is going to happen. Guan Zi (管子) said: "When focused in yi (i.e., wisdom mind) and keeping the xin (i.e., emotional mind) in the state of singularity, then consequently the ears and the eyes are sharp and know far." "When the four bodies (i.e., head, arms, legs, and torso) are in righteous condition (i.e., calm, relaxed, and peaceful), the blood and qi's circulation will be calm and smooth. With the concentrated yi and xin, the ears and the eyes are not turbid, and they see far as if it was near."[2] That means if you are able to use your wisdom mind to govern your emotional mind so it can be calm and steady, your sensitivity will be clear and reach far. This is because there is no disturbing thought to blur your feeling and judgment. This is the way of meditation. Meditation is one of the most effective ways to comprehend the root of the Dao.

In the book, *Li Ji* (《禮記·中庸》), it is said:

> *"Only those who are extremely sincere are able to develop their original human nature. If they are able to develop their human nature, then they are able to help other people to develop theirs. Once they are able to help others to develop their human natures, then they are able to help myriad objects to develop their original temperaments. If they are able to develop myriad object's temperaments, then they are able to help the world to nurture lives. If they are able to help the world to nurture lives, then they can be juxtaposed with heaven and earth as one of the three powers."* Thus, *"with extreme sincerity with the Dao, one is able to have prior knowledge of the incident coming."* *"Therefore, with extreme sincerity, the spirit can be enlightened."*[3] Ding, Fu-Bao (丁福保) *said: "It means that those sages' human natures are so content that their wisdom is able to reach myriad objects and there is no hidden secret not clear to them. Therefore, though the world is so big, they are able to know what is happening without leaving the house. Though the Dao of Heaven is so tenuous, they can see without peering through a window. This is because their desires are all repelled; thus, there is not even a tiny obstacle in front of them."*[4] *This means that once you are able to repel all human emotions and desires, your mind will be as truthful and simple as the day you were born. When this happens, you will be able to feel the energy change in the yin space. From this, you can already foresee the manifestation of this energy in yang space.*

Everything must have an adequate amount. Excess or deficiency may cause different results. Once you see the cause, you may be able to predict or foresee the future. There is a story in *Han Fei Zi* (韓非子). Han, Fei (韓非) said:

"The lord of Yue (越襄主) learned how to drive the carriage from Wang, Yu-Qi (王于期). Not too long after learning, he wanted to race with Wang, Yu-Qi. However, even if he changed his horses three times, still he was behind. The lord asked: 'I doubt that you have taught me all the skills of driving the carriage. Wang, Yu-Qi answered: 'I taught you all the skills already. However, you have overdone it. The most important thing in driving is that you must first assess the condition of the horses. The horses must feel comfortable with the carriage. In addition, the driver's mind must be calm, steady, and coordinate with the horses. Only then you can increase your speed and run them for a long distance. Today, the lord wanted to catch up to me. When you were ahead, you were afraid that I would catch up to you and when you were behind, you restlessly urged the horses to catch me. When two persons are competing, if one is not ahead, he will be behind. However, the lord's mind only considered being ahead and was not concerned for the feeling of the horses. That is why the lord lost."[5] Often we make the same mistake: letting our emotional desires take control of our thinking. However, if we allow our wisdom mind to govern the situation, then our actions will be rational and make more sense. Ding, Fu-Bao (丁福保) said: "Most humans are trapped and sunken in desires and thoughts of individual benefit. Their minds are tempted by external attractions; consequently, their wisdom is dazed (i.e., puzzled) by thoughts of what seems like benefits to them. Thus, their human natures part farther from them daily and the emotional demands thicken daily. When the emotional demands get thick, the heart (i.e., mind) will become darker (i.e., away from righteousness)."[6]

Qigong Interpretation

The Dao inside humans is the spirit. It is from this spirit that the actions and behaviors (the De) are manifested externally. When the Chinese refer to a person's thinking and behavior, they use the word "Dao De" (道德) and it means "moralities."

Chinese culture, which has been heavily influenced by *The Book of Changes* (《*Yi Jing*, 易經》), holds that there are two dimensions or spaces coexisting in this universe. One is the material world, called "yang space" (yangjian, 陽間), which can be seen. The other, called "yin space" (yinjian, 陰間), is the spiritual world that can only be felt or sensed. Although there are two spaces, they cannot be separated and are interdependent. They are just like two polarities of the universe and must coexist. Whenever there is any energy change in either dimension, the other will be affected and respond. Therefore, the Chinese believe that whatever you have done in your physical life, good or bad, will be recorded on the other side. Eventually, this energy will be manifested again in the physical dimension. This is called "cause and consequence" (yinguo, 因果), and in Hinduism it is called karma. Since the human body is constructed in these two dimensions, we are constructed with two lives, the physical life and spiritual life. The physical body will be recycled and return to nature while the spirit is able to continue for a long period of time. Normally, once a regular person's body dies, his spirit is no longer able to reside in the body, and will separate from the physical body and search for a new residence again. This is due to his spirit still being at a low level. This is the theory of reincarnation.

From past qigong experience, it is believed that if you are able to cultivate your spirit to a very high level and your spirit and the natural spirit can be reconnected, then you will be able to foresee what will happen in the yang world. This reconnection is called "unification of heaven and human" (tian ren he yi, 天人合一). In order to reach this reconnection, you must first reopen your third eye. The third eye is called "heaven eye" (tian yan, 天眼) (tian mu, 天目) in Daoist society. Once you have opened your third eye, you will be able to feel or sense the spiritual energy changes of the yin space. This is called "coherence of spirits" or "communication of spirit" (shen tong, 神通) and means "enlightened" since suddenly you are able to foresee, feel, and sense a lot of natural phenomenon that normal people cannot.

After making a spiritual connection with Nature, your spirit will be able to leave your physical body while your physical body is still alive. In Daoist society, when the third eye is reopened, the new spiritual baby (sheng ying, 聖嬰) is born. After that, it takes at least three years of nursing (san nian bu ru, 三年哺乳). That means the new baby must stay near the mother's body and receive its energy. After that, you will enter the final stage of "ten years of facing the wall" (shi nian mian bi, 十年面壁). That means it will take at least ten years of spiritual cultivation so your spirit can be separated from the mother's body without perishing. Therefore, this is a cleansing process for you to jump out of human emotional bondage. Only then can the spiritual baby grow up and become independent without the mother's body. When this happens, the spirit can decide to stay or leave. This spirit can survive in the yin space forever (eternal life) since you will have already known how to absorb the energy from Nature to keep the spirit alive. This is the stage of "Buddhahood" (Cheng Fo, 成佛) (Buddhist society) or "immortality" (cheng xian, 成仙) (Daoist society). This may be why those who have become enlightened and achieved Buddhahood or immortality seldom wrote down anything for later generations; they had jumped out of the human matrix and were no longer focused on mundane activities.

To reach the final stage of Buddhahood, you must first find and feel your spiritual center or residence that is located at the center of your head, the limbic system. This place is also where your subconscious mind is situated. Next, you must minimize the activities of your conscious mind, the human matrix. Only then will you be able to awaken your subconscious mind that is pure, innocent, and connected with your spirit. Since we humans created this emotional world (the human matrix), we have moved farther and farther away from the truthful spirit. We have become confused and emotionally trapped. Therefore, we have lost the root of the Dao and know less and less of the truth.

The *Yi Jing* (《易·繫辭上》) says: "The change is to change to: no thinking, no action, and quiet without moving. Through feeling and sensing, it is thus able to communicate with the universe (i.e., nature). If it is not from the extreme cultivation of spirit, how can one reach this?"[7]This means that when you are in a condition of no thinking and no action, then your subconscious mind will be in a state of higher alertness and awareness. Through feeling and sensing, you will be able to communicate with Nature and see the changes. Lie Zi (列子) said: "My body is harmonious with my heart (i.e., mind), my mind is in accord with my qi, my qi is concordant with my spirit, and my spirit is unified with nothingness. (In this case,) even if there is a very tiny matter or weak sound, though is so far as eight fields (i.e., long distance) or so close as next to my eyes, if they intrude, I will know."[8]

Gui Gu Zi (《鬼谷子·陰符》) said:

"Doing nothing to reach peace and quietness, (the qi in) the five internal organs and six bowels is transporting smoothly and harmoniously, and the essence and spirit are firmly staying at their centers without moving. In this case, I will be able to observe and listen to myself internally, to condense my spirit and stabilize my will, to meditate and ponder on the grand insubstantial (i.e., spiritual world), and wait for the spirit's passage to and fro. When this happens, I will be able to observe Nature's opening and closing (i.e., actions) and become acquainted with the creation and derivation of myriad objects, comprehend the beginning and the ending of the yin and yang changes, and understand the rules and routines of human affairs. Thus, I can 'know the world without leaving my house and see the Heaven Dao (i.e., Nature) without peering through windows.'"[9]

Guan Zi (管子) said:

"If a person is able to keep himself righteous and calm, his skin is smooth and healthy, the functions of the ears

and eyes are clear, and the tendons are stretchable (i.e., have endurance) and bones are strong. In this case, he will be able to keep himself upright, his observation will be very clear, his thinking and behavior will be cautious, and thus his good deeds will be increased daily. When this happens, he will be able to know things in every corner of the world. If he also cultivates his essence and qi to an abundant level internally, then it is called: 'acquirement internally.' However, some people cannot reverse their path to reach these; this is because of their wrong life-style."[10]

Hui Nan Zi (《淮南子·精神訓》) said:

"If the blood and qi can be gathered in five internal organs without leaking, then all internal organs' blood and qi will be abundant and, thus, the addiction to the desires will be reduced. When these organs are abundant and healthily functioning, then the ears and eyes are clear and the vision and hearing can be unimpeded and reach far. When the ears and eyes are clear, it is called: clarity. Thus, if all five internal organs' qi circulation can be governed by the mind and not be aberrant, then the thinking and will can be in charge and, thus, the actions will not be chaotic. When the thinking and will are in charge and the actions are not disordered, then essence and spirit (i.e., the spirit of vitality) will be abundant and qi will not be dispersed. When essence and spirit are not dispersed, then the entire body is in order and functioning healthily. When the body is functioning healthily, then it is uniform and harmonious. When the body is uniform and harmonious, then the spirit can be raised. When the spirit is raised, there is nothing that cannot be seen, nothing that cannot be heard, and nothing that cannot be accomplished. Consequently, disaster cannot fall upon you, and evil qi cannot invade you."[11]

Conclusions

The procedures for reaching Buddhahood (Buddhist) (Cheng Fo, 成佛) or "spiritual immortality" (cheng xian, 成仙) through meditation are:

1. Self-recognition (zi shi, 自識). Drop the mask on your face, face yourself, and recognize who and what you are. Face the true you.
2. Self-awareness (zi jue, 自覺). Wake up your subconscious mind so you can be aware of your past, present, and possible future. You also analyze your life and ponder its meaning.
3. Self-awakening (zi xing/zi wu, 自醒/自悟). You have awakened and see clearly the mission or purpose of your life. You are sure that you want to jump out of the human matrix.
4. Freedom from spiritual bondage (zi tuo, 自脫). Set yourself free from the bondage of human dogmas and the matrix.
5. Unification of heaven and human (tian ren he yi, 天人合一). Reopen your third eye so your spirit is able to reconnect to the natural spirit.
6. Becoming Buddha or an immortal (cheng fo/cheng xian, 成佛/成仙). Cultivate your spirit until it can be independent without mother's body. This is the stage of eternal spiritual life.

1. 孔子曰："吾道一以貫之。"
2. 管子說："專于意，一于心，耳目端，知遠之證。""四體既正，血氣既靜，一意摶心，耳目不渾，雖遠若近。"（《心術下》）
3. 《禮記·中庸》："唯天下之至誠，為能盡其性；能盡其性，則能盡人之性；能盡人之性，則能盡物之性；能盡物之性，則可以贊天地之化育；可以贊天地之化育，則可以與天地參矣。"故"至誠之道，可以前知。""故至誠如神。"
4. 丁福保說："謂聖人性真自足，則智周萬物，無幽不鑒。故天下雖大，可不出戶而知；天道雖微，可不窺牖而見。以其私欲淨盡，而無一毫障蔽故也。"
5. 韓非說："越襄主學御于王于期，俄而與于期逐，三易馬而三后。襄主曰：'子之教我御，術未盡也？'對曰：'術已盡，用之則過也。凡御之所貴，馬體安于車，人心調于馬，而后可以進速致遠。今君后則欲逮臣，先則恐逮于臣。夫誘道爭遠，非先則后也；而先后心在于臣，上何以調于馬？此君之所以后也。'"

6. 丁福保說：“若夫人者，沈瞑利欲，向外馳求，以利令智昏，故去性日遠，情塵日厚，塵厚而心益暗。”

7. 《易‧繫辭上》：“易，無思也，無為也，寂然不動，感而遂通天下之故，非天下之至神，其孰能與于此？”

8. 列子說：“我體合于心，心合于氣，氣合于神，神合于無。其有介然之形，唯然之音，雖遠在八荒之外，近在眉睫之內，來干我者，我必知之。”（《仲尼》）

9. 《鬼谷子‧陰符》：“無為而求安靜，五臟和通六腑，精神魂魄固守不動，乃能內視、反聽、定志，思之太虛，待神往來。以觀天地開闢，知萬物所造化，見陰陽之終始，原人事之政理，‘不出戶而知天下，不窺牖而見天道。’”

10. 管子說：“人能正靜，皮膚裕寬，耳目聰明，筋信而骨強，乃能載大圜，而履大方，鑒于大清、視于大明，敬慎無忒，日新其德，遍知天下，窮于四極。敬發其充，是謂內得。然而不反，此生之忒。”（《內業》）

11. 《淮南子‧精神訓》：“夫血氣能專于五臟而不外越，則胸腹充而嗜欲省矣。胸腹充而嗜欲省，則耳目清，視聽達矣。耳目清，視聽達，謂之明。五臟能屬于心而無乖，則教志勝而行不之僻矣。教志勝而行之不僻，則精神盛而氣不散矣。精神盛而氣不散，則理。理則均，均則通，通則神，神則以視無不見，以聽無不聞，以為無不成也。是故憂患不能入也，而邪氣不能襲。”

CHAPTER 48
Forgetting Knowledge—Maintaining the Dao
第四十八章
忘知—護道

為學日益，
　　　為『道』日損。
損之又損，
　　　以至於「無為」。
　　　「無為」而無不為。
取天下常以無事。
　　　及其有事，
　　　不足以取天下。

The more (knowledge) one learns, the more (desires) one increases
each day.
the more Dao one learns, the more (desires) one reduces each
day.
Reduces and more reduces,
till reaching the stage of wuwei (i.e., non-action).
When it has reached wuwei, then nothing cannot be accomplished.
The world is governed by constant noninterference.
If there are interferences,
then one is not qualified to govern the world.

General Interpretation

The more knowledge one acquires, the more he knows the methods to trick other people. The more he learns about the human matrix such as glory, dignity, pride, and misguided loyalty the more he will be confused and the more he will be trapped in the emotional bondage. Therefore, the more he learns and knows, the further away he is from the Dao.

If one learns about the Dao, follows it, and practices it, his attraction to human desires and emotions will be reduced each day. He Shang Gong (河上公) said: "Learning means the learning of politics, education, courtesy, music, etc. The more one learns, the more emotions, desires, and decorations (i.e., faking actions) will be increased each day. The Dao means the way of nature. When one follows the way of nature, all emotions, desires, and faking will be reduced."[1]

When one follows the Dao to a certain stage, one does not have to put any effort in it and emotions and desires are reduced until there is nothing to be reduced. He will has reached the stage of wuwei (無為) (doing nothing). When this happens, he will be able to accomplish anything without difficulty. Wang, Bi (王弼) said: "If there is doing, then there is a loss. Thus, when there is not doing, then nothing cannot be done."[2]

From this, you can see the learning of the Dao is from knowing, following, and practicing till one day all of the human emotions, desires, and faking are removed. This is the process of regulating. Once you practice to a stage where there is nothing to be regulated anymore, then you are following the Dao without even thinking about it. This is the stage of "regulating of no regulating" and means "wuwei" (doing nothing).

From this, you can see that if a ruler is able to follow the Dao till the stage where no regulating is necessary, then he does not have to do anything to rule the country since his examples have influenced the people. In this case, he will be ruling the country of no rulers. Therefore, he does not have to force or interfere in people's daily affairs to achieve his ruling. He is ruling without ruling. If there is too much interference, the peace and harmony of the country will be disturbed and become chaotic.

Mencius (孟子) said: "Those rulers who have acquired the Dao will receive abundant assistance while those who have lost the Dao will receive only very little help. When help is reduced to its minimum, even relatives will betray him. Those rulers with abundant assistance will have all the people in the country follow and obey him."[3] That means those rulers who rule the country with benevolence will receive support from the people while those rulers who tyrannize the people will be rebelled against even by their close relatives. Du, Guang-Ting (杜光庭) said:

> "If the ruler is doing nothing, there is nothing to be ruled in the country so all the people will have allegiance to him." "When there is nothing to be ruled, then the country will not be disturbed. When there is wuwei (i.e., doing nothing), people will be peaceful automatically." "When ruling the country without the Dao, then people will rebel and relatives abandon the ruler. Ruling the country with the Dao, people will have allegiance cheerfully. When there are rebellions and emigrations, then the country is dispersed, and when there is allegiance, then people are gathered happily. When people are gathering, the country will be peaceful and prosperous. When people are dispersed, then the country is empty and perishes." "Therefore, at the end of the Qin (秦) Dynasty, the laws were so strict and many were just like a net with frozen grease. People were crying and did not know what to do. Thus, the country dispersed and collapsed."[4]

Qigong Interpretation

This chapter talks about two things. First, in order to reach the stage of regulating of no regulating (wu tiao er tiao, 無調而調) (wuwei, 無為), you must first regulate until no regulating is necessary. Qigong practices include five fundamental regulating processes: regulating the body (tiao shen, 調身), regulating the breathing (tiao xi, 調息), regulating the mind (tiao xin, 調心), regulating the qi (tiao qi, 調氣), and regulating the spirit (tiao shen, 調神). For example, when you just begin to learn Five Animal Sports Qigong (Wu Qin Xi, 五禽戲), your mind pays attention to the physical movements with the coordination of stepping, relaxation, rooting, and balance. This is the stage of regulating the body. Once you have mastered the movements smoothly and harmoniously without the mind's attention, you are in the state of regulating without regulating. After that, you then regulate your breathing, emotional mind, qi, and, finally, spirit.

The most powerful qigong practice is to bring the training into your lifestyle. For example, once you have regulated your body to keep it upright, relaxed, and balanced, you will have established a habit to keep this body in the right posture all the time without thinking about it. This is the stage of wuwei.

Second, you maintain your body's healthy condition through a healthy lifestyle. For example, if you have already established a healthy lifestyle and go to bed a couple hours after sunset, then you have followed the Dao. However, if you frequently interfere in your daily routine with late night parties and alcohol, your body's qi will soon become chaotic and finally bring you sickness. When you have a healthy lifestyle, simply maintain it.

There are a few common purposes of qigong practice. The first one is to build up a habit of daily practice so that health can be maintained. The second is to condition the body so that health can be improved. For example, if you are losing strength in the legs, then you practice squatting qigong to recondition your legs. However, once you have established the daily routine, then you will be on the path of wuwei. The third is to treat special illnesses. For example, if you have liver qi deficiency or excess, then you learn special qigong to regulate the qi status of the liver. Once the liver's qi resumes its normal state, then you stop the daily routine and just practice it once in a while for maintenance. This is because some of the qigong for sickness is very aggressive. When you are sick, this kind of qigong practice serves the purpose, but when you are not sick, it can bring you more harm than help.

If you are interested in knowing more about the qigong five regulatings, please refer to the book: *The Root of Chinese Qigong*, by YMAA Publication Center.

Conclusions

The final goal of qigong practice is to reach the stage of regulating without regulating (wuwei). However, you need to regulate first until you have established a habit. Once you have established a good healthy routine, you should not interfere in this routine too often. Too much interference will just lead you to the unhealthy condition again.

1. 河上公說："學謂政教禮樂之學也。日益者，情欲文飾日以益多。道謂自然之道也，日損者，情欲文飾日以消損。"

2. 王弼說："有為則有所失，故無為乃無所不為也。"

3. 孟子說："得道者多助，失道者寡助。寡助之至，親戚叛之；多助之至，天下順之。"（《公孫丑下》）

4. 杜光庭說："無為無事，天下歸懷。""無事則天下不擾，無為則百姓自安。""為國失道，眾叛親離；為國以道，人必悅服。離叛則散，悅服則聚；聚則國泰而昌，散則國虛而亡。""所以秦之季年，法如秋察，網如凝脂，嗷嗷生民，無所措其手足，故土崩瓦解。"

CHAPTER 49
Trust in Virtue—Regulate the Mind
第四十九章
任德—調心

『聖人』常無心，
　　以百姓心為心。
善者吾善之，
　　不善者吾亦善之，
　　德善。
信者吾信之，
　　不信者吾亦信之，
　　德信。
『聖人』在天下，歙歙焉，
　　為天下渾其心，
　　百姓皆注其耳目。
　　『聖人』皆孩之。

Those sages never have a set mind,
  they regard people's mind as their mind.
Those who are good, I am good to them,
  and those who are not good, I am also good to them.
  This is the deed (i.e., virtue) of goodness.
Those who can be trusted, I trust them,
  and those who cannot be trusted, I also trust them.
  This is the deed (i.e., virtue) of honesty and trust.
Those sages in the world are cautious without bias,
  to teach the world to keep the mind innocent and simple,
  and people all pay attention to them with their ears and eyes.
  Those sages take care of all of them and make them innocent
  like children.

General Interpretation

Although those sages usually keep their mind in a neutral state of no desires, they are not selfish and still have a benevolent heart with concern for others. Wang, An-Shi (王安石) said: "The sages do not have xin (i.e., emotional mind); thus they don't think and don't act. Though, without thinking does not mean without thinking; and doing nothing does not mean without action. They share the fortune and misfortune with the people."[1] Dong, Si-Jing (董思靖) said: "Those sages do not think of themselves and their hearts are not allured by the objects (i.e., material attractions). So when the objects (i.e., situations) come, they just accord with them and follow them naturally."[2]

Since those sages have a benevolent heart and concern for others, they treat all people in the same manner. For those good people, they treat them well and for those bad people, they also treat them well. In this case, through their influences, they will be able to make all the people good. This is the manifestation of the Dao for goodness. He Shang Gong (河上公) said: "When people are good, sages treat them with goodness. However, for those people who are not good, sages will influence them and make them also good."[3] Not only that, those sages will trust those trustworthy people, but for those people who cannot be trusted, they also trust them. Again, through their influence, they will turn all the people trustworthy. He Shang Gong (河上公) also said: "When people are trustworthy, those sages will trust them. For those who are not to be trusted, those sages will influence them till they can be trustworthy."[4]

Those sage rulers are so careful about what they say and what they do, and treat everyone equally. In this case, all people will pay attention to them and follow them sincerely. Those sage rulers will treat and love their people like their own children and make them simple and innocent. Sages teach people by demonstrating their good deeds and the people are influenced automatically. There is a story in *Zhuang Zi* (《莊子·田子方》):

> "Tian, Zi-Fang (田子方) attended upon the lord of Wei (衛文侯), sitting next to him. He praised Xi, Gong (谿工) a few times. The lord asked: 'Is he your teacher?' Zi Fang

said: 'No. He is the person in my town. Because his speaking and doing follow the Dao, so I praise him.' The lord
asked: 'Then, don't you have any teacher?' Zi Fang said:
'Yes.' The lord ssked: 'Who is your teacher?' Zi Fang said:
'Dong Guo Shun Zi (東郭順子).' The lord said: 'But why
have you never praised him?' Zi Fang said: 'He is simple,
pure, and truthful, though his face looked normal like
others, but internally, the way he follows the Dao is insub-
stantially calm, and follows and protects myriad objects'
with genuine nature. His mind is so clear and distinct that
he is capable of comprehending myriad objects. When he
encounters those who don't follow the Dao, he just influences them with his righteous deeds till they comprehend
it and their evil thoughts vanish. I just don't know how to
use words to praise him.' After Zi Fang left, the lord felt
absentminded and lost, and went without speaking the
whole day."[5]

Song, Chang-Xing (宋常星):

"It is because of their inherited temperament that there
are many different varieties of cleanliness and turbidity.
Consequently, there are some good and some not good
and some trustful and some not trustful. Since there are
so many varieties, it is not easy to influence all of their
minds to become simple and innocent. Thus, those sages
are cautious and vigilant, and urgently try to influence
their mind to be simple and innocent."[6]

Since all sages have a concerned and benevolent heart, people will
pay attention to their actions and words, and follow and imitate their
deeds willingly. According to Kong Cong Zi (《孔叢子·抗志第十》): "The
king of Qi (齊王) said to Zi Si (子思): 'Sir, your reputation is so high in the
country so all the people in the country pay attention to you with their
ears and eyes.'"[7] Zi Si was Confucius' student. Zi Si was a good model
for others, so all the people liked to follow his words and actions by paying

attention to him with their ears and eyes. Su, Che (蘇轍) said: "Those who are good, evil, trustful, and hypocritical all believe they are right and criticize each other. However, sages will treat all of them the same way. So everyone's ears and eyes pay attention to see how those sages react to these various people. However, those sages treat everyone the same like babies (who act) without knowing what is like or dislike. Therefore, those good and trustworthy persons are not conceited and those who are not good will not be resentful. Thus, all of them relieve their tensions and, consequently, the country is stable and peaceful."[8]

Qigong Interpretation

In order to reach a high level of qigong practice, you must regulate your mind till your desires are eliminated and you are not allured by the temptations of the outside world. You should also keep your mind neutral, and be compassionate but not emotional. Thus, you will have a benevolent concern for other people's heart.

When you apply this attitude to the care of your body, you must love your body and treat the every part of the body as equally important. Often, people drink too much alcohol or eat too much spicy food that will trigger a liver problem. The entire body must be treated as a single harmonious unit. Proficient qigong practitioners always have a neutral mind to take care of the qi. When qi circulation is good, they maintain it, but when qi is aberrant, they correct it. Naturally, in order to have a sensitive feeling of the body, you must be able to feel it deeply. Building up this deep inner observation or feeling is very difficult. It is called "gongfu of internal vision" (nei shi gongfu, 內視功夫). The reason it is called gongfu is because it takes a lot of practice and patience to develop this inner feeling.

Conclusions

Build up an inner observation (feeling). Treat the entire body equally and take care of it like an infant. Establish a good lifestyle.

1. 王安石說：“聖人無心，故無思無為。雖然，無思也，未嘗不思，無為也未嘗不為，以‘吉凶與民同患故也’。

2. 董思靖說：“聖人無我，其心不滯于物，而物來順應。”

3. 河上公說：“百姓為善，聖人因而善之；百姓雖有不善，聖人化之使善也。”

4. 河上公說：“百姓為信，聖人因而信之；百姓為不信，聖人化之使信也。”

5. 《莊子·田子方》：“田子方侍坐衛文侯，數稱谿工。文侯曰：‘谿工。子之師耶？’子方曰：‘非也。無擇之里人也。稱道數當，故無擇稱之。’文侯曰：‘然則子無師耶？’子方曰：‘有。’曰：‘子之師誰耶？’子方曰：‘東郭順子’。文侯曰：‘然則夫子何未嘗稱之？’子方曰：‘其為人也真，人貌而天虛，緣而葆真；清而容物，物無道，正容以悟之，使人之意也消。無擇何足以稱之！’子方出，文侯儻然終日不語。”

6. 宋常星說：“只因稟受氣質，有清濁之不一，所以有善有不善，有信有不信，種種異樣，不能渾其心也。是以聖人在天下怵怵焉，急為天下渾其心。”

7. 《孔叢子·抗志第十》：“齊王謂子思曰；‘先生名高于海內，吐言則天下之士莫不屬耳目。’”

8. 蘇轍說：“天下之善惡信偽，各自是以相非，聖人則待之如一。彼方注其耳目，以觀聖人之予奪。而一以嬰兒遇之，無所喜嫉。是以善信者不矜，善惡者不慍，釋然皆化，而天下定矣。”

CHAPTER 50
Value Life—Nourish Life

第五十章
貴生—養生

出生入死。
　　生之徒，十有三；
　　死之徒，十有三。
人之生，
　　動之死地，亦十有三。
　　夫何故？
　　以其生生之厚。
蓋聞善攝生者，
　　陸行不遇兕虎，
　　入軍不被甲兵。
兕無所投其角，
　　虎無所措其爪，
　　兵無所容其刃。
夫何故？
　　以其無死地。

Coming into life and entering into death,
 three out of ten live from birth to adulthood,
 and three out of ten live from old age to death.
Among those who live to adulthood,
 three out of ten die early due to their manner of living (i.e., lifestyle).
 Why so?
 Because they feed their lives with too much excess.
It is heard that those who are good at cultivating life,
 traveling on land without encountering rhinos or tigers,
 entering an army without being harmed by weapons,
This is because rhinos have no place to gore their horns,
 tigers have no place to clasp their claws,
 and soldiers have no place to launch their weapons.
How so?
 Because they don't enter the places where death is caused.

General Interpretation

Coming means coming to life and entering implies entering into death. Han Fei Zi (《韓非·解老》) said: "Humans begin with birth and end with death. Thus, beginning means coming and ending is called entering. Thus, it is said: 'Coming into life and entering death.'"[1]

For every ten people born, only about three live to adulthood and three die early. Again, for those who live to adulthood, actually 30 percent of them will still die earlier than they should. The reason for this is because their lifestyles are poor; for example, they eat too much, lack exercise, consume too much alcohol, or smoke. Consequently, even though they should have a long life, it ends up a short life. The number ten was used as a logical result of having ten fingers for counting. Thus ten is considered a complete number. Dong, Si-Jing (董思靖) said:

> "Ten is the common complete number, and that is why it was commonly used. It is said that those developing from birth to maturity, whose qi is strengthening, are the growing group. Thirty percent of the population belongs to this group. Those who are old and entering into death, whose qi is returning to its beginning, are the dying group. Thirty percent of the population belong to this group. However, if those who are strong are restlessly engaging in actions and losing their righteous lifestyle, then they are abusing their strength, and all die due to too much action."[2]

Si, De-Qing (釋德清) said:

> "People in the world do not understand the natural law that the life of a life must be ended at the end. Thus, they worry too much about their lives and cause death. The reason why some die early is due to too much of concern for their lives. There are nine out of ten people like this. Those who do not belong to this kind are only one out of ten and people don't know how they do it. Actually the reason

some live long is because they know how to nourish and take care of their bodies and those who die early are addicted by desires and forget to take care of their bodies, allowing their fire of desire to go wild without restraint."[3]

However, those sages have already understood that coming and going are only the natural cycling process, and thus there is no emotional excitement or sadness for this natural occurrence. Zhuang Zi (莊子) said: "Those truthful persons (Zhen Ren, 真人) in ancient time were not cheerful for their birth and not fearful for their death. They were not happy for coming and did not reject entering; they just go and come naturally."[4] Daoists called themselves "truthful persons" (Zhen Ren, 真人) since they do not lie. They believe if they are not truthful, they will not be able to reopen the third eye. They also believe humans come and go just to borrow the physical body to learn and cultivate so the spirit can continue to grow.

Those people who know how to take care of their lives will not risk their lives getting involved in dangerous situations unless it is necessary. That is why they are able to avoid the chance of being killed.

Qigong Interpretation

This chapter advises that those who have not comprehended the theory of qigong should not rush in. Qigong is a time-consuming practice. The Chinese term "qigong" means "gongfu of qi." Gongfu means a pursuit or work that takes time to understand and practice to achieve a proficient level. Therefore, qigong means "the hard study and practice of qi."

Often we see that people do not take the time to understand qigong practices before beginning them, which ends up causing them problems. For example, small circulation meditation practice is one of the most dangerous qigong practices one can encounter. Many people who rush into practice without understanding or guidance from an experienced master end up with serious damage to the body.

There are two major categories of qigong practices, external elixir (wai dan, 外丹) and internal elixir (nei dan, 內丹). External elixir qigong practices are usually safer since they focus on physical stretching, massage, and exercises while internal elixir practices can be dangerous. Internal elixir qigong helps you build up an abundant storage of qi, which you can then control through the mind. Since there is a lot of qi that can be built up internally, if you don't have a clear understanding of theory and practice, you may lead the qi into the wrong path and your mind into fantasy. As we saw earlier, these phenomena are called "walking into the fire and entering into the devil" (zou huo ru mo, 走火入魔).

The safest qigong is learning how to be as soft, relaxed, and neutral minded as an infant so the qi can be circulate and distribute evenly and harmoniously by itself. Zhuang Zi (《莊子・庚桑楚》): "I asked you originally, 'Can you be like an infant?' Infants do not know why they move or where they go. The body is like a dried tree branch and the heart (i.e., mind) is like ashes. Like this, the calamity will not fall and the fortune will not arrive. If there is no calamity and fortune, where can the disaster come from?"[5]

From this, you can see as a qigong beginner, you should begin with simple and easy external elixir sets such as the Eight Pieces of Brocade (Ba Duan Jin, 八段錦) or The Five Animal Sports (Wu Qin Xi, 五禽戲). After you have acquired adequate experience from external elixir qigong practice, then you can step into the internal elixir. Naturally, you should first understand the theory and seek for a qualified and experienced teacher. Often, merely a couple of sentences from a teacher are better than wasting ten years trying to figure it out by yourself. The Chinese have a saying: "Teachers only show you the way. You are the one who has to walk."[6] For example, if you are lost someplace, all you need is to ask someone who knows the way to show you. Also another saying is: "Teachers only lead you to the door. You must enter and cultivate the contents by yourself."[7] This also means teachers only lead you to the entrance. Once you enter, it all depends on you to become proficient.

You should not risk your life with something you are not sure about. For example, if you don't know how to drive, don't drive on the freeway. If you don't know how to swim, don't go into the deep water. This is how you avoid dangers. A higher level of awareness and alertness is one of the goals of qigong practice.

Conclusions

Learn to take care of your body. Don't get into dangerous situations. Establish a healthy lifestyle until it has become a habit. Learn to keep your mind in a neutral state and avoid emotional disturbance. Seek the guidance of an experienced practitioner to avoid danger when studying internal qigong.

1. 《韓非·解老》："人始于生而卒于死,始之謂出,卒之謂入。故曰:'出生入死'。"
2. 董思靖說:"十乃成數,故舉為例。蓋謂自生至壯,乃氣之伸,生之徒也,于十分之中居其三焉。自老至死,乃氣之歸,死之徒也,于十分之中居其三焉。苟動失其正,則用壯從妄,皆動之死地矣。"
3. 釋德清說:"言世人不達生本無生之理,故但養形以貪生,盡為貪生以取死。是所以入于死者,皆出于生也,大約十分居其九;而不屬于生死者,唯有一焉,而人莫知也。生之徒者,養形壽考者也;死之徒者,汩欲忘形,火馳而不返者也。"
4. 莊子說:"古之真人,不知悅生,不知惡死;其出不訢(喜),其入不距;翛然而往,翛然而來而已矣。"（《大宗師》)
5. 《莊子·庚桑楚》："吾固告汝曰:'能兒子乎?'兒子動不知所為,行不知所之,身若槁木之枝,而心若死灰。若是者,禍亦不至,福亦不來。禍福無有,惡有人災也?"
6. "師父指明路,學生自走路。"
7. "師父引進門,修行在自身。"

CHAPTER 51

Nursing Virtue—Following Heaven

第五十一章
養德—順天

『道』生之,『德』畜之,
　　物形之,勢成之。
　　是以
　　萬物莫不尊『道』而貴『德』。
『道』之尊,『德』之貴,
　　夫莫之命而常自然。
故『道』生之,『德』畜之;
　　長之畜之;
　　亭之毒之;
　　養之覆之。
生而不有,
　　為而不恃,
　　長而不宰,
　　是謂玄『德』。

The Dao produces (all objects), the De raises them,
   objects are formed, and the (world's) environments are completed. Thus,
   the myriad objects respect the Dao and value the De.
The Dao is respected and the De is valued,
   because they don't interfere with life and always maintain it naturally.
Thus, the Dao produces them and the De raises them.
   Grows and develops;
   perfects and matures;
   nurtures and protects.
Producing but not possessing,
   acts but does not flaunt,
   grows them without dominating,
   This is called mystic virtue.

General Interpretation

From the first chapter, we know that we still don't know what the Dao is. We just know that the Dao creates all objects in this universe. When the Dao is manifested in actions, it is the De. From the De, all objects have an adequate environment to live and grow. So can we say the Dao is like God in Western society? All that the ancient Chinese philosophers know is that the Dao is the spirit of Nature. Then, what is the spirit? How do we define it? It remains a mystery.

After the Dao created all objects, it nourished and raised them with the De. So the Dao can be considered as the yin while the De, the manifestation of the Dao, can be considered as yang. With these yin and yang working together, lives are created and raised. Accordingly, all objects respect the Dao and appreciate the nourishment of the De.

Though the Dao gives birth to all objects and the De provides the best environment for them to grow, they have never claimed their ownership, dominated them, or flaunted them. This is how marvelous and great the Dao and the De are. Song, Chang-Xing (宋常星) said:

> "The Dao is shapeless and the De is traceless originally.
> The raising of objects is the application of the De. There
> is a Dao, then there is a De. There is a De then there is
> a development. All objects received from the Dao, is the
> De. When the De raises all objects, it is development. The
> myriad objects in this world will not be born without Dao
> and will not develop without De. What is development?
> It has the capability of moisturizing and nourishing so to
> assist the formalization of Nature. Thus, there is no limi-
> tation to the myriad developments. This is all because of
> the magnificent cultivation (of De). Consequently, every-
> thing can be accomplished. Thus, it is said: 'The De
> develops them.'"[1]

Wu, Cheng (吳澄) said: "Man's respect and nobility must be given by someone. For example, the heaven gives the respect to an emperor so he can be honored. The emperor gives nobility to the feudal lords so they can be valued. However, there is nothing that gives the Dao respect and the De nobility, but myriad objects will always respect and value them."[2]

Qigong Interpretation

Since humans are the products of the Dao and the De, we have become the copies of Nature. In Chinese qigong society, the nature (universe) that the Dao and the De have created and nourished is considered as "grand heaven and earth" (da tian di, 大天地) (grand nature) while the human is considered as "small heaven and earth" (xiao tian di, 小天地) (small nature). The human's spirit is the Dao while the behaviors are the De. A human being's thinking and behavior are called "Dao-De" (道德) and mean the moralities.

Even though we have not yet understood what the human spirit is, from Chinese qigong we already know that the spirit is related to our subconscious mind that resides in the limbic system of our brain. We have noted that from a qigong understanding, we have two minds, the conscious and subconscious minds. While the conscious mind dominates our thinking, is emotional, plays tricks, and is aggressive, our subconscious mind is natural, more truthful, soft, and gentle. From our conscious mind, the human matrix was created. However, our subconscious mind, through feeling, is still connected with Nature. Unfortunately, since we were born, our thinking and behavior have been dominated by the conscious mind and gradually we have lost our connection with Nature. Today, we have been separated from Nature by a long distance.

In order to reconnect with Nature, we must downplay our conscious mind and wake up our subconscious mind. From cultivation of our subconscious mind, we will be able to reconnect and return ourselves to Nature. Through embryonic breathing meditation (taixi jing zuo, 胎息静坐), we will be able to reach this goal.

Conclusions

We should subdue the activities of our conscious mind and allow the subconscious mind to wake up to be cultivated. Only then, will we be able to reconnect with Mother Nature and discover the meaning of our lives.

1. 宋常星說："道本無形，德本無跡。畜者，是德之用也。有此道，便有此德；有此德，便有此畜。物之得于道者，便是德；德之養于物者，便是畜。天地萬物非道而不生，非德而不畜。畜者，含蘊滋潤，輔翼陶成。飛潛動植，萬有不窮，皆是培植極厚，而無不遂者也。故曰：'德畜之'。"
2. 吳澄說："人之尊貴，必或命之。天子之尊，以上帝命之而后尊；諸侯之貴，天子命之而后貴。道尊德貴，則非有命之者，而萬物常自如此尊貴之也。"

CHAPTER 52

Returning to the Origin—Hold on to the Female

第五十二章
歸元—守雌

天下有始，
　　以為天下母。
既得其母，
　　以知其子；
既知其子，復守其母，
　　沒身不殆。
塞其兌，閉其門，
　　終身不勤。
開其兌，濟其事，
　　終身不救。
見小曰『明』，
　　守柔曰『強』。
用其光，復歸其明；
　　無遺身殃，
　　是為襲『常』。

There was a beginning in the universe
    that can be regarded as the mother of this universe.
Those who acquire the mother
    will also know her children.
Since (they) have already known her children, again return to
    guard the mother,
    (consequently, they will) live without danger their whole life.
Close the opening and shut the doors,
    live a whole life without toil.
Open the mouth and meddle in the affairs,
    then live a whole life without help.
Seeing detail is called clarity,
    holding on to the softness is called strength.
Using the light (i.e., soft strength of spirit), again return to clarity;
    leaving no disaster to the self.
    This is called practicing (truthful) routines.

General Interpretation

Where and how did the universe begin? Whatever produced the universe was the mother of this event. This mother was the Dao. He Shang Gong (河上公) said: "There was a Dao at the beginning. The Dao is the mother of myriad objects in the universe."[1] At the beginning, space was full of yin and yang energies (qi). Through interaction of these yin and yang energies, all objects were generated. After all objects were produced, these energies continued to nourish them and make them grow and become prosperous. These actions were the manifestation (the De) of the qi (or the Dao). Du, Guang-Ting (杜光庭) said: "Providing the qi is the beginning and then later giving the life is the mother. At the beginning, it is the interaction of yin and yang qi. This interaction has, thus, given birth to myriad objects. It has the De of nourishing and prospering and can be the mother of the universe."[2]

All objects are the children of the Dao (the mother). As humans, we were created in these interactions of yin and yang qi and received their nourishment (the De). From this, we can actually see we are the offspring of Nature. Therefore, we will be able to see the mother from observing ourselves (as her sons). Once we know ourselves, we should then return to protect our mother (qi of nature). Dong, Si-Jing (董思靖) said: "A human receives qi to live; qi is the mother. Essence resides in qi; thus the sons are produced. If one is able to keep guarding the mother, then the qi will be concentrated and the spirit will be peaceful."[3] This means that the qi is the origin of life. After birth, the essence of the physical life lives in the qi's nourishment. Thus, if you are able to protect the mother (qi), then you will be healthy and peaceful.

To protect your qi, you must first regulate your mind and keep your mind from outside allurements. You must also know how to control your emotions and desires. When this happens, the qi's circulation will not be aberrant and wasted. Huai Nan Zi (《淮南子·道應訓》): "If a king wants his kingdom to last long, then he must stop the people's openings."[4] "Openings" means the doors of desires: seeing, listening, tasting, smelling, and touching. That means if a king wants to rule the country effectively and keep the country peaceful and harmonious, he needs to keep people's minds simple, without emotional desires. This also implies that if the mind (the king) wants to keep its body (country) healthy and last long, it must first regulate its mind and stop the allurements that come from outside the body. You must also keep your mind in a state of simplicity and stop your desires and emotional turmoil. If you don't do this, you will damage your health and soon perish.

From qi point of view, if you understand how it is related to your life and comprehend how to manage your good and bad qi, then your mind is clear. In order to protect your qi (mother) so the qi can be stored at an abundant level, you must be strong internally and the qi must be led softly. Without this internal strength, you will become emotional with desires and allured by outside attractions. If you are able to regulate your mind until the point of no regulating in your daily life, then you have established a daily routine.

Zhang, Er-Qi (張爾岐) said:

> "This chapter is talking about comprehending the Dao. 'Beginning from mother' means the Dao. The sons mean myriad objects. Knowing the small (i.e., sons/myriad objects) and keeping the weakness (i.e,. softness) mean to guard the mother. Small and softness mean xi (希) (i.e., inaudible), yi (夷) (i.e., invisible), and wei (微) (i.e., fine formless). It is to describe the mystery of the Dao. When seen, it is invisible and implies small. If you are able to see the invisible, it means 'clarity.' To guard so that there is nothing to be guarded, means 'softness.' If you are able to guard this nothingness, it means 'strength.'"[5]

Wang, An-Shi (王安石) said:

> "When the light is used, the clarity can be returned. This light is the application of clarity and the clarity is the body (i.e., root or foundation) of the light. When talking about the strong, then it should be known that the softness is the body (i.e., root). When talking about clarity, then it should be known that the light is the application. Only

those who are able to use light to return to their root (i.e.,
clarity), throughout their entire life there will be no faults
and they will be able to harmonize with the Dao to achieve
longevity. Thus, it is said: 'Leave no disaster to the self.
This is called practicing (truthful) routines.'"[6]

This paragraph uses the light and clarity as an example. The light is
the application of clarity. When there is no light, there is no clarity that
can be seen. Lighting is to bring clarity; thus, the light is the application while clarity is the body. Similarily, strength is the application of
the softness while softness is the body. When your mind is strong, you
can lead the qi softly. However, if your mind is weak, the qi cannot be
led softly. Long-lasting health and longevity is from knowing the body
(softness) and also the applications (strength).

Qigong Interpretation

The Dao gives birth to all lives and the De is the manifestation of
the Dao that formalizes the world. The Dao is the spirit of Nature in the
yin dimension while the De is the material manifestation of the yang
dimension. When this concept is applied to a human body, the spirit is
the Dao that belongs to the yin dimension while the physical life is the
De that belongs to the yang dimension.

From the spirit, our lives are formed. In our lives, there are countless small lives that live within. These lives are cells and all cells have
their lifespan and require a specific amount of qi to live. For example,
the average lifespan of our skin cells is twenty-eight days. That means
all skin cells, after twenty-eight days, must be replaced. It is the same
for all other cells, though the lifecycles are different. This cell replace-
ment process is called "metabolism" and is the biochemical reaction
happening in the body so the new cells can be produced. From this,
you can see that the spirit (related to the mind) controls the entire body's
functioning and nourishes all cells with qi so they can survive.

In order to have a healthy life, your vital spirit must be high so it
can govern the body's energy and function effectively and efficiently.

That means you have to know the mother (spirit) and all the children (cells). Once you know their relationship and how much they affect each other, you then know how to build up a healthy lifestyle so the entire body can function smoothly.

One of the main keys of building a healthy lifestyle is to downplay your emotional mind and desires so you are not allured by the outside world. Once you have built up a healthy lifestyle, it is called "constancy." When your mind is clear of why and how to build a healthy lifestyle, it is called "clarity."

Conclusions

The spirit of our lives is the mother. From this mother, all cells will be nourished and functioning. To keep the body healthy and help it live long, you must stop all temptations generated from emotions and desires. This is called the clarity of your mind. Once you have built a healthy daily routine in your life, you will have health and longevity.

1. 河上公說："始有道也。道為天下萬物之母。"
2. 杜光庭說："資氣曰始，資生曰母。" "始者沖氣也，言此沖氣生成萬物，有茂養之德，可以為天下母。"
3. 董思靖說："人受氣以生，氣為母。精寓于氣，故為子。守母則氣專神安。"
4. 《淮南子·道應訓》："王者欲久持之，則塞民之兌。"
5. 張爾歧說："此章言體道之事。始于母，指道也。子萬物也。知小守弱，即守母也。小、柔即希、夷、微之意，形容道妙之辭。視而不可見者，小也；能見此不可見，是曰明。守之而無可守，柔也；能守此無可守，是曰強。"
6. 王安石說："用光復歸其明者，蓋光者明之用，明者光之體。言強則知柔之為體，言明則知光之為用。唯其能用其光，復歸其根，則終身不至于有咎，而能密合常久之道，故曰：'無遺身殃，是謂襲常。'"

CHAPTER 53
Increasing Evidence—Insubstantial Life

第五十三章
益証—虛世

使我介然有知，
　　行於大道，
　　唯施是畏。
大道甚夷。
　　而民好徑。
朝甚除，
　　田甚蕪，
　　倉甚虛；
　　服文綵，
　　帶利劍，
　　厭飲食。
財貨有餘，
　　是謂盜夸。
　　非道也哉！

Even if I have only a scrap of sense,
    like to walk on the Great Dao,
    only fear deviating from the path.
The Great Dao is smooth and plain,
    but people like the sidetracks.
While the courts are arrayed in luxurious splendor,
    the fields are barren,
    and the granaries are empty;
    officials wear embroidered clothes,
    carry sharp swords,
    overindulge themselves with food and drink.
They acquire excessive possessions,
    this is called robbery.
    This not the Dao!

General Interpretation

This chapter talks about stopping the temptation of the emotional desires and material enjoyments. All of these temptations will lead you away from the Dao. The path to the Dao is very simple and plain; however, most people like the excitement of life and this will take them away from the correct path.

One of the human emotions is selfishness. Those who have power and wealth will immerse themselves in the luxurious enjoyments and ignore those who are poor and need help. This is not the way of the Dao. Those sages will share whatever they have with others and feel natural and comfortable helping others. With this kind of benevolent heart, you will accumulate good deeds. When they see people also doing good things, they will check themselves if they are doing the same. However, when they see people are doing bad things, they will check themselves if they are also doing bad things. They will then be able to keep themselves on the correct path of the Dao. Xun Zi (荀子) said: "When seeing good deeds, take a sincere look at yourself. When seeing others' bad deeds, worry about how to conduct oneself. When I have done good deeds, I should make sure I continue to do them. When I have done bad deeds, I should despise myself and feel like disaster is going to fall upon me."[1]

Qigong Interpretation

When you are learning qigong, one of the most important elements is to keep yourself on the righteous path of the Dao. When you are on the right path, your mind will not feel guilty and uncomfortable. If you are on a wrong path, such as taking advantage of others, allowing yourself to be allured by desires, and being attracted by the material enjoyments, you will develop negative feelings that will lead you away from the path of the Dao. However, if you are able to keep your mind benevolent and neutral to help others, then you will build up good deeds. This good feeling within will make your spirit shine and your life enlightened.

Conclusions

There are two important things in qigong cultivation. One is keeping yourself on the righteous path so you are not allured by selfish emotions and desires. The other is having a benevolent heart so you can share what you have to help others. This will help you build good deeds.

---

1. 荀子說：「見善，修然必以自存也；見不善，愀然必以自省也；善在身，介然必以自好也；不善在身，菑然必以自惡也。」

CHAPTER 54

Cultivating Observation—Caring for Others

第五十四章
修觀—關心

善建者不拔，
　　善抱者不脫，
　　子孫以祭祀不輟。
修之於身，其『德』乃真；
　　修之於家，其『德』乃餘；
　　修之於鄉，其『德』乃長；
　　修之於邦，其『德』乃豐；
　　修之於天下，其『德』乃普。
故以身觀身，
　　以家觀家，
　　以鄉觀鄉，
　　以邦觀邦，
　　以天下觀天下。
吾何以知天下然哉？
以此。

Those well established cannot be uprooted,
    those things strongly held cannot be taken,
    the commemoration will be continued by the descendants
    forever.
Cultivate in yourself, the De (i.e., virtue) shall be true;
    cultivate in the family, the virtue shall be in surplus;
    cultivate in the home village, the virtue shall be lasting;
    cultivate in the nation, the virtue shall be prosperous;
    cultivate in the world, the virtue shall be universal (i.e.,
    harmonious).
Thus, observe other people with yourself,
    observe other families with your family,
    observe other villages with your home village,
    observe other nations with your nation,
    observe the world with your world.
From what do I know the world?
From this.

General Interpretation

Those who are good at cultivating their spirit and accumulating their good deeds by following the Dao will not uproot themselves and cannot be easily uprooted by others. They will not walk in the wrong path and no outside temptation will be able to allure their mind. He Shang Gong (河上公) said: "Establish means to build up. Those who are good at using the Dao to establish their lives or countries cannot be allured and uprooted (i.e., destroyed). Those who are good at using the Dao to embrace their spirit of vitality cannot be affected and separated (from the Dao)."[1] Fan, Ying-Yun (范應元) said: "Those who are good at establishing the De (i.e., deeds) will be so deep they cannot be uprooted. Those who are good at embracing the Dao will be so firm they cannot be allured."[2]

When those sages pass their philosophy of life to their offspring, their offspring will also follow the same path of the Dao and keep the family in the line. The next generations will then respect and worship their ancestors ceaselessly and thus last long. Han Fei Zi (韓非子) said: "As offspring, if he can comprehend the Dao, protect the imperial ancestral temple, and worship ancestors ceaselessly, this means endless worship."[3]

Those sages pass their way of life not only to their family but also to their villages. From there it will propagate to the country and then into the world. This is the way of the Dao. In *Li Ji* (《禮記・大學》), it is said:

> *"The great learning of the Dao is to pursue comprehension of the bright De (i.e., the manifestation of the Dao) and to influence other people until the ultimate goodness can be reached. Once you know, then your mind is steady without doubts. When the mind is steady, then you are able to acquire calmness. When you are calm, then you find peace. When you are at peace, then you are able to ponder. When you are able to ponder, then you gain. All objects have their initiation and ending and all matters have a beginning and expiration. If one knows the beginning and the end, then one is closer to the Dao."[4]*

The cultivation of the Dao is through learning. From cultivating good deeds, you can influence others until they are also good. Once you know this theory, your mind will be stable and this stable mind enables you to be calm. When you are calm, the mind is peaceful. When the mind is peaceful without disturbance or interference, you will be able to meditate and ponder deeply until you finally comprehend the meaning of the Dao. Song, Chang-Xing (宋常星) said: "Observe all people's bodies in the world as your own body, and observe your own body as all people's bodies in the world."[5] That means treat yourself and others the same without difference.

Often, if you put your mind into others' minds and your feeling into others' feelings, you will be able to see people's intentions and motivations. By observing others and analyzing the situation, you will be able to foresee the consequences. This can help you avoid future problems.

Qigong Interpretation

Cultivating your spirit is not an easy task. To be successful, you must have a strong will, perseverance, confidence, and patience. Only if you have firmly established these foundations will you not be influenced by others or allured by outside temptations. If you are influenced and allured by excitement and enjoyment, your spiritual cultivation will be held pulled back or even uprooted. The Chinese have a saying: "Learning is just like rowing a boat up stream: if not forward, it will be backward."[6]

Next, you should know that the best way of learning is through teaching others. There are two most common ways to teach others: through speaking or by example. Between these two, showing good examples is the most effective both for your own cultivation and for teaching. In order to show a good example to others, you must first cultivate yourself until you are in the stage of regulating of no regulating. Additionally, if people learn from observing your deeds and follow your manners, they will learn deeply in their hearts by themselves. This is more powerful and effective than teaching by speaking. The more you share, the more you learn. The Chinese have another saying, "Teaching and learning help each other to gain."[7]

Conclusions

To be successful in your qigong spiritual cultivation, you must have a firm mind that cannot be moved. Next, the best way of learning is being concerned for others and influencing them. Setting a good example is the best way of teaching. The Chinese have yet another saying: "To put yourself into other people's position."[8] That means to empathize with others. In this case, you will have a benevolent heart. This is a crucial key to reaching the Dao.

1. 河上公說："建，立也。善以道立身立國者，不可得引而拔也。善以道抱精神者，終不可拔引解脫。"
2. 范應元說："善建德者，深而不拔；善抱道者，固而不脫。"
3. 韓非說："為人子孫者，體此道以守宗廟，不滅之謂祭祀不絕。"
4. 《禮記·大學》："大學之道，在明明德，在親民，在止於至善。知止而后有定，定而后能靜，靜而后能安，安而后能慮，慮而后能得。物有本末，事有始終，知所先后，則近道也。"
5. 宋常星說："觀天下眾人之身，如自己之一身；觀自己之一身，即是天下眾人之身。"
6. "學如逆水行舟，不進則退。"
7. "教學相長。"
8. "推己及人。"

CHAPTER 55

Mysterious Talisman—Return to Childhood

第五十五章

玄符—返童

含『德』之厚，
　　比於赤子。
毒蟲不螫，
　　猛獸不據，
　　攫鳥不搏。
骨弱筋柔而握固。
　　未知牝牡之合而朘作，
　　精之至也。
終日號而不嗄，
　　和之至也。
知和曰『常』，知『常』曰『明』。
益生曰祥，
　　心使氣曰強。
物壯則老，謂之不『道』。
　　不『道』早已。

Those who contain the De (i.e., virtue) profoundly,
  are like newborn infants.
Poisonous insects do not sting them,
  ferocious beasts do not pounce upon them,
  predatory birds do not swoop down on them.
Their bones are pliable and their tendons are soft, but with a firm
  holding (of qi).
  They do not know of sexual union, but are able to manifest
  arousal,
  this is because their essence is at its optimum.
They may cry the whole day without being hoarse,
  this is because of an optimum of harmony.
Knowing to accord with harmony means constancy and knowing
  constancy means clarity.
Excessively increasing the lifespan is called inauspicious,
  the mind is aggressive when it overuses the qi.
When things are overstrengthened (i.e., overdone), then they grow
  old (i.e., degenerate) rapidly, this means they are contrary to the
  Dao.
  Not with the Dao, then soon perish.

General Interpretation

Those who have accumulated deep and profound deeds act as infants. They are so innocent and naïve they will not bring any harm to others. Thus, others will not harm them either. Wang, Bi (王弼) said: "Those infants do not have demands and desires, do not infringe upon other beings. Thus, poisonous insects will not infringe upon them either."[1] Since infants are so innocent without emotional demands or desires, they don't have ambitions or the intention to fulfill desires. They are pure and simple without knowing how to infringe upon other beings; thus, other beings will not disturb them either.

Although infants are soft and tender, and have pliable bones, their qi is abundant and firm. Therefore, even if they don't have sexual desire, their penises will raise automatically. He Shang Gong (河上公) said: "Infants do not know the intercourse of male and female; thus, yin is strong and furious. This is caused from abundant calm qi (i.e., yin qi)."[2] Infants have an abundant qi. When qi is manifested externally, they are active, and when qi is manifested internally, since there is no loss from sexual intercourse, their penises will raise automatically without them knowing it. Not only that, they can cry the whole day without being hoarse since their qi is harmonious. Wu, Cheng (吳澄) said: "The (infants') physical shape (i.e., physical body) is not yet completed, but the qi is condensed. The emotions are not touched yet, but the qi will respond automatically. This is because of the ultimate purification of essence and qi. (They can) cry long, but the qi is not harmed (i.e., reduced). This is because they are able to regulate the qi adequately to a harmonious state."[3]

Thus, those who follow the Dao will bring themselves to the infant stage so they are able to accord with the Dao. Then it can be said that they have known constancy and clarity. Pang, Ming (龐明) said: "If a person's cultivation in Dao and De (i.e., moralities) is very high and carries the infant's heart, then his human nature has accorded with the Dao. Consequently, his qi will be communicative with the qi of the Great Nature and receive abundant nourishment. In this case, his original qi in the body will be abundant and reach the stage of 'optimum of essence' and 'optimum of harmony.' These kinds of people will have a high exuberant vitality and acquire more wisdom and talent than normal people."[4] He Shang Gong (河上公) said: "If a person is able to know that the softness and weakness of harmonious qi is very beneficial to humans, then he knows the constancy of the Dao." "When a person is able to know the constancy of the Dao and always do it, then he will gain clarity daily and finally reach the mysterious truth of the Dao."[5]

Trying to increase lifespan irrationally with excess efforts will only cause the body to weaken faster. The growth of nature is a gradual process. If you push it too fast, the result can be reversed. In addition, the qi's circulation in the body is soft and smooth, and if you use your mind to abuse it aggressively, then the qi's circulation can be imbalanced and cause sickness. Su, Che (蘇轍) said: "If a person, in order to increase their lifespan, consumes too much qi so the qi is unable to follow Nature, though he is getting stronger daily, aging will follow. In this case, he has lost his human nature as an infant (i.e., pure heart of an infant which is in accord with the Dao)."[6]

There is a story in Zhuang Zi (《莊子·德充符》):

"Hui Zi (惠子) asked Zhuang Zi (莊子): 'Do humans have no emotions?' Zhuang Zi replied: 'Yes.' Hui Zi said: 'If humans do not have emotions, how can we call ourselves human?' Zhuang Zi said: 'The Dao gives us an outlook and the heaven gives us shape (i.e., physical body), so how can we say we are not human?' Hui Zi argued: 'Since you call us human, how can we be without emotions?' Zhuan Zi said: 'But this is not the same emotion that I am talking about. The 'no emotion' that I am talking about is the emotion not affected by good or evil that results in harming one's human nature. This is the emotion that always follows nature without adding anything else. Hui Zi asked: 'If there is no addition, how can we maintain our bodies?' Zhuang Zi answered: 'The Dao gives humans the outlook and the Heaven gives us shape. We should not bring harm to our human nature. Now, you expose your mind and spirit externally and waste your essence; lean on the tree to chant the poetry, and rest your head on the desk with eyes closed for napping. The nature offers a healthy shape (i.e., body) and you abuse it with 'hardness.' Still you proudly argue about your opinion!'"[7]

Qigong Interpretation

This chapter has pointed out a few important things about qigong practice. First, it has again emphasized the accumulation of good deeds and virtues. This will create in you a righteous, generous, peaceful, harmonious, and benevolent mind.

Second, it mentions that the key of keeping the qi at its residence (or center) is embracing singularity. This means to keep your mind at the lower real dan tian (center of gravity). When keeping the mind at the center, your mind is not actively leading the qi out of its residence. This practice is called "keep at singularity" (shou yi, 守一), "embracing singularity" (bao yi, 抱一), or "hold and firm" (wo gu, 握固). There are two ways of accumulating the qi to an abundant level. One is conserving the qi and the other is increasing it. However, even if you know how to increase the qi to a higher level, without knowing how to conserve it, the qi build up will be just wasted.

Third, you should not abuse your qi. Even if you know how to preserve your qi and keep it at the lower real dan tian, if you abuse your qi and your body, the qi will be depleted very quickly. For example, too much sexual activity (for males), too much alcohol, too much spices, and too much muscle development are some of the causes of abusing the body's qi.

Fourth, you must have a healthy routine. This routine is the constancy referred to in this chapter. If you can comprehend its benefits and effectiveness, then your mind is clear. Fan, Ying-Yuan (范應元) said:

> *"The Dao of life is doing nothing. How can we increase the lifespan? The integration of qi should be natural. How can we make it happen? Thus, Zhu Zhen Ren (朱真人) said: 'What is the Dao (in the body)? It is the qi (i.e., energy). The body of the Dao is insubstantial. What is insubstantial? It is to be natural. What is to be natural? It is wuwei. What is wuwei? It means the heart (i.e., mind) is not moved (i.e., touched). When the internal heart is not moving, then external phenomena (i.e., attraction)*

will not enter. When both internal and external are at peace and calm, then the spirit is steady and qi is harmonious. When spirit is steady and qi is harmonious, then the original qi will be righteous. When the original qi is righteous, then the qi in five organs will be smoothly circulated. When the qi circulation of the five organs is smooth, the essence and fluid are abundant. When essence and fluid are abundant, then there is no thinking of five tastes. When the five tastes are stopped, then there is no thirst and hunger. When there is no thirst and hunger, then the qi in three dan tians is full. When the qi in three dan tians is full, then marrow is stronger and bones are solid. Consequently, you can return your old to the original young. Cultivate like this, then you have accomplished the real Dao.' From this, how do we need to increase the lifespan?"[8]

Finally, I would like to offer a paragraph from Zhuang Zi (莊子) for you to ponder. Zhuang Zi (《莊子·在宥》) said:

"The refinement of reaching the Dao is deep and profound, vague and unconscious (i.e., a semisleeping state). The best way of approaching the Dao is with the subconscious and by being extremely calm. There is no seeing and no hearing; embrace the spirit with quietness, and the shape (i.e., physical body) will be righteous by itself. In order to be quiet, your mind must be clear; no over laboring of the physical body, and no losing of semen, then you can live long. When eyes see nothing, ears hear nothing, and the heart (i.e., mind) knows nothing, your spirit will guard your shape (i.e., physical body). Thus, the shape will live long. You must be careful of your thoughts internally and shut down the external temptations. Knowing too much is the cause of failure. In this case, you will be able to approach the great enlightenment and reach the origin of ultimate yang. You will also be able to enter

the door of the deep yin (dimension) and reach the origin of ultimate yin. There is a master of the world and there is a constancy of yin and yang's existence. If you cultivate your body carefully, you will be strong (spiritually and physically). I will embrace my spirit with calmness so I can unify and harmonize the essence, qi, and spirit. Thus, I can cultivate my body for one thousand and two hundred years and my shape is not weakening."[9]

In order to reconnect with the Great Nature, you must cut off all distractions from the material world. You must bring yourself to an extremely calm and quiet condition. When you reach this, you will be in a semisleeping state. In this state, the actions of your conscious mind have been downplayed to their minimum and the subconscious mind begins to wake up. It is known in qigong that your subconscious mind connects to your spirit. When the subconscious mind is awakened, through embracing and condensing your spirit to a certain level, your spirit and the natural spirit will be united into one (singularity). This is called "embracing singularity" (bao yi, 抱一) or "keep at singularity" (shou yi, 守一). Through feeling and sensing, you will be able to reach the natural spirit.

According to *The Book of Changes* (Yi Jing, 《易經》), there are two main dimensions coexisting in this universe. One is called "yang space" (yang jian, 陽間) (the De) and the other is "yin space" (yin jian, 陰間) (the Dao). Yang space is the material world while yin space is the spiritual world. It is understood that the energy and its manifestation in these two worlds must be balanced and harmonious with each other. Although there are two dimensions, actually it is two faces of the same body, the Dao and the De. The Dao is the origin and the force while the De is the manifestation of the Dao. If a person would like to be healthy and live long, he must cultivate his two lives, physical and spiritual. Though the physical life will perish at the end, the spiritual life can be eternal if you have cultivated your spirit to an independent stage. This is called "Buddhahood" (cheng Fo, 成佛) or "immortal" (cheng xian, 成仙).

Conclusions

Can you be as soft as a baby? Can you be as innocent and naïve as a baby? Can you be so pure and simple that you are without desires? Can your mind be neutral and not be allured by temptations? If you can, you have followed the Dao.

1. 王弼說："赤子無求無欲，不犯眾物，故毒蟲之物無犯之。"

2. 河上公說："赤子未知男女之合會，而陰作怒，由靜氣多之所致也。"

3. 吳澄說："形未完而氣自專，情未感而氣自應，由其精氣純一之極也。聲久費而氣不傷，由其和氣調適之甚也。"

4. 龐明說："如果人的道德修養很高，具備赤子之心，那麼他就從本性上與'道'相符，因而和大自然之氣相通，而獲其充分的供養。這樣，體內元氣充盈，就能達于'精之至'、'和之至'。這樣的人，一定是生機勃勃，并具備超乎常人的智能。"

5. 河上公說："人能知和氣之柔弱，有益于人者，則為知道之常也。""人能知道之常行，則日以明達于玄妙也。"

6. 蘇轍說："益生使氣，不能聽其自然，日于日剛強，而老從之，則失其赤子之性矣。"

7. 《莊子·德充符》："惠子謂莊子曰：'人固無情乎？'莊子曰：'然'。惠子曰：'人而無情，何以謂之人？'莊子曰：'道與之貌，天與之形，惡得不謂之人？'惠子曰：'既謂之人，惡得無情？'莊子曰：'是非吾所謂情也。吾所謂無情者，言人不以好惡內傷其身，常因自然而不益生也。'惠子曰：'不益生，何以有其身？'莊子曰：'道與之貌，天與之形，無以好惡內傷其身。今子外乎子之神，勞乎子之精，倚樹而吟，據槁梧而瞑；天選子之形，子以堅白鳴。'"

8. 范應元說："生道無為，豈可益之？沖氣自然，豈可使之？是以朱真人曰：'道者氣也。道體者，虛無也。虛無者，自然也。自然者，無為也。無為者，心不動也。內心不動，則外境不入；內外安靜，則神定氣和；神定氣和，則元氣自正；元氣自正，則五臟流通；五臟流通，則精液上應；精液上應，則不思五味；五味已絕，則飢渴不生；飢渴不生，則三田已盛；三田已盛，則髓堅骨實，返老還元。如此修養，則真道成矣。'以此證之，則何嘗益生？"

9. 《莊子·在宥》："至道之精，窈窈冥冥；至道之極，昏昏默默；無視無聽，抱神以靜，形將自正；必靜必清，無勞女形，無搖女精，乃可以長生。目無所見，耳無所聞，心無所知，女神將守形，形乃長生。慎女內，閉女外，多知為敗。我為女遂于大明之上矣，至彼至陽之原也；為女入于窈冥之門矣，至彼至陰之原也。天地有官，陰陽有藏，慎守女身，物將自壯。我守其一，以處其和；故我修身千二百歲矣，吾形未嘗衰。"

CHAPTER 56
Mysterious Virtue—Tranquility
第五十六章

玄德─坦然

知者不言，言者不知。
塞其兌，閉其門，
　　挫其銳，解其紛，
　　和其光，同其塵。
是謂『玄同』。
故不可得而親，
　　不可得而疏。
不可得而利，
　　不可得而害。
不可得而貴，
　　不可得而賤。
故為天下貴。

Those who know may not talk and those who talk may not know.
Close the mouth and shut the door,
blunt down the sharpness and untie the tangles,
harmonize the light (with others), and situate with dust.
This is called mystic unity.
This (i.e., mysterious virtue) cannot be acquired and become
    intimate,
      this cannot be acquired and become estranged,
This (i.e., mysterious virtue) cannot be acquired and be benefited,
      this (i.e., mysterious virtue) cannot be acquired and be harmed.
This (i.e., mysterious virtue) cannot be acquired and be valued,
      this cannot be acquired and be ignoble.
Therefore, they are honored by the world.

General Interpretation

Those who really know the Dao may not talk about it and those who do not know may talk a lot about it. Since the Dao is so great and mysterious, talking about it may just mislead listeners. It is better to shut the mouth, keep yourself at home, and continue to ponder it. Don't try to show how much you have understood, but continue to resolve confusion. Just be humble, hide your attainment, and humbly position yourself with the dust. Then you will be in accord with the Dao. According to *Zhuang Zi* (《莊子·外物》): "The purpose of a fish trap is to catch fish; after acquiring the fish, the trap is forgotten. The purpose of a rabbit trap is to catch rabbits; after acquiring the rabbit, the trap is forgotten. The purpose of a speaker is to transmit his meaning; once the meaning is transmitted, the words are forgotten."[1] The fish and rabbit traps are used to catch fish and rabbits. Once they are caught, traps are not important anymore. It is the same for speaking. The purpose of speaking is to pass the message. Once the message has been passed, the speaking is no longer important. For the same reason, the purpose of cultivating and regulating your nature is to reach final accordance with the Dao. Once the Dao is reached, all the cultivating and regulating processes will not be important anymore.

Those sages who follow the Dao are not governed by emotion and thus make no distinction between those close to or distant from them. It does not matter to them if someone or something can be beneficial of harmful to them. Furthermore, they do not care whether they are valued or degraded. Since they are neutral and selfless, they treat everyone the same. That's why people honor them. Su, Che (蘇轍) said:

"The object can be acquired and feel close, but it can also be acquired and feel distant. Some of what is acquired can be valuable, but some can also be degraded. Those who have comprehended the Dao will treat all myriad objects the same. Does it not matter what is close and what is distant? They will wait and see the consequences of those who follow or are against (the Dao). Who knows which one is beneficial or harmful? Without knowing glory or disgrace, does it not matter which ones are noble or ignoble? All the emotions and plots cannot approach them; thus they are honored by the world."[2]

That means that we don't know what the results will be in the future. Something seems close but, in fact, ends up distant. Something seems beneficial, but is actually harmful in the end. Some things seem attractive and noble, but the truth can be the reverse. All of these conditions are generated from emotions and desires. Since sages' minds are neutral and not affected or attracted by emotions and desires, they treat all objects and affairs the same way. For this reason, nothing is able to tempt them. Thus, they are valued and honored by the world. Si, De-Qing (釋德清) said: "This is because those sages, although they are living in the large domain (i.e., society), their hearts (i.e., minds) have seen through the external attractions of objects (i.e., the material world) and have not situated themselves in the middle of close or distant, benefit or harm, and noble or ignoble. This is why they are valued by the world."[3]

Qigong Interpretation

To many qigong practitioners, the final goal of spiritual cultivation is to reopen the third eye or heaven eye (tian yan, 天眼) so their spirit can reconnect with the natural spirit. This final goal of cultivation is called the unification of the heaven and human (tian ren he yi, 天人合一). Therefore, to them, the physical body is borrowed only temporarily for their spirits to learn, experience, and grow. After they have reached the goal, the physical body is no longer important and instead is useless.

Furthermore, they deeply realize that when you are trapped or suffering in certain situations, you learn more and get wiser. Whenever you make a mistake, once more you learn. The more mistakes you have made, the wiser you are. The more suffering you have undergone, the stronger you will be. The more failures, the more experience you have. Thus, qigong practitioners will not hesitate to face a challenge or suffering. They believe all the sense organs have a natural function and are to be used for learning instead of developing addiction to desire.

There is a saying in Chinese society: "When carrying the weight, you should carry the heavier weight. When climbing mountains, you should choose the higher mountains to climb."[4] This is because the more weight you carry, the stronger you will be, and the higher the mountain you climb, the greater challenge you will face. Ksitigarbha Buddha (地藏菩薩) said: "If I don't go to hell, who will? If hell is not empty, I swear that I will not become a Buddha."[5] That means if you are able to go to hell to help others so there are no more unfortunate persons in hell, then you have the heart of a Buddha. Sacrificing yourself for others is the best deed. Thus, serving people is an honor and an opportunity. This is the Dao of the benevolent heart.

Conclusions

Do not take mental and material enjoyment seriously. Knowing the meaning of life is not through personal enjoyment but from serving others; not for glory or honor, but for spiritual cultivation. If your goal is spiritual attainment, how can you become trapped in emotional desires?

1. 《莊子·外物》: "荃者所以在魚,得魚而忘荃;蹄者所以在兔,得兔而忘蹄;言者所以在意,得意而忘言。"
2. 蘇轍說: "凡物可得而親,則亦可得而疏;可得而貴,則亦可得而賤。體道者均覆萬物,孰為親疏?等觀順逆,孰為利害?不知榮辱,孰為貴賤?情計之所不及,此所以為天下貴也。"
3. 釋德清說: "以其聖人寄跡寰中,心超物表,不在親疏利害貴賤之間,此其所以為天下貴也。"
4. "挑擔要找重擔挑,爬山要找高山爬。"
5. 地藏菩薩曰: "我不入地獄,誰入地獄。地獄不空,誓不成佛!"

CHAPTER 57
Simplicity of Customs—Establishing a Model
第五十七章
淳風—楷模

以正治國，
　　　以奇用兵；
　　　以無事取天下。
吾何以知其然哉？
　　　以此：
天下多忌諱，而民彌貧；
　　　朝多利器，國家滋昏；
　　　人多伎巧，奇物滋起；
　　　法令滋彰，盜賊多有。
故『聖人』云：
　　　「我『無為』而民自化；
　　　我好靜而民自正；
　　　我無事而民自富；
　　　我無欲而民自樸。」

Govern a country with justice,
  deploy the military with surprise tactics,
  take the world with nonintervention.
How do I know this?
  By the following:
When there are more restrictions in the country, the poorer the
  people are;
  when there are more sharp weapons, the more chaotic the
  country is;
  when people are more clever and cunning, the more contriv-
  ances are created;
  when there are more rules and regulations, the more thieves
  and robbers have.
Therefore, those sages said:
  "Without my interference, people will transform themselves;
  I love peace and calm, and people will be righteous themselves;
  I do not intervene, and people will be prosperous themselves;
  I have no desires, and people will simplify themselves."

General Interpretation

A ruler can govern a country with justice and regulation and he can also deploy a powerful military with sophisticated strategies; however, all of these policies are not as good as not interfereing with the world. When the ruler does not interfere, the world will respect him and follow him willingly. Fan, Ying-Yuan (范應元) said: "Using justice to rule a country and using surprise tactics to deploy military force are not as good as taking the world with the Great Dao and without intervention."[1]

The reason for this is very simple. When a government has set up too many rules and regulations, people have less freedom and opportunities to find their own way to survive. However, if the government is calm, without interference, the people will follow righteous and prosperous paths by themselves. All a government should do is set up a good model without corruption, desires, and aggression. When this happens, people will follow the Dao and also make their lives simple without desires. He Shang Gong (河上公) said: "The world means whoever governs the world and the taboo means to guard and forbid. When the laws are superfluous and confusing, there will be cunning and when the bans are too many, then the people become fraudulent. These affect each other and result in poverty."[2]

Song, Chang-Xing (宋常星) said:

> "When a person has power, it is like he has a sharp weapon in his hands . . . When the ruler authorizes the power of his officials, they will use the power and over-execute the law even more than the ruler. Consequently, the rules and regulations, rewards, demotions, and promotions can be abused recklessly."[3]

He Shang Gong (河上公) said: "What people say about the rulers are those lords who govern hundreds of square miles, since they are cunning and smart, they will decorate the palace with carvings and paintings, carry engraved jewelry, and wear luxurious clothes. Strange objects are then created. The lower people will copy the top and also decorate their house with gold and jade and wear fancy and colorful clothes. Thus, this has become a fashion that grows fast daily."[4]

Wang, An-Shi (王安石) also said: "What the laws and rules are for is to ban those illegal things and deeds. It is, therefore, falsehoods that emerge. This is because when there are laws, the cunning thoughts and evil deeds are generated. When the orders are given, the deception begins. Thus, it is said: 'When the laws and regulations are widely carried out, the thieves and robbers are many.'"[5]

There is a story from the Chinese Han Dynasty (漢朝) (74–48 BCE) (《漢書·龔遂傳》):

> "After the Xuan emperor's (宣帝) accession, there were multiple robbery cases in the Bohai Sea (渤海) area. Local governors and officials could not catch the robbers and stop them from growing stronger. The prime minister recommended to the emperor that Minister Sui (遂) handle this case. Sui was already more than seventy years old at that time. The emperor summoned him and asked him to take over the case. Sui requested that he have complete authority to handle situations. The emperor agreed. When Sui arrived in the Bohai area, the local governor heard of the new minister's arrival; he came with soldiers to welcome him. However, Sui sent all of them back and gave an order to abolish all county officials' duties in handling the cases. Those who carried farm tools were good people and officials could not pursue them and question them. Those who carried weapons were robbers. Then, he traveled to his official residence by himself without escort. The county was peaceful with no signs of robbers."[6]

The Xuan emperor was the tenth one crowned in Han Dynasty.

There were a few emperors who ruled the country with the Dao. Yao (堯), Sun (舜), and Yu (禹) are the most well-known in Chinese history. Confucius (《論語·衛靈公》) said: "It was Sun who ruled the country without doing anything (wuwei, 無為). All he did was just face the south (i.e., reigned the country) himself with sincerity and righteousness."[7] According to tradition, the ancient ruler's seat in the palace court faced south. What this means is Sun simply showed himself to be a good model for people and people followed the model.

Qigong Interpretation

This is talking about regulating the mind. When you downplay the conscious mind, you can cease your emotional mind's activities and develop profound spiritual feeling through your subconscious mind. If you are able to follow your feeling and natural instinct from your subconscious mind, you will be in the state of doing nothing since you will take care of your body without putting too much effort into it. This is because once you have established daily routines and have reached the stage of "regulating of no regulating," you don't have to aggressively make it happen. This is the most powerful qigong practice, "doing of not doing."

Conclusions

The most powerful qigong practice is reaching the stage of "regulating of no regulating" (bu tiao er tiao, 不調而調). This is the stage of "wuwei" (doing nothing).

1. 范應元說："以正治國，以奇用兵，不若以大道無事而取天下也。"
2. 河上公說："天下謂人主也。忌諱者，防禁也。令煩則奸生，禁多則下詐。相殆故貧。"
3. 宋常星說："人之有權，如有利器在手一般，··· 君之權移于下，臣之權僭之于上，紀綱法度，行賞黜陟，皆可濫用，皆可以妄為也。"
4. 河上公說："人謂人君，百里諸侯也，多知技巧，謂刻畫宮觀，雕琢服章，奇物滋起。下則化上，飾金鏤玉，文繡彩色，日以滋甚。"
5. 王安石說："法令者，禁天下之非。因其禁非，所以起偽。蓋法出奸生，令下詐起。故曰：'法令滋彰，盜賊多有。'"

6. 《漢書·龔遂傳》：宣帝即位後，渤海一帶盜賊并起，郡守不能禽制。丞相御史荐龔遂。時遂已七十餘，上召見。遂請一切便宜從事，上許之。至渤海界，郡聞新太守至，發兵以迎，遂皆遣還，下令："屬縣一律廢除捕盜官吏。持農具者，皆為良民。官吏不得追問。持兵者乃盜賊也。"遂單車獨行至府，郡中安然，盜賊無影無蹤。

7. 《論語·衛靈公》："子曰：'無為而治者，其舜也歟？夫何為哉？恭正南面而已矣'。"

CHAPTER 58
Transform in Accordance to (the Dao)—Proper Living (Lenient Governing)
第五十八章
順化—正居（寬政）

其政悶悶，
　　其民淳淳；
其政察察，
　　其民缺缺。
禍兮，福之所倚，
　　福兮，禍兮所伏。
　　孰知其極？
　　其無正？
正復為奇，
　　善復為妖。
　　人之迷，其日固久。
是以『聖人』：
　　方而不割，
　　廉而不劌，
　　直而不肆，
　　光而不耀。

When the government is lackluster,
　　people are simple and genuine.
When the government is scrutinizing,
　　people are shrewd and crafty.
When there is a misfortune, fortune is next to it,
　　when there is a fortune, misfortune may hide beneath.
　　Who knows what is the ultimate end?
　　Isn't there a determined outcome?
When justice has become injustice,
　　goodness has become wicked.
　　People have been deluded for a long time.
Thus, those sages are:
　　Righteous, but without being scathing,
　　incorruptible without being harsh,
　　straightforward without being ruthless,
　　and brilliant without being dazzling.

General Interpretation

When a government governs its people with leniency, without too many laws, the people will become simple and honest. However, if a government is harsh and scrutinizing, then people will become cunning and guileful. Wang, An-Shi (王安石) said: "What is lackluster? It means there is no distinction. Because there is no distinction, people will not have desirous ideas. Therefore, people are simple and genuine."[1] This means when people do not compare themselves with others, their desires will be weak, and thus they will be simple, honest, and always appreciative of what they have. Wang, An-Shi (王安石) again said: "What is scrutinizing? It means there are distinctions. Because there are distinctions, people will not be innocent and without desires. Thus, people become cunning and fraudulent."[2] When people have comparisons and see differences, then desires are generated. When this happens, they become sneaky and tricky.

Who knows if, when there is bad luck, there will not be subsequent good luck? Or when there is good luck if there will be bad luck hidden behind it. Therefore, since we don't know the future, how will we know what is genuine good luck or bad luck? Since there is no method to decide or predict what is genuine good luck or bad luck, people become confused. Cheng, Yi-Ning (程以寧) said: "When superiors do it, the lower people follow. This influence will occur quickly. The Dao of Heaven always bounces back (i.e., every action has a consequence); there is nothing that doesn't return to itself."[3] This means when leaders favor something, the followers will copy and soon what the leaders favor becomes fashion. When this happens, the harmony and peace of society will be disturbed and disordered. Consequently, these disturbances and disorders will eventually cause problems for the leaders.

Han, Fei (韓非) said:

> "When a person has good luck, then wealth and grandeur arrive. When wealth and grandeur arrive, then there are fancy clothes and tasty food. When there are fancy clothes and tasty food, then pretension grows. When pretension grows, then bad habits are developed and righteous

principles are disregarded. When bad habits are devel-
oped, then people die wicked. When righteous principles
are disregarded, then there is an internal disaster of dying
young and no reputation of external success. This is a big
disaster and this disaster originated from good luck origi-
nally. Thus, it is said: 'when there is good fortune, misfor-
tune may hide beneath.'"[4]

Since ancient times, nobody has known what the real outcome
would be of anything that happened. Good luck may result in bad fortune and, conversely, bad luck may result in good fortune. We are all
confused about the future since there is no rule or principle that allows
us to see it or predict it. Han, Fei (韓非) said:

"All people wish to be wealthy, noble, and live long; how-
ever, there are some people who cannot avoid the misfor-
tune of being poor, lowly, and dying young. Though the
mind wishes to be wealthy and live long, it dies young
with poverty and lowliness. These are cases of unfulfilled
desire. Whoever has lost the path of their original desired
dream is called 'in delusion.' When deluded, they will not
be able to acquire what they wish for. Today, many people
cannot acquire what they wish for; thus, they are called
"deluded.' Since ancient times people cannot acquire
what they wished for; thus, it is said: 'People have been
deluded for a long time.'"[5]

Therefore, those sages will choose the center: not too strict or tough
and not too loose or soft. This is called "the Dao of moderation" (Zhong
Yong Zhi Dao, 中庸之道) or "The Dao of the center" (Zhong Zheng
Zhi Dao, 中正之道). Song, Chang-Xing (宋常星) said:

"The Dao of the center is the greatest foundation (i.e., guide-
line) of the world and the original root of myriad method-
ologies. Those who are cultivating the Dao are able to keep
themselves at the center; the Dao will always accommodate

them. Those who are governing the family, if acquiring the center; no family cannot be governed. Those who are ruling countries, if acquiring the center; no country cannot be ruled. The Dao of the center does not allow witty cunning and prevents personal desires from being generated. The principle of keeping at the center is not too excessive and not too deficient. Therefore, the reason those sages can be sages is because they are able to fulfill 'the Dao of the center.'"[6]

Qigong Interpretation

From a qigong point of view, the government referenced in this chapter refers to your mind's governing of the body's functions. Actually, this implies the importance of regulating your lifestyle and how to do so.

Lifestyle is the result of a repeated cycle of daily activities that become habitual. The accumulated effects of our lifestyle choices can lead us to become either healthier or sicker. For example, if you smoke or overconsume alcohol, your lungs and liver will have to bear an extra burden to manage the stresses tobacco and alcohol put on them. In time, you may have health problems. However, if you have a healthy lifestyle, you may not avoid such problems.

Health problems may be triggered by too much excitement or depression. The best way to maintain the body's function is to keep the mind and the qi's manifestation at the middle. Keep emotions at the neutral state so the qi's circulation is smooth and harmonious. However, if your mind is in an extreme emotional state, your qi circulation will be imbalanced. For example, if you are typically depressed or have chronic unexpressed feelings, you may develop an ulcer.

Therefore, as a qigong practitioner, you should always regulate your mind and keep it at the center. Since you are not governed by the emotional mind, you will be calm, peaceful, and clear thinking. This will provide you with a good state of mind from which to establish your moderate and healthy lifestyle and qigong practice routines. When you blend your qigong practice into your daily lifestyle to reach the stage of "regulating of no regulating" (wuwei), this is the most powerful qigong practice you can cultivate.

Conclusions

Keeping your mind in the neutral state is the key to regulating your emotional mind. Since we don't know the future and cannot foresee the consequences of our present actions, we should not sink into unnecessary emotional turmoil. If you can keep your mind in a neutral state, you will be able to see things more clearly, analyze situations calmly, and remain balanced.

1. 王安石說:"悶悶者,無所分別。唯其無所分別,則常使民無知欲,故其民淳淳。"
2. 王安石說:"察察者,有所分別也。有所分別,則民不能無知無欲,而常缺缺也。"
3. 程以寧說:"上行下效,捷如影響;天道好還,無往不復。"
4. 韓非(《解老》)說:"人有福則富貴至,富貴至則衣食美,衣食美則驕心生,驕心生則行邪僻動棄理。行邪僻則身死妖,動棄理則無成功。夫內有死夭之難,而外無成功之名者,大禍也。而禍本生于有福,故曰:'禍兮福之所伏。'"
5. 韓非(《解老》)說:"人莫不欲富貴全壽,而未有免于貧賤死夭之禍也。心欲富貴全壽,而今貧賤死夭,是不能至于其所欲至也。凡失其所欲之路妄行者之謂迷,迷則不能至于其所欲至矣。今眾人之不能至于其所欲至,故曰:'迷'。眾人之所以不能至于其所欲至也,自天地剖判以至于今,故曰:'人之迷也,其日故以久矣'。"
6. 宋常星說:"中正之道,是謂天下之大本,萬法之元宗也。修身者,得其中,道無不就。齊家者,得其中,家無不齊。治國者,得其中,國無不治。中正之道,不容機智之巧,不生人欲之私。中正之理,無太過,無不及。是故聖人之所以為聖者,只是全此中正之道也。"

CHAPTER 59

Guarding the Dao—Accumulating Good Deeds

第五十九章
守道—積德

治人，事天，
　　莫若嗇。
夫唯嗇，
　　是以早復。
　　早復，謂之重積德。
重積德則無不克。
　　無不克則莫知其極。
莫知其極，
　　可以有國（之母）。
有國之母，
　　可以長久。
是謂
深根固柢，
　　長生久視之道。

When governing people and serving heaven (i.e., Nature),
    there is nothing to do but to be frugal (i.e., conservative).
Because of frugality,
    thus, recovery to the origin will be sooner.
    Recover sooner, is called "accumulate good deeds."
If the accumulation of the De (i.e., deeds) is emphasized, then
    nothing cannot be subdued.
    Nothing cannot be subdued, then nothing is limited.
If there is no limitation,
    one can possess the sovereignty.
When there is possession of sovereignty,
    then the maternal leadership can be long lasting.
Thus,
a deep root with firm foundation,
    is the long lasting vision of longevity.

General Interpretation

You must know how to conserve your energy and protect your body when you govern people and serve Nature. If you know how to conserve your energy, you can recover soon and return to your original healthy state. Han, Fei (韓非) said:

> *"What the book (i.e., Dao De Jing) said about 'governing people' is when there are activities, (you) should know how to properly regulate between movement and stillness and do not waste too much energy in contemplation. What is said about 'serving the heaven' means to not exhaust your wisdom and deplete your knowledge. If you exhaust your wisdom and put all your effort (into all of these), then spirit will have too much of consumption (i.e., be wasted). When the spirit is consumed too much, the disaster of blindness, deafness, and craziness will fall upon you. Therefore, you should conserve. Conservation means loving your spirit of vitality and being frugal with your wisdom and knowledge."[1]*

We have often seen talented and knowledgeable people exhaust their energy and wisdom without knowing how to conserve it, and get sick or even die young. If you know how to conserve your energy, even though you consume some of it, you can soon recover your energy easily. This means you know how to protect your energy and body. If you know how to protect your body, then you have no limitations when it comes to accomplishing what you want to do. You will have a firm mind in governing your body. Your mind will be like a ruler who knows how to take care of the country.

The book *Lü's Spring and Autumn* (《呂氏春秋·情欲》) says: "Those ancients who acquired the Dao lived long and were able to enjoy sounds (i.e., music), colors (i.e., seeing), and taste for a long time. Why? It is because they know to control early (i.e., conserve). Knowing to control early so the essence was not exhausted."[2] This saying implies that if one knows how to control his sexual desires and conserve his qi, then he will have a long happy life. If one overindulges in sexual activities, he will soon be exhausted and die. Wu, Cheng (吳澄) said: "The shape (i.e., physical life) of a human is from receiving the qi of the heaven. Know how to govern and serve it so that life can be cultivated and nourished. If conserving, then what we have acquired will not be easily wasted; thus, there is no excessive consumption. This is the important technique of maintaining health and treasuring qi."[3]

Qigong Interpretation

When the mind governs and cultivates the qi to harmonize with Nature, what is most important is to cultivate your spirit and conserve your qi. When the spirit is cultivated and raised up to a high level, your spirit and qi will be able to unite with Nature. This is called "unification of the heaven and the human."[4] When you know how to conserve and protect your qi efficiently, then the qi can last long. With these two elements, spirit and qi, you will be able to handle unforeseen misfortunes easily.

In order to govern the qi so it can be manifested efficiently, you must have a calm and steady mind. That means your conscious mind (emotional mind) must be downplayed so it can be calm and not active. This will allow the subconscious mind residing at the limbic system (center of your head) to awaken. When this happens, you may reopen your third eye so your spirit can reconnect to the natural spirit.

As we have noted, in qigong society, the body is considered as a "small universe" (xiao tian di, 小天地). In the small universe, the mind is the equivalent of the Dao while the manifestation of the mind is the equivalent of the De. Once you have a strong spirit and abundant qi circulation, then you will be able to manage your body's health problems effectively. This is the manifestation of the Dao and thus is the De. Han, Fei (韓非) said: "When thinking and worry are calm, the De will not depart. When the conscious mind is empty, then harmonious qi will enter. Thus, it is said: 'emphasizing deeds' accumulation.'"[5] When your conscious mind is regulated with calmness and peace, your feeling in the subconscious mind will be enhanced. When this happens, the mind is in the insubstantial state and the harmonious qi will be developed. When harmonious qi is developed, the manifestation of the Dao will be significant. Dong, Si-Jing (董思靖) reports that Cheng, Yi-Chuan (程伊川) said: "The reason that (spiritual) cultivation is so attractive to people is because it can bring a long-lasting good blessing to a country (i.e., body) and normal laymen (i.e., qi) up to the level of a sage. When gongfu has reached this level, then there is a such response (i.e., consequence)."[6]

Cheng, Yi-Ning (程以寧) said:

> "The upper dan tian (上丹田), Ni Wang Gong (泥丸宮), is the residence of spirit (shen). This spirit is not the spirit after birth, but before birth. Lower dan tian (下丹田), shui jing gong (水精宮) (i.e., water and essence palace), is where the essence is stored. When the root of a tree is deep, it cannot be uprooted. For a human, when the essence is complete (i.e., preserved and protected), it means the root is deep. This is not the essence received after birth, but the essence of pre-birth. The middle dan tian (中丹田), huang ting gong (黃庭宮) (i.e., yellow yard palace) is where the qi is stored. When the flower pedicle is firm, the fruit produced will be firm and solid. For humans, when the qi is complete (i.e., abundant) means the pedicle is firmed. This is not because of the post-birth qi, but pre-birth qi. Thus, this is the Dao of deep root and firm pedicle, long vision of longevity."[7]

The upper dan tian is the brain (including the limbic system) and Ni Wan Gong (Mud Pill Palace) is at the center of the head, the limbic system. It is understood from qigong that Ni Wang Gong is the residence of the spirit (shen shi, 神室) and also where the subconscious mind developed. If you are able to lead the qi from the brain cells (conscious mind) to the center of the head, you may calm down the brain's activities, especially emotions. Thus the subconscious mind can be awakened. The subconscious mind is connected to the spirit via feeling. Shui Jing Gong (水精宮) (Water and Essence Palace) means the kidneys.

Some qigong practitioners in ancient times believed that the kidneys are the lower dan tian (xia dan tian, 下丹田) that stores the essence (jing, 精) of qi. From this essence, the qi can be developed. They also believed that Huang Ting Gong (黃庭宮) (Yellow Yard Palace) (center of gravity), the middle dan tian (zhong dan tian, 中丹田), is the dwelling place of qi (qi she, 氣舍). Therefore, if you are able to strengthen and firm your spirit and conserve the qi to an abundant level, then you have built a healthy root for your longevity. (Note: Actually, today it is understood more accurately that the kidneys store the original essence (yuan jing, 元精) and the guts (center of gravity) are the dwelling place of the qi (qi she, 氣舍).)

From this, you can see the spirit and qi are considered as the "mother" of your health and longevity. As a qigong practitioner, you should always keep this in mind; raise up your spirit and conserve your qi. Then, you will have a firm foundation of health and longevity.

Conclusions

The major keys of successful qigong practice are "conserving your essence and loving your qi."[8] When you have acquired these two keys, your spirit can be raised up to a high level. High spirit is one of the crucial keys of health and longevity.

1. 韓非說：“書之所為‘治人’者，適動靜之節，省思慮之費也。所謂‘事天’者，不極聰明之力，不盡智識之任。苟極盡則費神多，費神多則盲聾悖狂之禍至。是以嗇之。嗇之者，愛其精神，嗇其智識也。”
2. 《呂氏春秋‧情欲》：“古人之得道者，生以壽長，聲色滋味能久樂之，奚故？論早定也。論早定則知早嗇，知早嗇則精不竭也。”
3. 吳澄說：“人所成之形，天所受之氣。治、事，修之養之也。嗇，所入不輕出，所用不多耗也。留形惜氣要術也。”
4. “天人合一。”
5. 韓非（《解老》）說：“思慮靜，故德不去；孔竅虛，則和氣入。故曰：‘重積德’。”
6. 董思靖說：“程伊川曰：‘修養之所以引人，國祚之所以祈天永命，常人之至聖賢，皆工夫到這裡，則有此應矣。”
7. 程以寧說：“人身上丹田泥丸宮樓神也，非后天之神，乃先天之神也。下丹田水精宮藏精也。樹根深則不拔，人以精全為根深，非后天之精，乃先天之精也。中丹田黃庭宮藏氣也。花蒂固則堅實，人以氣全為固蒂，非后天之氣，乃先天之氣也。是謂深根蒂固長生久視之道。”
8. “惜精愛氣。”

CHAPTER 60

Harmonization—Positioned in the Right Place

第六十章
調和—居位

治大國，
　　若烹小鮮。
以『道』蒞天下，
　　其鬼不神；
非其鬼不神，
　　其神不傷人；
非其神不傷人，
　　『聖人』亦不傷人。
夫兩不相傷，
　　故『德』交歸焉。

To rule a big kingdom,
    is just like cooking small fish.
Using the Dao to (rule) the heaven and the earth (i.e., country),
    those evil doings will not rise up.
This is not because those evils cannot rise up,
    it is because the spirit (of the Dao) will not allow them to harm
    people.
This is not because the evil spirit cannot harm people,
    it is because those sage rulers also will not allow it to harm people.
Therefore, both (sage rulers and people) are not mutually harming
    each other,
    then "the De" (i.e., manifestation of the Dao) will be returned
    (i.e., harmonize) to each other.

General Interpretation

Small fish are not easy to cook. If you are not careful, it will become a mess. It is the same as ruling a big country. The kings or sages on the top must be careful. If they are not cautious, the country will become chaotic and disordered.

Han, Fei (韓非) said: "If workers change their jobs frequently, then the accomplishment will be lost. If leaders keep shifting their decisions, then the merits will be destroyed. If one person lost a half day of his work each day, then five persons' achievement will be lost in ten days. If there are one hundred thousand persons working and each lost a half day, then fifty thousand achievements will be lost. When there are more people, the more will be lost . . . When ruling a big kingdom while changing the laws frequently (i.e., stirring the fish), the people will suffer."[1]

However, if a king or sage rules a country with the Dao, then those evil deeds will not be performed. This is not because there is no evil. It is because the spirit of the Dao forbids evil from rising up. Additionally, if the spirit of the king or sage is not good and righteous, this evil spirit can still be harmful to the people. However, since those sages have a high level of spirit, evil deeds cannot be manifested.

Wu, Cheng (吳澄) said: "The King who has the Dao will use the Dao to rule the kingdom: simple and calm without disturbing people. Therefore, the atmosphere among people is peaceful which fills up two places (i.e., the heaven and the earth) that correspond with each other (harmoniously). In this case, the qi between the heaven and the earth will not become chaotic; consequently, the evil-doings will not be able to rise up."[2]

The book Li-Ji (《禮記・中庸》) also says: "When a country is growing prosperous, that must be a good sign (i.e., harmony); when a country is going to end, there must have been evildoing."[3]

When the king or sage has this good spirit, then the manifestation of the Dao (the De) can return to its origin.

Qigong Interpretation

Following the Dao (Nature) has always been the most important guideline for a qigong practitioner. When your mind (the king) is managing the qi (the people), you must follow the Dao carefully; otherwise, the qi circulation will be aberrant and chaotic. The mind is considered as yin and qi's manifestation is yang. That means the qi's behavior (the De, yang) is the manifestation of mind (the Dao, yin). If the mind is able to follow the Dao, the spirit will be calm, focused, and harmonious. Then the spirit and qi can be harmonized and unified. This is called "the unification of spirit and qi" in qigong practice.[4] This is also called "spirit and qi return to their root."[5] When this happens, the body's five yin organs' qi will return to their origin. This is called "five qi return to their origins."[6] Naturally, all sicknesses can be prevented. The five yin organs include: heart, lungs, liver, spleen, and kidneys.

Song, Chang-Xing (宋長星) said:

> *"Therefore, (if we) think that a human body is like a kingdom under the heaven and the earth (i.e., world), the mind (i.e., xin) is the master of the body and is just like the king of a kingdom. If the yin qi (i.e., evil qi or chaos qi) (commonly) extends (i.e., grows) without bending (i.e., yielding), then this is the Dao of the body's evil-doings. If (one is) able to recognize that the Dao (i.e., mind or spirit) is the root of the human temperament and the temperament is the origin of the mind, (one is) further able to use the Great Dao (大道) to establish the foundation of temperament and life, and use the spirit and qi to manage the variations of yin and yang, and thus prevent disaster before it happens. Ruling a kingdom (i.e., body) is then just like cooking small fish."[7]*

This means that in order to maintain the body's health, you must first harmonize your mind and qi. In order to have this harmony, you must have a peaceful mind that follows the natural Dao. Only then will the qi's circulation not be chaotic and cause problems. However, most important of all is your temperament, the foundation of your mind. If your temperament does not follow the Dao, then your mind will be disordered. The temperament is your human nature that is closely connected to your spirit. In order to reach a high level of spirit, you must follow the Dao and cultivate your temperament. All this cultivation is just like ruling a kingdom or cooking small fish; you must be careful and the mind should not be allured by external temptations, which are obstacles to cultivating the spirit.

Conclusions

Evil qi (xie qi, 邪氣) (imbalanced qi) always exists in the body. This is the way of the Dao. Whenever your mind has become disordered and chaotic, the evil qi will grow stronger. However, if the mind is able to be calm, peaceful, and govern the body's qi by following the Dao, then the evil qi will not rise up. Wu, Cheng (吳澄) said: "The reason that (the imbalanced qi) cannot harm a person is not because it is like that naturally. It is because the sage (i.e., the mind) is able to make the qi peaceful without damaging the (harmony of) the heaven and the earth's qi (i.e., the body). When the heaven and the earth's qi are peaceful and harmonious, there is no harm to the people."[8]

When we use the Great Dao to cultivate our mind, we should first cultivate our temperament. Consequently, our mind will be peaceful, calm, and harmonious. Whenever our mind is agitated by our emotions, our body's qi will be chaotic. Understanding this relationship and cultivating our temperament can set our spirit free from emotional bondage and thus contribute to a healthy and long life.

1. 韓非曰：“工人數變業則失其功，作者數搖徙則亡其功。一人之作，日亡半日，十日則亡五人之功矣。十萬人之作，日亡半日，十日則亡五萬人之功矣。然則其人彌眾，其虧彌大矣。···治大國數變法，則民苦之。”
2. 吳澄曰：“有道之主，以道臨蒞天下，簡靜而不擾其民，故民氣和平，充塞兩間，相為感應，而天地之氣，無或乖戾。故鬼不為靈怪興妖災也。”
3.《禮記·中庸》：“國家將興，必有禎祥；國家將亡，必有妖孽。”
4. “神氣相合。”
5. “神氣歸根。”

6. "五氣朝元。"

7. 宋長星曰："以是思人之有身,即如天下之有國;心為一身之主,即如皇王是一國之主。身中之陰氣伸而不屈,即是身中鬼神之道。果能認的道為性之本,性之心之源,以大道立性命之根基,以神氣施陰陽之造化,進大防危,未嘗不是烹小鮮而治大國也。"

8. 吳澄曰："所以不傷害人者,非自能如此也,以聖人能使民氣和平,不傷害天地之氣;天地之氣亦和平,而不傷人也。"

CHAPTER 61
Virtue of Humility—Lead Qi with Yi

第六十一章
謙德—意引

大國者下流，
　　　　天下之交，
　　　　天下之牝。
牝常以靜勝牡，
　　　　以靜天下。
故大國以下小國，
　　　　則取小國；
小國以下大國，
　　　　則取大國。
故或下以取，
　　　　或下而取。
大國不過欲兼畜人，
　　　　小國不過欲入事人。
夫兩者各得其所欲，
　　　　大者宜為下。

(If) a large country positions itself at the lowest stream,
  it will become the converging place of the world,
  (and) also be the female (i.e., mother) of the world.
The female always overcomes the male with serenity,
  (thus), is able to maintain serenity (i.e., peace) in the world.
Therefore, a large country wins over small countries,
  by placing itself below small countries.
Small countries win over a large country,
  by placing themselves under the large country.
Consequently, (a large country) positions itself in a low place to
  absorb (small countries),
  (small countries) position themselves in a low place to be
  subsumed (i.e., protected).
This is because a large country wants to protect others,
  while small countries want to join and serve (a large country)
  (i.e., be protected).
Thus, both receive what they wish.
  It is appropriate for a large country to position itself at the
  lower place.

General Interpretation

If a large country is able to be humble and treat other small countries with humility, all of the small countries will treat it as a leader of the world. In this case, the large country will be just like a mother taking care of and protecting children. Wang, Bi (王弼) said: "The male is usually restless, moving, aggressive, and anxious while the female usually maintains her serenity. Consequently, the female is able to win over the male. This is because (the female) is able to keep her serenity and also position herself in a lower position. Consequently, all things are going her way."[1]

If a large country positions itself in a low place, it will become a leader and protector of the world. Small countries will also position themselves at a lower place to serve the large country and be protected. Mencius (《孟子·梁惠王》) said: "A large (country) likes to serve small (countries) because it is happy to do so; (small countries) like to serve large (countries) because they are afraid. Those (large countries) happy to serve (small countries) will protect the world while those (small countries) fearful of (big countries) are able to secure their countries."[2]

From this, you can see that a large country should be humble and treat small countries with respect and kindness, thus becoming a leader and a mother of the world. At the same time, small countries should be humble and respectfully serve a large country. They will then be protected. It is said in *Li Ji* (《禮記·中庸》): "Those who rule countries of the world should have nine rules to follow: self-cultivation, respect the talented, love relatives, respect chancellors, sympathize with all officers, love people like their own children, attract various skillful experts, kindly treat those who come from afar, and placate the lords of all nations (i.e., treat all lords with generosity)."[3]

Qigong Interpretation

From a qigong point of view, a large country is the yi (意) (wisdom mind) that must be logical, wise, and calm. Small countries are just like the xin (心) (emotional mind) that is emotional and restless. In qigong society, yi (wisdom mind) is compared to a horse while xin (emotional mind) is compared to monkeys. Although a horse (wisdom mind) is calm and strong, it must respect and be concerned with the monkey's disturbed mind (emotional mind) so he is able to govern it. However, the emotional mind is chaotic, confused, and in need of the wisdom mind to guide and govern it. As you can see, the wisdom mind is serene like a female, calmly managing your body's functions.

In Chinese qigong, it is said: "Use your yi to lead the qi."[4] In order to lead, the yi must be low since qi is like water that can be led. That means the yi, though firm, is soft and gentle. In this case, not only the qi can be led, but also the xin can be governed.

Conclusions

To have a peaceful and harmonious country (body), everyone in the country (every portion of the body) must know his position and cooperate with others. The lord (the mind) must be sincere and humble to pay attention to the people (the body and qi).

1. 王弼說："雄躁動貪欲，雌常以靜，故能勝雄也。以其靜，復能為下，故物歸之也。"
2. 《孟子·梁惠王》："以大事小者，樂天者也；以小事大者，畏天者也。樂天者保天下，畏天者保其國。"
3. 《禮記·中庸》："凡為天下國家有九經，曰：修身也，尊賢也，親親也，敬大臣也，體群臣也，子庶民也，來百工也，柔遠人也，懷諸侯也。"
4. "以意引氣。"

CHAPTER 62
Practice Dao—Value Dao

第六十二章
為道—貴道

『道』者，萬物之奧。
　　善人之寶，
　　不善人之所保。
美言可以示尊，
　　美行可以加人；
　　人之不善，
　　何棄之有？
故立天子，置三公，
　　雖有拱璧，
　　以先駟馬，
　　不如坐進此『道』。
古之所以貴此『道』者何？
　　不曰：求以得，
　　有罪以免耶？
故為天下貴。

What is the Dao? It is the mystery concealed in myriad objects.
    It is the treasure of good people,
    and the sanctuary of bad people.
Admirable words are able to gain esteem,
    admirable deeds are able to receive respect;
    those bad people,
    how can they be abandoned?
Therefore, when crowning the emperor and installing the three
    ministers,
    though there are large jades offered,
    before four horses,
    none can be compared with the settlement of the Dao.
Why did the ancients value the Dao this much?
    Didn't they say: "Seek, and you will find,
    the sins of the guilty can be forgiven"?
Thus, (the Dao) is the treasure of the world.

General Interpretation

The Dao is vast and unlimited. It conceals everything in this universe. He Shang Gong (河上公) said: "Ao (奥) means conceal. The Dao conceals myriad objects in this universe, nothing cannot be contained."[1] Xiao, Tian-Shi (蕭天石) said:

"'The Dao conceals myriad objects.' This is just like the ancient saying: 'The Great Dao in this universe is shapeless, and (in a state of) quietness and solitude. It can be the master of myriad objects and does not wither with the four seasons.' It transcends this universe, independent, and goes beyond time and exists alone. It is able to protect everything and also support everything. It contains everything and is also far above everything. Therefore, myriad objects respect and obey nothing but the Dao."[2]

Those people who have done good deeds by following the Dao treasure the Dao as most precious. However, for those who have done bad deeds by not following the Dao, if they can learn to follow the Dao, the Dao can be a sanctuary for them.

Those who are praised and have done good deeds are always rewarded with esteem and respect. However, we should not abandon those who have done bad things. If we are able to lead them to the Dao, they can be changed into good persons and avoid sin. Wu, Cheng (吳澄) said: "'Value the Dao as most precious' means what is concealed within is precious. If good persons have gained the Dao, they will obtain these treasures. However, if bad persons have followed the Dao, their lives can be protected. Since ancient times, why has the Dao been valued as most precious? Isn't it because when good people value the Dao, they are able to receive what they want? Isn't it because when bad people have followed the Dao, they are able to prevent themselves from being sinful? Thus, the Dao is most precious to the world."[3]

To keep a country in order, an emperor is chosen and three ministers with different duties are assigned. These people are honored with big jade and precious horses; however, how can these compare with ordering the country according to the Dao?

In ancient times, people believed and valued the Dao because they knew if they looked for it, they would find it. They also understood that if those guilty persons were able to follow the Dao, all the bad deeds they have done can be forgiven. From this, we can see how the Dao can be so precious in this world. Xiao, Tian-Shi (蕭天石) said:

> *"The Dao, when asking for it, you acquire it. When you abandon it, you lose it. When you ask for happiness, you receive happiness. To those who are guilty, they can be absolved. Those who ask for happiness, acquire it, because they are seeking for it. Those guilty persons are exempted, because they get rid of bad deeds and are able to automatically neutralize into the Dao. In this case, how can they be guilty anymore? Therefore, it is said: 'Disaster is because I make it happen; happiness is because I seek for it. Fortune is because I am able to turn it around.' Chun Yang Zi (純陽子) said: 'My life depends on me not by heaven, my fortune depends on me not by divinity.' How true is this saying. This is why Lao Zi concluded this chapter with 'Thus, (the Dao) is the treasure of the world'"[4]*

Qigong Interpretation and Conclusions

The Dao treats all objects the same in this universe. However, whoever follows it will benefit. Even for those who didn't follow the Dao and have committed sinful deeds, if they can follow the Dao again, they can escape from their misfortune. For example, the body's qi circulation follows the sun, the moon, and the earth's natural timing (the Dao). According to Chinese medicine, our entire body's qi circulation and distribution all have a timing that has been set due to the influence of the sun, moon, and the earth. This influence is called "zi wu liu zhu."[5]. Zi (子) means "midnight," wu (午) means "noontime," and liu zhu (流注) means "the main qi flow." When we practice qigong, if we are able to follow this natural qi flow pattern (follow the Dao), then we can gain health due to improvement of the qi's circulation. But if we interfere in this natural qi flow pattern, we will become sick. However, if we have already been sick, when we are able to correct the mistakes and follow the Dao again, the body can heal rapidly. That's why it implies that, to those good people (healthy people), the Dao is supremely precious since it offers them health and longevity. To those who are bad (sick people), if they are able to correct their lifestyle and follow the Dao, the Dao can bring them back to health.

When people practice qigong, they often set up practice routines (installing ministers) and hope that through this effort, the body can be made healthy. In some ways this is true. Without these practices, the qi's circulation may become imbalanced (disorder of the country). However, the most powerful qigong practice is having a healthy lifestyle that follows the Dao. You should not wait until problems appear and then practice qigong. However, if you have already had problems with your health and can correct your poor lifestyle and follow a natural healthy lifestyle, you will be able to reestablish your health.

1. 河上公說：“奧，藏也。道為萬物之藏，無所不容也。”

2. 蕭天石說：“‘道者，萬物之奧’正古德所謂‘大道之天地，無形本寂寥；能為萬物主，不逐四時凋’者是。以其超宇宙而獨立，超時空而獨存；用能庇蔭一切又護持一切，涵蓋一切又超越一切。故萬物莫不唯道是尊，唯道是從也。”

3. 吳澄說：“貴此道，言萬物之奧；求以得，言善人之寶；罪以免，言不善人之所保。自古所以貴此道者，何也？豈不曰善人以此道為人所寶，得遂所求邪？不善人以此道保其身，免陷於罪邪？道所以為天下貴也。”

4. 蕭天石說：“斯道者，求則得之，捨則失之。求福得福，而有罪得免。求福得福者，自求多福也。有罪得免者，自去其不善，自化于道，何罪之有？故曰：‘禍自我作，福自我求，命自我立，運自我轉。’純陽子不云乎：‘我命由我不由天，我運由我不由神。’旨哉其言也。是以老子于本章結之曰：‘故為天下貴’。”

5. “子午流注。”

CHAPTER 63

Think of Beginning—Advance Gradually

第六十三章
恩始—漸進

為「無為」，
　　事「無事」，
　　味「無味」。
大小多少，
　　報怨以德。
圖難於其易，
　　為大於其細。
天下難事，必作於易；
　　天下大事，必作於細。
是以『聖人』終不為大，
　　故能成其大。
夫輕諾必寡信。
　　多易必多難。
是以『聖人』猶難之，
　　故終無難矣。

(The goals of pursuing the Dao are) to do things without doing,
   to conduct affairs without conducting,
   and to taste flavor without tasting.
Whether big or small, many or few,
   requite hate with kindness.
Handle the difficulty while it is still easy;
   manage the big while it is still small.
All difficult tasks in the world must begin while it is still easy.
   All great achievement in the world must begin while it is still
   small.
Thus, those sages never strive for greatness and,
   therefore, achieve greatness.
Those who make a promise easily are surely seldom trusted.
   Taking matters lightly will surely result in more difficulty.
Therefore, those sages always see difficulties when it seems easy,
   thus, they never have difficulties.

General Interpretation

The Nature has always developed gradually. For those who are cultivating the Dao, the final goal is "doing without doing" (wuwei, 無為). However, to reach this level, you must begin with the easy and small. Only after you are able to take care of easy and small matters should you then gradually advance into more difficult and bigger matters.

Keep your mind gentle, kind, and generous. This is the first step in cultivating your temperament. It does not matter how big or small the offence; you should treat them equally, with kindness and fairness. There will then be no enmity and no disturbance of your peaceful and harmonious mind. Song, Chang-Xing (宋常星) said:

> *"(We should) follow Nature (i.e., the Dao) without insisting on our own opinion, correspond to the event with feeling, and have no concern for the self (i.e., no bias or selfishness). However, even if there are some complaints about me, big or small, many or few, which cause people's resentments, since these resentments are from the people, how can I have resentment myself? If I also have resentment about others and find the way to repay the coming resentment equally, then, the big and small thoughts will be merged and more or few self-opinions will be generated. In this case, those resentments that fall upon me will not cease and my thought of revenge will not end. Then, it is not only others fault, but also my fault. Only if we ignore those resentments falling upon us and don't payback the resentment . . . I will be able to influence others and finally there will be no problems. Therefore, it is said: 'It does not matter if it is big or small, many or few; just repay the resentment with good virtue.'"[1]*

You should not give your promise easily without profound consideration. With every initiation of an event, there is a consequence. If you are not able to fulfill your promise, then you have lost others' trust. It is the same when someone makes his promise too easily without thinking it over. Very often, this promise cannot be trusted. After a few untrustworthy promises, you will eventually not be able to trust this person anymore. Song, Chang-Xing (宋常星) said: "For example, if those shallow people (i.e., people who do not think deeply) who talk carelessly, whose mind is not firm, just brag about their capabilities, and give promises lightly and, in the end, cannot fulfill their promises, with their actions not matching their words, and there is no result from what they said, they will receive little trust from others."[2]

Next, in order to achieve a great task, you must begin with the fundamentals. You must think deeply and plan far ahead so you can foresee the future. Often, those who do not see far and make promises easily cannot be trusted. Those who do not take matters seriously at the beginning may end up with a huge disaster at the end. Confucius said: "If a person does not think into the distance, he will soon encounter worry."[3] This means it is necessary to have forethought and precaution. When you see far and plan ahead, you will not worry about the present since you will have already prepared for what obstacles you may encounter.

Han Fei (韓非) said:

> "Bian Que (扁鵲) (a famous doctor in ancient times) came to see Cai Huan Gong (蔡桓公) (a lord of Cai). He stood there for a while. Then Bian Que said: 'You are sick. It shows on your skin. If you don't treat it, I am afraid it will get more serious.' Huan Gong said: 'I am not sick.' After Bian Que left, Huan Gong said: 'Those doctors like to treat those without sickness and receive credit.' After ten days, Bian Que again saw Huan Gong: 'Your sickness has entered from the skin into the muscles. If you don't treat it, it will go deeper.' Huan Gong did not respond. After Bian Que left, Huan Gong was again not happy. After another ten days, when Bian Que saw Huan Gong, he turned his back and left quickly. Huan Gong sent someone to ask him the reason. Bian Que said: 'When the sickness showed on the skin, herbs could have treated it. When the sickness showed in the muscles, acupuncture

could have treated it. When the sickness reached the intestines and stomach, the internal fire was initiated. When the sickness reached the marrow, it was hopeless to save his life. Now, I cannot do anything to help since the sickness has reached the marrow. This is why I did not ask him to undergo further treatment.' After five more days, Huan Gong experienced serious bodily pain. He sent people to look for Bian Que, but it was in vain since Bian Que had already escaped to Qin. Finally, Huan Gong died."[4]

Those sages always think far ahead, plan far ahead, and treat matter seriously and cautiously. Since all difficulties are seen, predicted, and prepared for, the sages can avoid them. Song, Chang-Xing (宋常星) said:

"When an affair is about to happen, I don't think about it before, nor worry about it at the beginning or the end, without knowing the seriousness of the problem, and not gauging how it can be accomplished. I just think there is nothing I cannot do and there is no time restraint for what I want. I use multiple minds, ignorant, shallow, uneasy thinking, without knowing the possibility of success. This will result in the possibility becoming an impossibility. Often that which can be accomplished has become unobtainable. That which was easy will change and become difficult."[5]

Qigong Interpretation

This chapter has pointed out three important concepts of qigong practice. First, the final goal of qigong practice is to reach the stage of "wuwei" (無為) (doing nothing). This means the "regulating of no regulating" in qigong practice.[6] When you practice qigong to a certain level and it has become a daily routine, a part of your lifestyle, you will practice it without even knowing it. For example, if you sit too often and too long in front of a computer, you commonly will develop a deformed torso. Your torso becomes curved and the neck stretches forward. This is very harmful since the qi can be trapped at the front chest area and can trigger heart problems and cause the heart to be on fire. Furthermore, due to the trapping or stagnation of qi in the front chest area, smooth breathing can become hindered and cause sickness such as asthma or other breathing difficulties. In addition, due to the constant forward stretching of the neck, the qi and blood circulation from the torso to the head will be stagnant. Naturally, this will affect your brain's normal functions as well. Once you know what problems you have, you can begin to practice qigong to correct them. After you have practiced for a long time and a new healthy habit has been established, you won't have to use your mind to make it happen. This is called "regulating of no regulating." When you have reached this stage, you will have a more powerful qigong solution for your problem. That means you will practice qigong subconsciously. This is the final goal of qigong practice. Huang, Shang (黃裳) said: "When gong (i.e., qigong) has been practiced to a stage that your insubstantiality (i.e., subconscious mind) has harmonized with the Dao (i.e., become natural), it is the stage of 'doing of not doing'; following Nature and dealing with the matter without dealing with it. Since it is so insipid (i.e., plain, common, and natural), and is nothing exciting, how can we have taste (i.e., special feeling, excitement, or effort) at this stage?"[7]

Second, in order to reach the final goal of "regulating of no regulating," you must begin with a simple and easy practice. Only after you have mastered the basic skills should you then step into the more difficult ones. For example, if you use qigong exercises to condition your physical body, since your body cannot be rapidly conditioned, you must be patient and take it easy, advancing slowly and gradually. If you push yourself too fast, you will cause injury.

Third, before your get involved in qigong practice, you must know your problem or goal. You must know the theory behind the practice, you must know your body, you must analyze your capability, and you must determine how much time it will take to reach the goal. You also need to set up a plan so you can reach the stage of "regulating of no regulating." For example, if you want to practice qigong for breast cancer prevention or even treat it, you must first recognize and analyze the problem (what), why these qigong practices will help (why), and the methods of practice (how). Once you have these clearly in mind, you may set up the plan. As we all know, we are lazy. At the beginning of any project, we often get excited. However, once the honeymoon period is over, we become lazy and finally quit. If you have a plan and set up a rule and routine, then you must place a whip behind you to achieve your plan. For example, you may set up a rule that when evening TV news is on, instead of sitting down, you begin to swing your arms while you are watching. When the news is over, you stop and you have already practiced thirty minutes.

A wise person will know himself and find the way to conquer himself. If you are able to do so, without doubt, you are a person who can keep his commitment and be successful.

Conclusions

The final goal of qigong practice is "wuwei" (regulating of no regulating). The method of reaching this goal is advancing gradually until you have established a subconscious habit. The key to success is knowing what, why, and how. However, the most important key of success is conquering your laziness and impatience.

---

1. 宋常星說：「順其自然，不立己見，因感為應，不生有我。即令人之加于我者，或大或小，或多或少，為人心可怨者，然可怨在彼，而我何怨哉？若因其可怨，而報之必欲相稱，則大小之念無所不起，多少之見無往不生。由是而人之加我者不已，我之欲報人者不盡，是人之失，而我亦失也。唯忘乎可怨，報之如無怨，‧‧‧‧ 在人亦可感化，而成歸于無事矣。故曰：『大小多少，報怨以德。』」

2. 宋常星說：「譬如淺陋之人，言不謹慎，意無一定，只圖妄誇大口，妄自輕諾，以言語輕易許之于人，事至竟而不能踐其言，言行不能相顧，所言終無著落，必然寡信矣。」

3. 子曰：「人無遠慮，必有近憂。」

4. 韓非說：「扁鵲見蔡桓公，立有間，扁鵲曰：『君有疾，在腠理，不治將恐深。』桓公曰：『寡人無疾。』扁鵲出，桓公曰：『醫之好治不病以為功。』居十日，扁鵲復見曰：『君之病，在肌膚，不治將益深。』桓公不應。扁鵲出，桓公又不悅。居十日，扁鵲望桓公而還走。桓公使人問之，扁鵲曰：『疾在腠理，湯熨之所及也；在肌膚，箴石之所及也；在腸胃，火齊之所及也；在骨髓，司命之所屬，無奈何也。今在骨髓，臣是以無請也。』居五日，桓公體痛，使人索扁鵲，已逃秦矣。桓公遂死。」

5. 宋常星說：“事之將行，不思前后，不慮始終，不知事之輕重，不審事之可否，以為無事不可任我作，無時不可隨我便，以多易之心，而輕忽淺躁，事之機會不知，往往可行者皆成為不可行，往往能行者皆成不能行，多易必變而為多難。”

6. “無調而調。”

7. 黃裳說：“功至煉虛合道，為無為也；順應自然，事無事也；平淡無奇，何味之有？”

CHAPTER 64
Mind the Insignificant—Prevention

第六十四章
守微—防治

其安易持，其未兆易謀；
　　　其脆易泮，其微易散；
　　　為之於未有，治之於未亂。
合抱之木，生於毫末；
　　　九層之臺，起於累土；
　　　千里之行，始於足下。
為者敗之，執者失之。
　　　是以聖人無為，故無敗；
　　　無執，故無失。
民以從事，常幾於成而敗之；
　　　慎終如始，則無敗事。
是以『聖人』
　　　欲不欲，不貴難得之貨；
　　　學不學，復眾人之所過；
　　　以輔萬物之自然，而不敢為。

When peaceful, it is easy to maintain. Without omens, it is easy to plan.

　　If brittle, it is easy to shatter. If too small, it is easy to scatter.

　　Handle matters before indications of chaos. Organize it before it becomes disordered.

A tree that can be embraced begins from a tiny sapling.

　　A tower with nine stories starts from a heap of dirt.

　　A journey of a thousand miles begins with one's feet.

Whoever meddles, will fail; whoever persists will lose.

　　Thus, sages do not meddle, thus they do not fail;

　　they do not persist, thus they do not lose.

People, when handling affairs, often fail when they are about to succeed.

　　(If they are) careful in the end as in the beginning, then they will not fail.

Thus, those sages,

　　desire to have no desire, value no goods that are hard to acquire;

　　learn what is unlearned, not to repeat the faults of the people;

　　this is to assist myriad objects return back to nature without reluctance.

General Interpretation

When everything is in order, things are easy to maintain. When there is no sign of problems, it is also easy to make a plan since there is no problem or the problems are unnoticeable. When objects are brittle, it is easy to break them. If different small objects are together, it is easy to mix them or scatter them. All these sayings are just to remind us that prevention is more important than solving problems after they have happened. It is also wiser to organize things before they become chaotic.

The Chinese have a saying: "When there is a cause, there must be a consequence."[1] Han Fei (韓非) (《喻老》) said:

> "In the past, the lord of Jin (晉), Chong Er (重耳), was a fugitive from Jin. When he passed through Zheng (鄭), the lord of Zheng did not welcome him with courtesy. Zheng's officer, Shu, Zhan (叔瞻) admonished the lord of Zheng and said: 'This is a sage lord; the lord should treat him with great politeness. By doing this, you will accumulate a good deed.' But the lord of Zheng did not accept the advice. Shu, Zhan again admonished: 'If the lord does not want to treat him with great politeness, then it is better to kill him so there is no worry of future trouble with him.' Again, the lord of Zheng did not listen. Later, when the lord of Jin, returned to Jin, he sent troops to attack Zheng and decisively defeated it, taking over eight cities. Also (another example), the lord of Jin, Jin Xian Gong (晉獻公), used a very precious piece of jade to borrow the passage from Yu (虞) so Jin was able to attack Guo (虢). The officer Gong, Zhi-Qi (宮之奇) admonished the lord of Yu and said: 'We should not allow this. When the lips are dead, the teeth will suffer from cold, Yu and Guo mutually protecting each other is not just for establishing mutual good deeds (i.e., for favor). When Jin exterminates Guo today, Yu will follow and die tomorrow.' The lord of Yu did not listen and accepted the jade for allowing

Jin's troop to pass (through) Yu's territory. Later, after Jin had taken over Guo, Jin exterminated Yu on their way back. These two officers (i.e., Shu, Zhan and Gong, Zhi-Qi) advised their lords because they had foreseen the future problems. Thus, these two officers can be compared with Bian, Que (扁鵲). Due to the refusal of the advice of these two lords, both Zheng and Yu were destroyed. Thus, it is said: 'When peaceful, it is easy to maintain. Without omens, it is easy to plan.'"[2]

A big tree began very small. A tall building started from the foundation at ground level. A long walk started off with a few steps. Learn to intervene early before a minor situation gets worse. Li, Jia-Mo (李嘉謨) said:

"The reasons that people, when following the Dao, find things hard to accomplish and find it easy to fail are because they have put forth too much intention and overpersisted with their minds. When they began, there was nothing that could affect their diligence and at the end, they could not avoid being lazy. All these faults are due to overintention and overpersistence. If they do not have these from the beginning to the end, how can one ask them to be diligent first and later become lazy?"[3]

A lot of people, even they know how to follow the Dao, begin a new undertaking with excitement and enthusiasm, fully engaging their minds and putting in maximum effort. However, after this honeymoon period is over, they gradually become lazier and lazier and finally quit and fail. If they would have planned carefully with the wisdom mind instead of the emotional mind, then they would have been able to last long.

Most people lack patience and discipline; thus, when they undertake some project, they often fail at the end. If they are able to handle things with caution, patience, discipline, and enthusiasm from the beginning until the end, they will no doubt be successful. Wu, Cheng (吳澄) said: "If one thinks it is difficult at the beginning and will not be difficult at the end, and again, does not dare to be arrogant at the beginning but becomes arrogant at the end, then often they fail at the end. Therefore, one must be as careful at the end as in the beginning, and also must treat a task as seriously at the end as in the beginning. In this case, one is not arrogant at the beginning nor at the end, so consequently one will not fail."[4]

Sages will not disturb peace and harmony or take advantage of others. In this way, they also gain peace and harmony.

Qigong Interpretation

This chapter has pointed out many key points of qigong practice. First, you must be careful and advance your practice gradually and slowly. If there is any sign that the qi is being misled in a way that causes a problem, you must stop it from getting worse. The way of preventing problems in qigong practice is to have a high level of awareness and alertness. You must be able to sense the initiation of a problem before it gets serious. For example, when you sense some qi stagnation in your lower back when you meditate, you must correct the posture before it gets worse and causes physical injury.

Second, when you practice qigong, you must be patient. Usually, people quit before they reach the goal and see the result. Although you should not be stubborn in persisting with special routines, you must still have a will to complete your practice until the end.

Third, when you practice qigong, you should not let your emotional mind dominate your thinking and actions. The emotional mind can get you excited easily but can also make you lose patience and quit. However, if you allow your wisdom mind to govern your practice, you will surely see your practice to its completion.

Fourth, qigong training aims to improve physical health and cultivate the spirit. Therefore, you should pay attention to these subjects and not be attracted by the outside world or material luxury. The fewer material desires you have, the more your mind can focus.

Fifth, in order to reach a higher level of qigong practice, you must be humble and willing to learn. If you are humble, you can learn a lot from other people's mistakes. Then you should ponder the solutions. Finally, you will be able to help people back to the Dao. The best way of teaching is by your own example.

Conclusions

Five keys for successful qigong practice are:
1. Advance practice gradually and cautiously.
2. Be patient from the beginning till the end.
3. Govern your emotional mind.
4. Don't be allured by the luxuries of the material world.
5. Maintain an attitude of humility.

1. "有因必有果。"
2. 韓非說："昔晉公子重耳出亡,過鄭,鄭君不禮。叔瞻諫曰:'此賢公子也,君厚待之,可以積德。'鄭君不聽。叔瞻又諫曰:'不厚代之,不若殺之,無令有后患。'鄭君又不聽。及公子返晉邦,舉兵伐鄭,大破之,取八城焉。晉獻公以垂棘之璧假道于虞而伐虢,大夫宮之奇諫曰:'不可。唇亡而齒寒,虞虢相救,非相德也。今日晉滅虢,明日虞必隨之亡。'虞君不聽,受其璧而假之道。晉已取虢,還返滅虞。此兩臣者,皆爭于腠理者也。然則叔瞻、宮之奇亦虞、鄭之扁鵲也。而二君不聽,故鄭以破,虞以亡。故曰:'其安易持,其未兆易謀也'也。"(《喻老》)
3. 李嘉謨說："世之為道所以難成而易壞者,由其有意于為之執之。方其始若無所容其勤,及其終又不免于怠,皆為執之之咎也。使其始終不為且執,則求其勤且不可得,而況乎其怠歟!"
4. 吳澄說："始雖以為難,至終而不以為難;始雖不敢以為大,至終而至以為大。則事幾成而敗歟終者有矣。故必慎終如始。始以為難,而終亦以為難;始不為大,而終亦不為大,則終無敗事也。"

CHAPTER 65
Genuine Virtue—The Virtue of Simplicity

第六十五章
淳德—朴實

古之善為『道』者，
　　　非以明民，
　　　將以愚之。
民之難治，
　　　以其智多。
故以智治國，國之賊；
　　　不以智治國，國之福。
知此兩者亦稽式。
　　　常知稽式，
　　　是謂『玄德』。
『玄德』深矣，遠矣；
　　　與物反矣！
　　　然後乃至大順。

Those ancients who were good at the Dao,
    would not brighten people (i.e., teach them to be wise and
    cunning),
    but teach them to be simple and truthful (return to nature).
People are hard to rule
    because they are too wise and cunning.
Therefore, those who rule the country with cleverness are the
    thieves (i.e., harmful persons) of the country.
    Not ruling the country with cleverness is a blessing for the
    country.
Knowing these two principles will develop a standard of ruling.
    Always know this standard;
    it can then be called "xuan de" (profound manifestation of
    Dao).
"Xuan de" is deep and profound.
    From this, all objects can be returned to their original nature,
    then finally to the great harmony.

General Interpretation

As a ruler, you should teach your people to be truthful and simple. If you teach people how to use the wisdom and cunning mind to play tricks, then the country will soon enter a disordered and disastrous situation. If you teach your people to be truthful to each other, then there is no criminal that can be hidden among the people. If you teach people to be simple, then desires for power, dignity, glory, and material wealth will be minimized. In this case, the country will be in a harmonious and cooperative situation. This is the good fortune of a country. He Shang Gong (河上公) said: "Those ultimate good ancients (i.e., sage rulers) who used the Dao to cultivate themselves and rule countries, would use the Dao and the De to teach their people and make them be simple and not cunning."[1] Du, Guang-Ting (杜光庭) said: "If a lord knows to use wisdom (to rule the country), then he is a harmful person (i.e., thief) of a country. If (a lord) does not use wisdom (to rule the country), then it is a blessing. Therefore, one should repel the harm and acquire the blessing. In this case, he can be a model for ruling a country."[2]

Truthfulness and simplicity should be considered as rules of ruling. Only those who understand these rules and the theory behind them can comprehend the Dao at a profound level. Once people have returned to their simplicity and truthfulness in life, can they then follow the Dao and be reunited with it. He, Shang Gong (河上公) said: "If those rulers are able to apply the Dao to themselves and to rule the countries, then they can be said to have the same De (virtue) as nature."[3] Therefore, they will be able to return myriad objects to their original nature. Xiao, Tian-Shi (蕭天石) said: "Objects means myriad objects. Reverse means to return. Great Smooth (Da Shun, 大順) means the Dao (i.e., Great Nature). The last sentence means the marvelous De is far and profound. When humans and myriad objects all return to their true origins, this is the unification with the Dao."[4]

Qigong Interpretation

When you practice qigong, your mind must be clear and simple. Only then will the qi be lead smoothly and stay in its correct path. Too much thinking can only make the mind chaotic and lead the qi to the weird and wrong paths. Consequently, the body will become sickened. This is called "walking into the fire and entering the devil" in qigong practice.[5]

When you keep your mind simple and truthful, the entire body's qi will be harmonized. The way to reach this goal is to calm down the chaotic thinking generated from the conscious emotional mind and bring your mind to the limbic system where the spirit and truthful feeling reside. When this happens, your spirit will be able to reunite with the natural spirit. Knowing this is simple, but doing it is difficult. If you are able to make it happen and put it into action, then you have reached "xuan de" (profound manifestation of Dao).

Conclusions

Simplicity and truth are the foundation of the Dao. Though understanding these rules is easy, manifesting it in daily life is difficult. If one is able to apply these rules in action, then one one's life is a profound manifestation of the Dao (the De).

1. 河上公說："古至善以道治身治國者，將以道德教民，使質樸不詐偽。"
2. 杜光庭說："人君知用智則為賊，不用智則為福。當去賊取福。如此者可為理國之楷模法式也。"
3. 河上公說："能知治身及治國之法式，是謂與天地同德也。"
4. 蕭天石說："物，指萬物。反，借為返。大順，指道而言。此言玄德深遠，人主與萬物皆返于真，然后乃同至于道也。"
5. "走火入魔。"

CHAPTER 66

Putting Oneself Behind (Humility)—Guiding and Leading

第六十六章
後己（謙讓—導引）

江海所以能為百谷王者，
　　以其善下之，
　　故能為百谷王。
是以『聖人』，
　　欲上民，
　　必以言下之；
　　欲先民，
　　必以身后之。
是以『聖人』，
　　處上而民不重，
　　處前而民不害。
是以天下樂推而不厭。
以其不爭，
　　故天下莫能與之爭。

The reason that rivers and seas be the lords of hundreds of valleys,
  is because they are adept at staying low,
  thus, they can be the lords of hundreds of valleys.
Therefore, those sages,
  who wish to be over people,
  must first speak humbly to them;
  who wish to lead the people,
  must place themselves behind them.
Thus, those sages,
  though they are positioned above people, people do not feel
  burdened,
  though situated in front, people do not feel harmed.
Consequently, the people in the world are happy to push (sages)
  forward without resentment.
Because they do not contend,
  the world cannot contend with them.

General Interpretation

This chapter is talking about humility. As a leader, humility is the most important prerequisite to lead the people. The book *Shu* (《書·大禹謨》) said: "(Those) satisfied will cause damage and (those) humble will acquire benefits."[1] This is because those who are humble can take a low position, be open-minded, and be willing to learn; thus they gain. Those who are satisfied and proud of themselves will not listen and learn from others; thus they lose. *The Book of Changes* (《易·謙》) said: "Those who are humble and again humble always use their modest personality to restrain themselves."[2]

The reason that great rivers or oceans are able to gather so much water is because they position themselves in a low place. Those wise sage rulers know if they wish to be above the people and lead, they must be humble. When they are humble, people will love them and their leadership from the bottom of their hearts. When rules are humble and modest, people will also not feel burdened and pressured from the rulers. Wei, Yuan (魏源) said: "Only if you are not conceited, will the world not contend with you. Only you do not compete, will the world not compete with you. Make people forget that you are above and in front of them, and people are happy to push you above and in front of them. Then this Dao can be said great."[3] Gao, Heng (高亨) said: "When people support their ruler, but feel a big burden, that is a great heaviness. It is not just heavy but also cumbersome. When people do not feel heavy, this means the people will not become tired."[4] The work *Huai Nan Zi* (《淮南子·主術訓》) says:

> "It is plenty if using the many people's wisdom to take care of the world's need (i.e., business). However, if one just focuses his mind to handle (matters), then he cannot even protect himself (i.e., solve his own problem). Thus, those masters of people will cover (i.e., protect) the people with virtue and not use their wisdom. Consequently, myriad people will benefit. Since rulers follow people benefits, thus, people will support the rulers to be above them

and feeling no burden and position them in front without feeling harmed."[5]

Mencius (孟子) (《公孫丑上》) said:

"When people told Zi Lu (子路) (i.e., Confucius' student) about his faults, he was happy. When Yu (禹) (i.e., Xia emperor) heard good advice, he bowed with appreciation. Great Shun (舜) (i.e., second ancient Chinese ruler) is even greater. He treated himself as others, followed others instead of insisting on his own way, and was happy to take other people's advice. As an emperor, he cultivated the land, farmed, made pottery, and fished himself; he took nothing from others. He took advice from others so that he was able to offer them what they needed. Therefore, a gentleman's greatest virtue is doing good things for others."[6]

Du, Guang-Ting (杜光庭) said:

"When Yao (堯) (i.e., first ancient Chinese ruler) governed the world (i.e., country), all six directions (i.e., everywhere) were harmonious and all lives were lived together peacefully. All lives came to him like clouds. When they looked at him, he was like a sun; thus, without weariness, they supported him as the leader. Later when Yao died, all the people in the country felt so sad, just as if they had lost their own parents."[7]

Qigong Interpretation

Humility is the most important requirement for learning. It is the same when you learn qigong. My White Crane master, Zeng, Jin-Zao

(曾金灶) always told me: "In front of a teacher, you have no dignity."[8]. He also told me once: "The taller the bamboo grows, the lower it bows."[9] These sayings have been my mottoes since I was fifteen years old. I have received so much benefit in my life from them. Often, just a concept or an idea can change the whole world.

Qigong has been practiced for more than four thousand years. During this period, an enormous amount of knowledge and experience has been developed and accumulated. This knowledge and experience have been passed down to us and have become our precious guides for life and spiritual development. The spiritual world is just like a huge beautiful garden that, though it cannot be seen, it can be felt. Since we don't know too much about the spiritual world, we have treated it as mysterious. Understanding the Dao offers a possible key to unlock the door. Through meditation, our subconscious mind can be awakened, grow, and finally reconnect to the natural spirit.

Most religious qigong was studied and developed in Buddhist and Daoist monasteries. Their main goal of this cultivation is the final stage of "unification of heaven and human" (tian ren he yi, 天人合一). That means Nature is us and we are Nature.

In order to reach this goal, we must remain humble. When you are humble, your cup will always have space to receive more. However, if you keep your cup full, then you are satisfied and there is no more space for you to learn and receive. From long experience, one key practice for us to awaken our subconscious mind and feeling is embryonic breathing meditation. If you are interested in this subject, please refer to the book: *Qigong Meditation—Embryonic Breathing*, by YMAA Publication Center.

Conclusions

Humility is the crucial key to learning. Without a humble mind, your learning will be limited and shallow. Thus, you should always consider other people's thinking and feelings before your own. Then you will have a benevolent heart.

1.《書·大禹謨》：“滿招損，謙受益。”

2.《易·謙》：“謙謙君子，卑以自牧。”

3. 魏源說：“汝唯不矜，天下莫與汝爭能；汝唯不伐，天下莫與汝爭功。使天下忘其上且先，而爭樂推之使上，推之使先，斯道也可謂大矣。”

4. 高亨說：“民戴其君，若有負重以為大累，即此文之所謂重。故重猶累也。而民不重，言民不以為累也。”

5.《淮南子·主術訓》：“乘眾人之智，天下之不足有也；專用其心，則獨身不能保也。是故人主，覆之以德，不行其智，而因萬人之所利。夫舉踵天下而得所利，故百姓載之上弗重也。錯之前弗害也。”

6. 孟子說：“子路人告之有過則喜。禹聞善言則拜。大舜有大焉，善于人同，捨己從人，樂取于人以為善。自耕稼陶漁以至為帝，無非取于人者。取諸人以為善，是與人以為善者也。故君子莫大乎與人為善。”（《公孫丑上》）

7. 杜光庭說：“堯之理天下也，六合群生，就之如雲，望之如日，推崇為主，而無厭倦。及其棄世也，天下之人，如喪考妣。”

8.“師尊前，無尊嚴。”

9.“竹高必躬。”

CHAPTER 67
The Three Treasures—Follow the Dao
第六十七章
三寶—順道

天下皆謂我道大，似不肖。
　　夫唯大，故似不肖；
　　若肖，久矣其細也夫！
我有三寶，持而保之：
　　一曰慈，二曰儉，
　　三曰不敢為天下先。
慈，故能勇；儉，故能廣；
　　不敢為天下先，
　　故能成器長。
今舍慈且勇；
　　舍儉且廣；
　　舍后且先；死矣。
夫慈，以戰則勝，
　　以守則固。
　　天將救之，以慈衛之。

Everyone in the world says the Dao is great, but it seems that it is
    beyond comparison.
    It is because of its greatness that it cannot to be compared.
    If it can be compared, it would already have become insignifi-
    cant a long time ago.
I have three treasures that I keep and cherish:
    the first, compassion; the second, conservation;
    and the third, daring not to be ahead of others.
Whoever is compassionate can thus be brave; whoever conserves
    can thus can be wide (i.e., abundant);
    whoever dares no be ahead of others, can thus assume leader-
    ship.
If one has bravery, but discards compassion,
    reaching wide, but discards conservation,
    being ahead, but discards being behind, then follows death.
When fighting is done with compassion, then there is victory.
    Use it for defense, then secure firmly.
    Heaven will save them and guard them with compassion.

General Interpretation

Many people think they already know the Dao and how great it is. However, the Dao is so great that nothing can be compared with it. If it could be compared with, in ancient times it would have already become insignificant.

Confucius (孔子) (《禮記·中庸》) said: "I have already known that the virtue of the Dao cannot be carried out. Those clever persons have overdone it while those innocent people cannot (even) reach it. I have (also) known that the understanding of the Dao is vague. Those wise persons have overinterpreted it and those who are not wise cannot (even) touch it."[1]

If, while living in this world, you are able to keep the three treasures of compassion, conservation, and humility, then you will always be in a great position in your life. If you are benevolent, you will have friends and people who support you. From a benevolent heart, you will have courage. If you are conservative, you will have plentiful and abundant material necessities. If you are humble and righteous, you will become a leader of society. Su, Che (蘇轍) said: "Today's customs value bravery, admire the wide and great, and praise those who advance aggressively. However, my treasures are enduring compassion, frugal conservation, and humble righteousness. These three are not valued by the common customs."[2]

Wang, Bi (王弼) said: "Compassion, originated from the Dao and is acquired from benevolence. It is the leader of the three treasures."[3] Han Fei (韓非) (《解老》) said:

> "When a loving mother loves her weak children, she will try her best to make them happy. To make them happy, she must first protect them from disaster. To protect them from disaster, her thinking will be profound. When her thinking is profound, she will know how to arrange affairs. When she acquires the way of managing affairs, she will surely be successful. When she is surely successful, she will not have doubts. When there are no doubts, she will have courage." "Therefore, wise people are frugal with their

use of money and so become wealthy. Those sages love and treasure their spirit so their essence is abundant. Those rulers treat their soldiers preciously; therefore they have numerous people. Thus, it can be said: 'Whoever conserves can thus can be wide.'" "All myriad objects have their orders. Those consultant advisers meet to discuss regulations. Those sages just follow all of the rules and regulations; thus, 'not daring to be ahead of others in the world.' If not daring to be ahead of others (i.e., humble), then there is nothing that cannot be accomplished. Because they have achieved merits without asking for credit, their achievements will be matchless. In this case, even if they don't have a desire to be great officers, can they not be accepted? When you are in the position of a great officer, it means you are a leader of achievement. Thus, it says: 'daring not to be ahead of others' one can thus assume leadership."[4]

He Shang Gong (河上公) also said: "Those who are compassionate, all people will be close and attached to them, sharing the same heart and will. Use this to fight, then victory will come, and use it for defense, then strength and solidy will follow."[5]

Qigong Interpretation

The Dao of qigong practice is so wide and great that there are many theories and practices we don't even know of. If we try to compare it with anything, it will be misleading. However, there are three keys that can be used to approach it. The three key treasures are: compassion, conservation, and following Nature.

When you have compassion, your heart will be wide open and benevolent. You will have concern for other people's feelings and be able to share what you have with others sincerely. This is the mind of generosity, righteousness, and kindness. With this mind, you will be able to build up a good deed. This is the manifestation (De) of the Dao.

In qigong practice, you must treat your qi (people) with compassion. With this mind, you will be able to pay attention to any qi disorder and regulate it so as to bring it back to the correct path. Compassion provides you awareness and alertness to observe your qi internally. This is called "the gongfu of internal observation."[6] Without this foundation, the mind will be narrow for qigong development.

Next, you need to know how to conserve your qi. Conserving qi is one of the most important practices in qigong. If you don't have abundant qi's storage and circulation in your body, you will not be healthy, live long, and have a high spirit. There are two ways to increase your qi's storage. One is conserving it and the other is learning how to make more qi. It is just the same as living. If you wish to be wealthy, you must first conserve your money and not waste it. You must also know how to make more money so you have more income. That is why you need to know how to conserve your qi. The way of reaching this goal is practicing embryonic breathing meditation. Embryonic breathing meditation teaches you how to govern your emotional mind and wake up your subconscious mind. When the mind is effectively governed, the mind will be calm, peaceful, and steady. When this happens, since the qi is not led or made chaotic by the emotional mind, you can preserve the qi to an abundant level.

Then, to reach to a higher level of qigong practice, you must have the right attitude: be humble and yielding. When you are humble, you will learn modesty. There is so much knowledge that even if you spend a few lifetimes, you still cannot finish your learning. However, if you remain humble, you will always be inspired and learn. Additionally, you must be able to yield and follow the Dao. If you stubbornly insist upon your own ideas, you will channel yourself into a corner like a frog trapped in the well trying to gauge the dimension of the sky. If you are able to follow the Dao, you will be able to lead the qi efficiently and effectively.

Conclusions

Three important keys of qigong practice are compassion, conservation, and humility.

1. 子曰：“道之不行也，我知之矣。知者過之，愚者不及也。道之不明也，我知之矣。賢者過之，不肖者不及也。”《禮記·中庸》

2. 蘇轍說：“今夫世俗貴勇敢，尚廣大，誇進銳，而吾之所寶則慈忍，儉約，廉退。此三者皆世之所謂不肖者也。”

3. 王弼說：“慈者，生之道，仁之得，為三寶之首。”

4. 韓非說：“慈母之于弱子也，務致其福，務致其福則事除其禍，事除其禍則思慮熟，思慮熟則得事理，得事理則必成功，必成功則其行也不疑，不疑之謂勇。”“是以智士儉用其財則家富，聖人愛寶其神則精盛，人君重戰其卒則民眾，民眾則國廣。是以舉之曰：‘儉，故能廣。’”“而萬物莫不有規矩。議言之士，計會規矩也。聖人盡隨于萬物之規矩，故曰：‘不敢為天下先。’不敢為天下先，則事無不事，功無不功，而議必蓋世，欲無處大官，其可得乎？處大官之謂為成事長。是以故曰：‘不敢為天下先，故能為成事長。’”《解老》

5. 河上公說：“夫慈仁者，百姓親附，并心一意，以戰則勝敵，以守衛則堅固。”

6. “內視功夫。”

CHAPTER 68

Complying with Heaven—Follow the Dao

第六十八章

配天—順道

善為士者不武，
　　善戰者不怒，
善勝敵者不與，
　　善用人者為之下。
是謂不爭之『德』，
　　是謂用人之力，
是謂配天，
　　古之極。

The great commanders are not warlike,
    the great warriors do not get angry.
Those who are skillful in defeating opponents do not engage them,
    those who have expertise in managing others position them-
    selves low.
This can be called the virtue of noncontention
    and also called the effectiveness of managing people.
This is the way of harmonizing with Heaven,
    the ultimate principle of the ancients.

General Interpretation

Wise and great commanders will not use force to conquer an opponent. Those who use force, even if they win, will not last long. However, if they use kindness and compassion to defeat their enemies, they will keep good relations with them and, thus, last long. It is important that when you defeat your opponents, you defeat their hearts instead of bodies. Gao, Heng (高亨) said: "If opponents are defeated through battle, then it is not consummate. Those who are skillful in winning do not use troops and weapons, yet their enemies will surrender and submit themselves. Thus it is said: 'Those who are skillful in defeating opponents do not engage them.'"[1] Sun, Wu (孫武) also said: "To defeat opponents without war is the best among the best."[2]

In addition, as good commanders, they should always be humble and concerned with their people's safety, living standards, and happiness before their own. People or soldiers will then fight for them bravely in battle. *The Book of Changes* (《易·兌》) says: "When people are delighted to be led, they forget their fatigue; when people are happy encountering a difficulty, people forget their deaths."[3] This is the way of managing people by following the Dao. Xue, Hui (薛惠) Said: "The Dao of Heaven, victory without contention, achieve by doing nothing. If those sages are able to match their virtues with Heaven, it is called: 'harmonizing with Heaven.' This was the Dao that ancient rulers used. Thus, it is said: 'the ultimate principle of ancients.'"[4]

Qigong Interpretation

This chapter reminds you that when you practice qigong, you must be humble and soft. You should get rid of ego and expectations. What will happen, will happen as long as you provide adequate conditions for it to happen. Therefore, in order to created these conditions, you must know your qi's status (the people) and and take loving care of it. If you are getting sick, your qi will be strengthened to boost your immune system and raise up the spirit to fight against your sickness. However, if you abuse your qi and often use it improperly then, when you need it, it will be weak and dispersed.

You take care of your health by taking care of your body. Establish a healthy lifestyle until you don't need to put effort into it. This is the stage of "regulating of no regulating," the stage of "harmonizing with heaven."

Conclusions

The Dao of Nature is soft without contending. To follow the Dao, you must have a humble mind. With a humble mind to take care of your body, both your mental and physical bodies will be strong. Consequently, bad fortune such as sickness or disaster will not fall upon you. The best way of reaching this goal is by establishing a healthy lifestyle.

1. 高亨說：“夫對鬥而后勝敵，非善也。善勝者，師旅不興，兵刃不接，而敵降服。故曰：‘善勝者不與也。’”

2. 孫武子說：“不戰而屈人之兵，善之善者也。”（《孫子兵法‧謀攻》）

3. 《易‧兌》說：“說（悅）以先民，民忘其勞；說（悅）以犯難，民忘其死。”

4. 薛惠說：“天之道，不爭而勝，無為而成，聖人德合于天。故曰‘配天。’此上古極致之道。故曰‘古之極。’”

CHAPTER 69
Indisputable—Cautious in Action?

第六十九章
不爭—慎行

用兵有言：
　　「吾不敢為主而為客，
　　不敢進寸而退尺。」
是謂
　　行無行，
　　攘無臂，
　　執無兵，
　　扔無敵。
禍莫大於輕敵，
　　輕敵幾喪吾寶。
故抗兵相加，
　　哀者勝矣。

In using military action, strategists have a saying:
    "I dare not be the aggressor, but the defender,
    dare not advance an inch, but prefer to retreat a foot."
This is called:
    act as if not taking action,
    raise arms as if not raising arms,
    confront enemies as if they are not enemies,
    wield weapons as if unarmed.
There is no disaster greater than underestimating the enemy,
    underestimating the enemy made me almost lose my treasures.
Thus, when a battle is in process,
    The side with compassion for sorrow will win.

General Interpretation

Wise military strategists believe that the way to defeat an enemy is not by aggression but by defense. Those who advance aggressively, even if they win temporarily, will soon be defeated. The energy behind the aggression will not last, but the minds of the opponent will grow stronger and stronger each day. Sooner or later, the situation will be reversed, and the opponent will have the upperhand. Those who fight with compassion and not aggression, even if they are initially in a defensive position, will win in the end. Du, Guang-Ting (杜光庭) said: "When troops are fighting against each other, those who attack are the host while those who respond to the aggression are the guest. Those who demonstrate their aggression imply that they like to make trouble and are greedy. Those who are in the guest position and respond to the aggression show their kindness for defending themselves."[1] Su, Che (蘇轍) said: "The hosts are trouble makers; the guests are responding against the enemy. The aggressors have the intention of contending while those retreating do not have the intention of contending."[2] The Chinese word "martial" (wu, 武) is constructed of two words: "止" (zhi) means "stop" and "戈" (ge) was an ancient weapon that was commonly used in battle. Therefore, "martial" means "to stop weapons." From this, you can see that using force or arms is not desired. Arms are used only to stop aggression or fights. Therefore, those who use arms should have compassion for the sorrow they create. There is an enemy, but it is as if there is none.

Ye, Meng-De (葉夢得) said:

> "Da Si Ma (大司馬) (i.e., ancient title of a high rank officer), Fa (法) said: 'When attacking, use the sounds of drum and bell to warn the enemies about their sins. The army stops at the border, just to convince the other side of their sins; there is no necessity for aggression.' Thus, it is rare to advance for an inch but common to withdraw for a foot. Therefore, though there is an action, it seems like no action. Though arms are raised, it seems as if there are no arms, seeing enemies as if there are no enemies, and holding weapons as if there are no weapons."[3]

Fan, Ying-Yuan (范應元) said: "When encountering enemies, if I am forced to fight, then I have a sorrowful heart. When there is a sorrowful heart, the heaven and the people will help you. Even when you do not wish to win, you cannot avoid it."[4] Gao, Heng (高亨) also said: "When two armies are battling against each other, there is one side that is cheerful and there is the other side that feels sorrow. Those who are cheerful will fail and those who feel sorrow will win. This is because those who feel sorrow cannot bear the mind of killing and are, without a choice, placed in the position of defense. In this case, with the help of the Dao of heaven and the people, they will win for sure."[5]

Qigong Interpretation

When encountering an illness, you have to face it in order to get well. You must first understand the causes and conditions of the sickness. Then, with compassion, you can find the way to enhance the qi's circulation. If you try to deal with the problem aggressively, you may end up causing an aberrant qi circulation and make things worse. However, while taking precautions, if you use your loving heart to take care of it, you will find the way to solve the problem. For example, if cancer has started to develop in your body and you aggressively attack the cancer cells, this may just end up making things worse, with the cancer spreading to other areas. However, if you just find the qigong way to boost your immune system and improve your natural defensive mechanisms, eventually, the results can be outstanding. According to Chinese medicine, cancer develops in the body because of abnormal qi circulation in the area. However, if you keep your mind calm and peaceful, you will feel and find the problem. Once you have developed the feeling, then you will be able to lead the qi and improve qi circulation there.

When you treat your sickness, you must be cautious not to under-estimate your condition. Often, people get sicker due to ignorance. However, the most important element in dealing with your sickness is the love and compassion you have for yourself. You should face the sickeness and find the way to solve make yourself well.

Conclusions

Keeping defensive capability strong is the best and benevolent way to deal with aggression. In order to have a strong defense, you must build up your strength, be confident, and be firm. When you are strong and powerful, aggression will not be able to harm you. Therefore, keeping your qi abundant, your immune system strong, and your spirit high are the keys to preventing sicknesses.

1. 杜光庭說：“吾者用兵之人也。先唱為主，后應為客。主先唱示生事而貪，客后應示以慈自守。”
2. 蘇轍說：“主，造事者也；客，應敵者也。進者，有意于爭也；退者，無意于爭也。”
3. 葉夢得說：“大司馬法曰：'伐者以鼓鐘聲罪而告之，止于境上，服其罪則已，不必進也。'故進以寸則常寡，退以尺則常多。此雖行而若無行也，雖攘而若無臂也，不見可敵若無扔也，雖執之若無兵也。”
4. 范應元說：“兩敵相加，而吾出乎不得已，則有哀心。哀心見則天人助之。雖欲不勝，不可得矣。”
5. 高亨說：“抗兵相加，有樂之者，有哀之者。樂之者敗，哀之者勝。蓋哀之者，存不忍殺人之心，處不得不戰之境，在天道人事皆有必勝之理也。”

CHAPTER 70

Knowing Difficulty—Handling Affairs
第七十章
知難—處事

吾言甚易知，
　　甚易行；
天下莫能知，
　　莫能行。
言有宗，
　　事有君。
夫惟無知，
　　是以不我知。
知我者希，
　　則我者貴。
是以『聖人』
　　被褐懷玉。

My words are easy to understand,
    and easy to practice.
Yet no one in this world understands them,
    and practices them.
My words have their basis (i.e., origin),
    and my actions have their principles.
Because people do not understand this,
    they don't know me.
Since few people know me,
    I am valued highly.
Therefore,
    those sages wear plain clothes, and hold the jade inside.

General Interpretation

Even though what I said about the theory and the methods of practicing the Dao are easy to understand and do, still, very few people are really able to comprehend it and put it into action. This is because people are often affected by emotional desires. Wang, Bi (王弼) said: "(You) don't have to leave the house or peek through a little window to understand; thus, it is said it is easy to know. (You) can do it without doing it (i.e., wuwei); thus, it is said, it is easy to practice. (People are commonly) puzzled by impatience and desires; thus, it is said, it is hard to understand. (They are) bewildered by achieving glory and benefits; thus, it is said, it is hard to practice."[1]

Lao Zi tried to teach people that practicing the Dao involved softness, weakness, and humility. People should be able to understand these easily. Wu, Cheng (吳澄) said: "Lao Zi only teaches people; soft, weak, and humble. These words are easy to understand, and it's also easy to put them into action. However, people commonly follow the traditional customs so there is no one able to understand the preciousness of his words and practice softness, weakness, and humility."[2]

Lao Zi believed that softness, weakness, and humility can be a foundation for all people and also can be the masters of a country. Wu, Cheng (吳澄) said: "Softness, weakness, and humility can be said to be the summary of all sayings. It is just like the root (i.e., ancestors) of a family. They can be the masters of all affairs just like the king of a country. Lao Zi sighed that the people at that time were ignorant and innocent and therefore did not know the preciousness of his words."[3]

Sages usually do not pay attention to their outside looks, but take their inner spiritual cultivation seriously. That's why it is said, "those sages wear plain clothes, but hold the jade inside." Yan, Jun-Ping (嚴君平) said: "Wearing plain clothes means treating the body lightly and holding the jade means taking spiritual cultivation."[4] Wu, Cheng (吳澄) said: "People do not know those sages. They only see them wearing plain clothes and not displaying anything precious externally. They don't know the jade-like preciousness of what they embrace internally."[5]

Qigong Interpretation

Following *The Book of Changes* (《*Yi Jing*, 易經》), the Chinese believe that there are two spaces (or dimensions) coexisting in this universe. One is calley Yin space (yin jian, 陰間) and the other is called yang space (yang jian, 陽間). Though there are two dimensions, actually, they are two faces of the same thing (Nature). Yin space is the spiritual world while yang space is the material world. Yin space is the Dao while yang space is the De. The De (yang space) is the manifestation of the Dao (yin space). Thus, the Dao is the mother of the De. Although we still don't know the Dao (spiritual world), from the manifestation of the Dao (the De) we are able to see some rules and functions of the Dao.

When we are alive, our body has two lives, a physical life and a spiritual life. This is because humans are propagated from the combination of these two worlds. That is the reason there are two lives coexisting in our body. Once the physical body is dead, the spiritual body will return to the yin space (origin) and wait to be reborn. This is the concept of reincarnation.

Buddhists and Daoists are always searching for the way to strengthen the spiritual body so that when the physical body is dead, they don't have to be reincarnated and can instead exist forever spiritually. This is the stage of Buddhahood. To them, although the physical body is important since it provides you physical health and longevity so you have more time for spiritual cultivation, it is more important to cultivate spiritual life.

Similarly, our mind includes two minds, a conscious mind and a subconscious mind. The conscious mind is in a matrix of illusion that society has imposed on us since we were born. Thus, we learn how to put masks on our faces and do what society expects us to do. We continuously lie to ourselves and other people in order to fit into this masked society. However, our subconscious mind is more truthful and connected to our spirit. The whole idea of spiritual cultivation is downplaying our conscious mind and awakening our subconscious mind. The spiritual side of our existence has always been a part of Nature. It is our conscious mind that has led us away from Nature and into traditional dogmas and bondage. Our spirits have been restricted.

To reach the spiritual side, we have to downplay our material desires and learn to govern our conscious emotional mind. The emotional mind makes us confused and irrational. When we downplay our conscious mind, we can slowly awaken our subconscious mind. The way of reaching awakened state is through softness, gentleness ("weakness"), and humility. This is the nature of our spirit.

Once you are able to reconnect your spirit with the natural spirit, you will be able to enter the spiritual garden of Nature. When you have acquired this, you will know its feeling and its marvelousness. It is this preciousness that those people who do not awaken the subconscious mind will never know and feel.

Conclusions

Softness, weakness, and humility are the three foundations of the Dao's practice. Although it can be easily understood, it is not easy to put them into action.

1. 王弼說：“可不出戶窺牖而知，故曰甚易知也。無為而成，故曰甚易行也。惑于躁欲，故曰莫能知也。迷于榮利，故曰莫之能行也。”
2. 吳澄說：“老子教人，柔弱謙下而已。其言甚易知，其事甚易行也。世降俗末，天下之人莫能知其言之可貴，莫能行柔弱謙下之事者。”
3. 吳澄說：“柔弱謙下，可以為眾言之統，如族之有宗；可以為諸事之主，如國之有君。老子嘆時人愚而無知，是以不知我言之可貴也。”
4. 嚴君平說：“被褐者薄其身，懷玉者厚其神。”
5. 吳澄說：“人不知聖人，但見其外知之所被如褐而不貴，不知其中之所懷如玉之可貴也。”

CHAPTER 71

Know the Sickness "of Not Knowing"—Know What Is Known

第七十一章

知病—知知

知不知，
　　上；
不知知，
　　病。
『聖人』不病，
　　以其病病；
夫唯病病，
　　是以不病。

Knowing that you don't know,
   is the best.
Not knowing, but thinking (you) do,
   is a sickness (ill mind).
The sages are without a sick (mind),
   since they recognize that the sick (mind) is a sick (mind).
Because they consider it as a sick (mind),
   thus, they are without a sick (mind).

General Interpretation

If you know that you don't know, you will be able seek the knowledge you lack and, thus, know. However, if you don't even know that you don't know, then your mind is not clear (this is what it means to have a "sick mind"). Confucius (孔子) (《論語·為政》) said: "If one knows what he knows and also knows what he does not know, then it is wisdom."[1]

Sages know what they know and what they don't know, and thus there is no confusion. Fan, Ying-Yuan (范應元) said: "The reason that those sages are not sick minded (i.e., confused) is because they realize that there is a sickness of not-knowing, but pretending to know in heaven and earth (i.e., world). Thus, they will stop pretending (i.e., recognize) to know what they don't know, so they will not be sick (confused)."[2]

Qigong Interpretation

Theory is the foundation of any practice. Correct theory is just like a map that leads you to the right path. Keep practicing without knowing the theory and you will only be misled into the path of confusion. In order to comprehend the theory behind the practice, you will need an experienced teacher or authoritative writings that can lead you to the entrance to the right path. After that, through pondering and practice, you will be able to comprehend the theory behind the practice.

It is the same in qigong practice. In order to accomplish the goal you have chosen, you need to know what, why, and how. That means: What are you looking for? Why does it work? And how do you reach the goal? Once you have a clear mind and then pursue your goals, you will have no doubt about your qigong practice.

The attitude for reaching a clear mind is to recognize what you know and don't know. You must have confidence in what you know and also humbly ponder and learn what you don't know. If you pretend you know, then you will be easily misled onto the wrong path.

Conclusions

Knowing what you don't know is the key to pursuing knowledge. The sages know what they don't know and what they know, so they are wise and don't have confusion in their practice of following the Dao.

1. 孔子說：“知之為知之，不知為不知，是智也。”（《論語・為政》）
2. 范應元說：“聖人所以不病者，以其病彼天下有妄知之病，是以知止其所不知，而不吾病也。”

CHAPTER 72

Loving Yourself—Knowing Yourself

第七十二章
愛己—自知

民不畏威，
　　則大威至。
無狎其所居，
　　無厭其所生。
夫唯不厭，
　　是以不厭。
是以『聖人』，
　　自知不自見，
　　自愛不自貴。
故去彼取此。

When people are not afraid of awe,
  then the big awful threat will happen.
Do not limit people's living space,
  do not meddle with people's livelihood.
Because they are not persecuted,
  they do not reject the ruler.
Therefore, those sages
  know themselves, but do not glorify themselves,
  love themselves, but do not value themselves.
Thus, they discard those (i.e., glory and self-importance) and take
  these (i.e., know and love themselves).

General Interpretation

A ruler should not use fear to control people. If he continues to use fear to rule, one day people will not be afraid of him anymore. When this happens, a big threat will come upon the ruler. Therefore, as a ruler, he should not restrict people's living space and meddle with their livelihood. When people are happy and harmonious, they will respect and obey the ruler.

Wang, Bi (王弼) said: "(When a ruler) parts from serenity and tranquility, carries out his desires with impatience, and gives up his modesty and humility, then society will be disturbed and people decimated. When awe cannot control people, and people cannot stand and fear no more the ruler's awe, then the whole country from the top (i.e., ruler) to the bottom (i.e., people) will have a great collapse. The heaven's massacre (i.e., disaster) will fall upon them. Therefore, it is said: 'when people are not in fear of awe, a big threat will arrive.'[1] Zhang, Song-Ru (張松如) also said: "This heaven's massacre and disaster are referring to the ruler. In fact, the truth is that 'the ruler forces people to turn against him.'"[2]

Therefore, wise rulers will remain humble without glorifying themselves. Not only that, they will pay more attention to people's feeling and not treat themselves as special. Xun Zi (荀子) recorded a conversation between Confucius and his students:

> "When Zi Lu (子路) enters the room, Confucius asks: 'You (由) (Zi Lu's nickname), how should a wise person be? How should a benevolent person be?' Zi Lu replies: 'Those wise persons will let people know them and those benevolent persons will make people love them.' Confucius says: 'In this case, you can be a scholar.' When Zi Gong (子貢) enters the room, Confucius asks: 'Si (賜) (Zi Gong's nickname), how should a wise person be? How should a benevolent person be?' Zi Gong replies: 'Those wise persons know others, and those benevolent love others.' Confucius said: 'In this case, you can be a gentleman.' When Yan Yuan (顏淵) enters the room, Confucius asks: 'Hui (回) (Yan Yuan's nickname), how should a wise

person be? How should a benevolent person be?' Yan Yuan replies: 'Those wise persons know themselves and those benevolent persons love themselves.' Confucius says: 'In this case, you can be an intelligent gentleman.'"[3]

This represents three levels of the cultivation of temperament. Those who are wise will know and love themselves first before they are able to love someone else or make others respect them and love them. Usually, it is easier to ask someone else to know and love you. It is also easy to know and love someone. But there are not too many people who will cultivate themselves and really know and love themselves. It is easier to demand of others than to demand of yourself. My White Crane master, Zeng, Jin-Zao (曾金灶) always said: "Conquering an enemy is easy and conquering yourself is hard. If you are able to conquer yourself, there is nothing you cannot conquer in the world."[4]

Qigong Interpretation

This chapter has pointed out two important things. When you practice qigong, your mind (ruler) has to be soft and gentle. If your mind has too much egoism and emotional disturbance, the qi's circulation will become imbalanced and chaotic. You should proceed in your practice gradually and patiently. Too much ego will only cause problems. Eventually, this abnormal qi circulation will bring you sickness or harm in some other form.

Secondly, to love your body and qi, you must cultivate your temperament first. You must be patient, humble, and enduring. Only if you know yourself first will you be able to regulate your body, breathing, mind, qi, and spirit. To reach a high level of qigong practice, especially internal elixir (nei dan, 內丹), you will need a lot of patience and have a calm and peaceful mind.

Conclusions

Success in qigong practice comes through self-cultivation. If you cannot first cultivate your temperament to a profound stage, your achievement will be shallow. Those who have reached higher level of temperament cultivation will also reach the deeper level of spiritual development. And, naturally, they will be able to reach a higher level of qigong practice.

1. 王弼說："離其清靜，行其躁欲。棄其謙后，則物擾而民僻，威不能復制民，民不能堪其威，則上下大潰矣。天誅將至，故曰民不畏威，則大威至。"
2. 張松如說："此天誅、禍亂。自是對統治者說的。實則是'官逼民反'之謂也。"
3. 荀子錄："子路入。子曰：'由，知者若何？仁者若何？'子路對曰：'知者使人知己，仁者使人愛己。'子曰：'可謂士矣。'子貢入。子曰：'賜，知者若何？仁者若何？'子貢對曰：'知者知人，仁者愛人。'子曰：'可謂士君子矣。'顏淵入。子曰：'回，知者若何？仁者若何？'顏淵對曰：'知者自知，仁者自愛。'子曰：'可謂明君子矣。'"（《子道》）
4. 曾金灶說："克敵易，克己難。能克己，則天下無不能克矣。"

CHAPTER 73
Daring to Act—Following Heaven

第七十三章
任為—順天

勇於敢則殺，
　　勇於不敢則活。
此兩者，
　　或利或害。
天之所惡，
　　孰知其故？
　　是以『聖人』猶難之。
天之道，
　　不爭而善勝，
　　不言而善應，
　　不召而自來，
　　坦然而善謀。
天網恢恢，
　　疏而不失。

Those bold and daring will be killed,
   those bold but not daring will live.
Of these two,
   one may be beneficial and the other may be harmful.
Who knows what heaven detests?
   Even for the sages it is difficult to see the answer.
The Dao of Heaven,
   does not contend yet it always wins,
   does not speak yet it gets a good response,
   does not summon and yet comes on its own,
   is naturally calm (i.e., not aggressive), yet it excels in planning.
The net of heaven is vast,
   though loose, yet nothing is able to slip through.

General Interpretation

Theoretically speaking, those who dare to accept challenges and take risks in life often get killed. Those who avoid danger and challenges usually survive. Du, Guang-Ting (杜光庭) said: "Those strong and decisive enough to accept challenges are brave, and those who dare to face the consequences have courage." He also said: "Those who are strong and rude, and advance with a sharp will, will enter disaster. Those who are humble and cautious, and know how to withdraw themselves, should be safe. These two ways to either be killed or survive are clear and can be verified."[1]

However, since we don't know the future and our personal destiny, it is hard to judge which decisions will be beneficial and which will be harmful. Heaven has its own arrangement. Occasionally, those taking risks and accepting challenges gain more experience in life while those who avoid challenges have less meaningful lives. Not only that, those who have taken on challenges and risks actually live longer while those who avoid challenge die younger. From this, how can anyone say who is wrong and who is right? Si, Ma-Guang (司馬光) said: "Even those sages dare not say what will be the decision of the Dao of Heaven."[2] Su, Che (蘇轍) said:

> "Those bold and daring will die and those bold but not daring will survive. It seems this is the natural rule. However, often those bold and daring survive and those bold but not daring cannot escape from death. It is often seen that personal luck may make this happen and is against the natural rule. However, the Dao of heaven is so deep and profound, it may have some luck involved, but who knows what goodness and evil will result later on? Therefore, though those sages use the natural rules as a guideline, and as for bravery, it is still hard for them to make a judgment. Laymen in this world observe heaven with ears and eyes, but can only see one part and not the complete Nature. Some people have seen those who have done good

*deeds but encounter disaster and those who have done
evil deeds but gain fortune. They suspect that the net of
heaven is too loose so the consequences of these events are
misplaced. Actually, one should know that, although
heaven's net is wide and loose, nothing can slip through
without consequences. One has to wait until the very end
to see the variations (i.e., consequences)."[3]*

As we know, every event initiated has its consequences. We may not
see it right away. However, when time passes, it will become clearer.
The Chinese have a saying: "Those who have done good deeds will be
rewarded with goodness while those who have done bad deeds will
receive bad things in return. If the retribution is not yet seen, it is
because the time has not arrived yet."[4] For example, Wang, Chong (王充)
said: "Li, Si (李斯) (Qin's prime minister) was jealous of Han, Fei's (韓非)
(a well-known scholar) talent, so he imprisoned him and killed him at
Qin (秦). Later, he was punished with death by splitting his body (by
horses). Shang, Yang (商鞅) (also Qi's prime minister) took advantages
of his old friend, seized Wei's (衛) prince, Yang (卬), with a trick, and
later was killed by the Qin emperor."[5]

The Dao of Nature is doing nothing, but things always happen. If
a person follows his consciousness to follow the way of the Dao, has a
good heart, and is involved in good deeds, then heaven will set up a
favorable path for him. However, if a person has evil thoughts and does
evil deeds, then heaven will also repay him with evil consequences.
There is karma in your every thought and deed.

The net of heaven is vast, and even though the mesh is wide open,
nothing can slip through. In Chinese society, it is said: "Planting melon
seeds produces melons and planting bean seeds produces beans."[6]

Qigong Interpretation

We can never know the future. However, we all know that what
we have planted is what we will harvest. Nobody is able to tell you

what is right and what is wrong. Every event or incident bears its consequence.

All we can do is follow Nature with a righteous mind and benevolent heart. This will help you gain a peaceful and calm mind. Whenever you feel guilty and have resentment in your heart, your mind will be disturbed. Your spiritual cultivation will then be hindered. Our subconscious mind is connected with our spirit. If our subconscious mind is truthful and we follow the Dao, our spirit will grow following the correct path. Where there is an incident in the yang world (the material world), there is karma established in the yin world (the spiritual world) and it eventually affects the yang world again.

In order to reconnect our spirit with Nature, we must be truthful. Without truth, we will continue to keep our third from reopening. When the third eye is reopened, our telepathy can be resumed. Only when our third eye is reopened can we then reconnect with the natural spirit and reach the goal of "unification of heaven and human" (tian ren he yi, 天人合一). The third eye is called "heaven eye" (tian yan, 天眼) in qigong society because we are able to reconnect with heaven through this eye. I believe that when all humans have opened their third eyes and have the power of telepathy, there will be no evil thoughts or deeds that can be carried out or hidden. When this happens, humans will reach final harmonization and peace.

Conclusions

The way of following the Dao is treating others with a righteous and benevolent heart. In this way, you will build good deeds or karma in the yin space (spiritual dimension).

---

1. 杜光庭說："剛決為勇，必果為敢。""強梁者銳志而前，自投禍患；謙慎者奉身而退，必保安真。殺活二途，昭然可驗矣。"

2. 司馬光說："聖人之于天道，亦不敢易言之。"

3. 蘇轍說："勇於敢則死，勇於不敢則生，此物理之常也。然而敢者或以得生，不敢者或不免死，世常僥倖其或然，而忽其常理。夫天道之遠，其有以或然者，熟知其好惡所以來哉！故雖聖人猶以常為正，其于勇敢未嘗不難之。世以耳目觀天，見其一曲而不睹大全，有以善而得禍，惡而得福者，未有不疑天網之疏而多失也。唯能要其始終而盡其變化，然后知其恢恢廣大，雖疏而不失也。"

4. "善有善報，惡有惡報；不是不報，時辰未到。"

5. 王充說："李斯妒同才，幽殺韓非于秦，后被車裂之罪；商鞅欺舊交，擒魏公子卬，后受誅死之禍。"
   《論衡·禍虛》

6. "種瓜得瓜，種豆得豆。"

CHAPTER 74

Restraining Delusion—Stop Abuse

第七十四章
制惑—止濫

民不畏死，
　　　奈何以死懼之？
若使民常畏死，
　　　而為奇者，
吾得執而殺之，
　　　孰敢？
常有司殺者殺，
　　　夫代司殺者殺，
　　　是謂代大匠斲。
夫代大匠斲者，
　　　希有不傷其手者矣。

If people are not fearful of death,
  how can they be threatened with death?
If people are made to always be afraid of death,
  then, for those unlawful persons,
  I capture and kill them.
  How many would then dare (to be unlawful)?
There is a master who executes prisoners.
  If we let someone else do his job of execution,
  it is like letting someone other than a great carpenter cut the
  wood.
Those who let someone other than a great carpenter cut wood,
  rarely avoid injuring their own hands.

General Interpretation

If people are not afraid of death, then even if there are laws, people will not be afraid. Su, Che (蘇轍) said: "If a government causes agony, punishes people heavily, and people are disordered and helpless, then they will not be constantly afraid of death. Even threatening them with death is useless."[1]

However, if a government knows how to take good care of people and make them happy and harmonious, they will be afraid of death. Under these circumstances, if there are some unlawful persons and the government seizes and kills them, who would dare not to obey the orders of the rulers? Su, Che (蘇轍) said: "If people are at peace with the way they governed, they will be happy in life and fear death. When there are unlawful people creating a disturbance, they should be captured and killed. Who would then dares not obey?"[2]

In a kingdom, every officer has his duty and responsibility. If any ruler interferes with the officers' duties and authority, then the government will become chaotic and disordered. It is the same if you are not an expert in carpentry and you pretend you are an expert. Often, you will injure yourself. Yan, Zun (嚴遵) said: "Thus, the Dao as a great king, is engaged in nothing and doing nothing. But, there is nothing that cannot be accomplished. (However) if officers overpower the ruler's authority, his life will perish, and if a ruler takes over an officer's job, then the country will be harmed."[3]

Qigong Interpretation

This chapter talks about two important qigong training principles. As we mentioned earlier, the body is like a country, the mind is the ruler of the body, the breathing is policies or strategies for governing the body (the country), the qi is the people, and the morality or morale is the spirit of the country. From this, you can see how important it is to be a ruler or a king since the ruler (the mind) has the authority and power to control the entire body's functioning.

First, our mind should not be addicted to bad habits. According to qigong, we have two minds, one is called yi (wisdom mind) and the other is called xin (emotional mind). The wisdom mind, as we saw, is compared to a horse: strong, yet able to be calm and intelligent. The emotional mind is compared to a monkey: though small and less powerful than a horse, it is able to create an annoying disturbance. This is called "xin ape and yi horse" (xin yuan yi ma, 心猿意馬). In qigong training, you are learning to make your wisdom mind stronger and more rational so it can govern the emotional mind's action. If you fail to do this, you can be influenced by or addicted to bad habits. Once a bad habit takes root, your subconscious mind will be negatively affected, and this will hinder your spiritual cultivation.

For example, if your wisdom mind fails to govern the emotional mind and you become addicted to alcohol or drugs, your subconscious mind will develop a memory of this which may spread to the entire body. This memory eventually will affect the entire body's normal qi function. As time passes, the abnormal qi circulation will affect your health. Naturally, when this happens, your spirit will also be negatively affected as well.

Second, the mind should not interfere with the internal organs' functioning unless necessary. Internal organs are just like officers who help the ruler govern the country. All officers have their responsibilities and duties and should not be interfered with. For example, the heart receives a proper amount of qi to maintain its normal function. If the mind (the ruler) overpowers the heart's function, disaster may happen. This is because when you focus your mind on the heart, the extra qi will be led to the heart and cause excess qi. When this happens, the heartbeat will be faster, blood pressure will increase, and the heart's normal functioning may be interrupted. This may trigger a heart attack and bring serious harm to the heart.

In another example, if the mind leads you to drink a lot of alcohol, this will put more pressure and stress on the liver and make it more yang. You may get angry more readily and acutely which may promote excessive qi in the liver, causing an excess fire condition (too yang) as well. All of these are examples of the ruler interfering with the officers' duties.

As a ruler or a king, you should pay attention to the entire body's harmonization and coordination but without interfering with them. When a ruler has a calm, logical, and peaceful mind, he will provide the most suitable environment (the proper lifestyle) for the entire kingdom. Then all officers (internal organs) can function normally and healthily.

Conclusions

Every part and organ in the body has its qi requirement and duties. They should not interfere with each other's functions. This is especially important for the mind since the mind governs the entire body's function. The mind should pay attention to the body's condition without interfering with their normal function.

1. 蘇轍說：“政煩刑重，民無所措手足，則常不畏死。雖以死懼之，無益也。”
2. 蘇轍說：“民安于政，故樂生畏死，然后執其詭異亂群者而殺之，孰敢不服哉！”
3. 嚴遵說：“是故帝王之道，無事無為，無所不克。臣行君道，則滅其身；君行臣事，則傷其國。”

CHAPTER 75

Harmed by Greediness—Nourishing Life

第七十五章
貪損—養生

民之飢，
　　以其上食稅之多，
　　是以飢。
民之難治，
　　以其上之有為，
　　是以難治。
民之輕死，
　　以其上求生之厚，
　　是以輕死。
夫唯無以生為者，
　　是賢於貴生。

The people's hunger,
    is because of the ruler's excess taxation;
    thus, they starve.
People are hard to govern,
    because the ruler's meddle too much,
    they are difficult to govern.
People disregard their death,
    because of the ruler's glutinous living;
    thus, they disregard their death.
Only those (i.e., sage rulers) who do not strive for living
    are wiser than those (i.e., regular rulers) who value living
    seriously.

General Interpretation

When a ruler collects too much in taxes, though the ruler is rich, people become so poor they cannot afford to feed themselves. If a ruler abuses his power, interferes with the normal functioning of the country, and frequently changes the country's laws and policies, then people will have difficulties following the rulers' orders. The society will become chaotic and hard to control. Wu, Cheng (吳澄) said: "When the top (i.e., the ruler) wants to display his power and use his witty skills to govern his subordinates, his subordinates will also use their guile to deceive the ruler. Thus, it is hard to govern."[1]

When a ruler treats his own life as more precious than the lives of others, is attached to luxurious living, and ignores people's lives and suffering, soon people will not value their own life and will turn against the ruler. However, those rulers who do not overvalue their own lives and live too luxuriously will be respected and loved. They will be better than those who value their lives greatly. Gao, Heng (高亨) said: "Don't take life seriously means don't care about what could happen in life. This means they don't value their lives. If rulers value their lives preciously and treat themselves with luxurious living, then in order to satisfy their luxuries, the ruler will be oppressive in governing. When the ruler is oppressive, then the people suffer. When people suffer, they value their lives lightly. Therefore, those rulers who have a tranquil thrifty life are wiser than those who value their lives preciously."[2]

Qigong Interpretation

This chapter is about how to manage your qi with your mind. The mind (the ruler) leads and controls the qi (people). If the mind abuses the qi, the qi's storage and circulation will become disordered. For example, if the mind continues to challenge the body's tolerance and pushes it beyond its limit, eventually there will be a qi deficiency and imbalanced qi circulation. The way of cultivating and nourishing the body is to know how to protect qi and keep yin (the qi body) and yang (the physical body) balanced.

From a qigong point of view, the body includes two parts: the physical part (yang) and the energy or qi part (yin). Both should be balanced. Putting too much demand on the physical will cause an inner deficiency of qi, and too little physical exercises will cause weakening and degeneration of the body. The right way of cultivating and taking care of the body is to know how to apply the right amount of qi to condition the physical body and also how to conserve and build up abundant qi to supply the body's needs.

Once you have established a healthy lifestyle, you should keep it so your body can get used to it. If you keep changing your lifestyle, your body will not be able to adjust itself easily and comfortably. The qi's circulation will then become aberrant. However, once you have established a healthy lifestyle, keep up with a correct routine. You should only make minor modifications that do not interfere with the entire body's function.

Conclusions

Adequately managing your qi with your mind is the crucial key of keeping the body's yin and yang balanced and harmonious with each other.

1. 吳澄說：「上有為，以智術御其下，下亦以奸詐欺其上，故難治。」
2. 高亨說：「無以生為者，不以生為事也，即不貴生也。君貴生則厚養，厚養則苛政，苛政則民苦，民苦則輕死。故君不貴生，賢于貴生也。」

CHAPTER 76

Abstaining from Strength—Approaching Softness

第七十六章
戒強—致柔

人之生也柔弱，
　　　其死也堅強。
萬物草木之生也柔脆，
　　　其死也枯槁。
　　　故
堅強者，死之徒；
　　　柔弱者，生之徒。
　　　是以
兵強則不勝，
　　　木強則折。
　　　強大處下，
　　　柔弱處上。

When a man is born, he is soft and weak;
  when dead, he becomes stiff and hard.
Myriad objects such as grass and trees, when alive, are supple and
  soft;
  when dead, they become brittle and dried.
  Therefore,
those hard and stiff accompany death;
  those soft and weak accompany life.
  Thus,
a strong army will not have victory,
  when the wood is hard, then it can be broken.
  Strong and big are positioned low,
while those weak and soft will be situated on high.

General Interpretation

When a person is born, he is weak and soft. However, once he is dead, he becomes stiff and hard. It is the same for myriad objects, such as grasses or trees: when alive they are supple and soft, and when dead they become brittle and dried. He Shang Gong (河上公) said: "When a person is alive, he has the harmonious qi circulating within, and the spirit is embraced; thus, soft and weak. When a person is dead and qi is exhausted, the spirit of vitality is perished; thus, stiff and hard."[1] Du, Guang-Ting (杜光庭) also said: "Grasses and trees, due to the gathering of qi, are alive; consequently, leaves and branches flourish, and are soft and supple. Once the qi is exhausted and there is death, then the branches become withered, brittle, and dried."[2]

From this, you can see that those who are stiff, strong, and hard will soon find death while those who are soft, gentle, and weak will survive. Wu, Cheng (吳澄) said: "Ponder: from these principles, we can see that those who are strong and hard will not die peacefully. They belong to the group of death. Those who are soft and weak will embrace their lives preciously. This is the group with life."[3] This is because those who are strong and powerful will not hesitate to use their strength when intending to conquer or subdue others. When this happens often, they will encounter another strong opponent and eventually both die. However, those who are weak and soft, recognizing that they are not strong, will conserve their energy, be kind and gentle, and thus, get along with others and survive.

It is the same when this theory is applied to the army. Those who often use their strength and power to fight and control others will eventually be conquered and perish. Those who are gentle and kind to neighbors will be peaceful and survive. From this, you can see that those who are strong are actually in the low positions of human society while those who are soft are in the high positions.

Qigong Interpretation

When you lead qi to circulate in the body, your mind must be soft. When your mind is soft, your body will be relaxed. When you are relaxed, your gentle mind will be able to softly and smoothly lead the qi to the deepest places in the body. On the contrary, if your mind is stiff, strong, and has too much ego, the body will be more tense. When this happens, the qi will be stagnant and cause sickness.

It is the same when you manage a business or other people. A soft and flexible attitude will allow you to take care of things smoothly and get along with others in a friendly way. However, if you are strong, stiff, and stubborn, you will fail in your friendships and business. Using softness to conquer the hard is the key principle of taijiquan practice. This is the reason that practicing taijiquan is so beneficial for one's health. So enable the qi to circulate smoothly in the body.

Conclusions

Softness is the crucial key to using your mind to lead the qi. When your mind is soft, your body is relaxed. When your body is relaxed, the qi can circulate smoothly.

1. 河上公說："人生含和氣，抱精神，故柔弱也；人死和氣竭，精神亡，故堅強也。"
2. 杜光庭說："草木氣聚而生，故枝葉敷榮而柔脆；氣竭而死，則條干變衰而枯槁。"
3. 吳澄說："推此物理，則知人之德行。凡堅強者不得其死，是死之徒也。柔弱者善抱其生，是生之徒也。"

CHAPTER 77
The Dao of Heaven—Balance
第七十七章
天道—平衡

天之『道』，
　　　其猶如張弓歟？
高者抑之，
　　　下者舉之；
有餘者損之，
　　　不足者補之。
天之『道』，
　　　損有餘而補不足；
人之道，則不然，
　　　損不足以奉有餘。
孰能以有餘奉天下？
　　　唯有『道』者。
是以『聖人』為而不恃，
　　　功成而不處。
　　　其不欲見賢邪！

The Dao of the Heaven,
     is it just like drawing a bow?
The high is lowered,
     and the low is raised higher.
Reduce what has excess,
     and add it to what is lacking.
Take away from those who have excess,
     give to those who are lacking.
The Dao of Heaven,
     always takes away from excess and gives it to those are lacking.
(However), the Dao of humans is not the same,
     take away from those who are lacking to give those who already
     have excess.
Who is able to offer his surplus to the world?
     Only those who have the Dao.
Thus, sages do things without conceit,
     achieve the goal claiming no credit.
They do not wish to display their superiority.

General Interpretation

The Dao of heaven (Nature) is just like drawing a bow. The goal of drawing the bow is to hit the target. You must raise and lower the bow as necessary. Without the correct angle and adequate strength, you will not be able to hit the target. A high-power bow, moreover, requires a strong string while a weaker bow requires a less strong string to work properly. Yan, Jun-Ping (嚴君平) said: "The use of a bow relies on its harmonization. If the string is too tense and urgent, then loosen it up; when the string is too loose and relaxed, then tense it up. What is too much, reduce it to lower it and what is too little, add to raise it. When the string and the bow are mutually balanced, the harmony between them can be achieved. Therefore, the bow can be used and the arrow can be shot."[1] Du, Guang-Ting (杜光庭) also said:

> "The use of a bow should be decided by the bow's material and also the adequacy of string's tension and loosening. When you shoot, if it is too high, lower it, and when it is too low, raise it up. This is decided by the target. Too much, reduce it and too little, add it. This decides the distance of the shooting, and then the target can be hit. The Dao of heaven is the same. Every day and month passes so the winter and summer come and go. When it comes, it reduces its excess and when it goes, it adds it to its deficiency. In this way, the yearly cycle is completed. A ruler should follow this Dao of heaven, suppressing the strong and helping the weak. Reduce who has excess and support those who have nothing. Thus, move surplus to the deficient. This is for the balance of the distribution."[2]

However, most wealthy humans are greedy and unwilling to share with the poor. Only sages, when they have surplus, share with others without hesitation. It is the same for a wise ruler: though he is wealthy, he still saves and conserves his wealth so he can share his wealth with the people. We, Cheng (吳澄) said: "Those rulers who have the Dao, though noble as an emperor and rich with the four seas, are not proud of themselves for their grandeur and wealth; eat simple food, are sick of lux-urious clothes, make humble their palace, and save the money for the world without wasting it. Systematize and divide the land with the people, teach them how to grow plants, and charge low taxes, so the people have enough for their living. This is the case of offering his excess to the world."[3]

Those sages or rulers who have the Dao conduct their actions with-out conceit and achieve their goals without claiming credit. They remain humble without displaying their superiority. When this hap-pens, they will eventually earn good repute and credit without asking for it. They will also receive recognition of their superiority without demanding it. In the book, *Shang Shu* (《尚書‧大禹謨》), it is said: "Only if you don't show off your superiority, will the people of the world not strive with you for superiority. Only if you don't flaunt yourself, will the people not contend with your achievement."[4] Wang, Li (王力) also said: "Those who are in the top position often greedily think the achievements of heaven (i.e., Nature) are their achievements. Since they believe they have accomplished such an achievement, they should be the masters of the people. This is because they feel arrogant, but actu-ally, we can see that they are small. Lao Zi said: 'Those sages do not want their superiority to be seen.' It is also because they don't want to be seen that their nobility is seen by itself."[5]

Qigong Interpretation

This chapter has pointed out two important qigong training con-cepts. The first is that yin and yang must be balanced and harmonious with each other in your practice. For example, practicing a lot of physical qigong will usually raise up your body's energy status, called li (fire) (離). When this happens, your body will become more energized and hot. This makes your body more yang. This training is called "charging" or "nourishing" (bu, 補). This is to build up the qi potential difference.

However, after physical exercises, you should relax your mind and physical body with deep breathing. This will allow the qi to circulate and distribute the built-up qi to the entire body. When this happens, the body begins to cool down and is considered as kan (water) (坎). This will make your body more yin and finally, yin and yang will balance each other.

It is the same for muscle/tendon changing and brain/marrow washing qigong. Muscle/tendon changing makes your body more yang while brain/marrow washing makes you more yin. If you train only muscle/tendon changing without training brain/marrow washing, you may experience the body becoming too yang and cause "energy dispersion" (san gong, 散功).

The second concept this chapter has pointed out is the importance of your mind. Too much ego or expectation can only make the qi's circulation become more imbalanced or chaotic. Your mind is the king or ruler of the body (kingdom) and the qi represents the people. The mind must be gentle, kind, open, and in a neutral state. Only then, will the mind have a correct feeling so the excess qi can be led to those areas where the qi is deficient. For example, if there is too much qi trapped in your upper body, such as the head, this can trigger high blood pressure or a headache. If your mind is able to feel this imbalance and lead the excess qi from the top to the lower part of your body, the heartbeat will slow down and the blood pressure and headache can be regulated.

Conclusions

The mind and its ability to lead the qi is yin while the expressed action (manifestation of yin) is yang. This yin and yang should be balanced. This is the natural law. If imbalanced, problems can occur. The best way of dealing with imbalance is providing the right conditions and environment to allow the qi to regain its balance. You should keep your mind humble with a high level of awareness so you can see the possible problem. Too much ego will cause the disorder in the qi.

1. 嚴君平說：“夫弓之為用也，必在調和。弦高急者，寬而緩之；弦弛下者，攝而上之；其有餘者，削而損之；其有不足者，補而益之。弦質相任，調和而常，故可用而矢可行。”

2. 杜光庭說：“夫弓之為用，當合材定體，弛張調利。高者抑之，下者舉之者，為架箭之時准的也。有餘者損之，不足者與之，為發矢之時近遠也。如此則能命中矣。天道亦然。日月寒暑，一往一來。來者損其有餘，往者與其不足，則成歲功矣。人君者當法于天道，抑強扶弱，損有利無，故舉虧盈益謙，欲令稱物平施爾。"

3. 吳澄說："有道之君，貴為天子，富有四海，而不自有其富貴，菲飲食，惡衣服，卑宮室，為天下惜財而不苟費，制田里，教樹藝，薄稅斂，使民家給人足，是以己之有餘而奉天下也。"

4. 《尚書·大禹謨》："汝唯不矜，天下莫與汝爭能，汝唯不伐，天下莫與汝爭功。"

5. 王力說："為民上者，往往貪天之功以為己功，自念有此大功，足為民之主宰；此其自大，適足以見其小耳。聃所謂'不欲見賢，'即不欲顯示其賢，不自為大，故能成其大也。"

CHAPTER 78
Trust in Faith—Follow Softly
第七十八章
任信—柔順

天下莫柔弱於水，
　　而攻堅強者莫之能勝，
　　其無以易之。
弱之勝強，
　　柔之勝剛，
天下莫不知，
　　莫能行。
是以『聖人』云：
　　「受國之垢，是謂社稷主；
　　受國不祥，是為天下王。」
　　正言若反。

Nothing in the world is softer and weaker than water,
   yet nothing is better (than water) in attacking the hard and
   strong,
   nothing is able to replace it.
Weak is able to defeat strong,
   soft is able overcome hard.
Everyone in the world knows,
   but nobody is able to carry it out in action.
Therefore, those sages said:
   "Those who are able to accept the humiliation of the country
   can be the lords of countries.
   Those who are able to accept the misfortune of the country can
   be the kings of the kingdoms."
   But, the truth seems opposite.

General Interpretation

Everyone knows that water is one of the most yielding substances in the world. But, water's power is able to penetrate hard stone and corrode steel. Nothing can replace this power. Du, Guang-Ting (杜光庭) said: "Water, though soft, is able to penetrate a hole in stone. But stone, though strong, cannot damage water. If strong is used to attack strong, then both are damaged. Use water to attack stone, then stone is damaged, but water remains intact."[1]

Though everyone knows that the weak is able to defeat the strong and the soft can overcome the hard, very few are able put this concept into practice. Du, Guang-Ting (杜光庭) said: "Everybody knows that softness and weakness are able to overcome hardness and strength. Though they know this, who is able to comprehend the importance of softness and use it to cultivate his temperament and use (the Dao of) softness to move his heart (from emotional allurement), defeat its tenacity, and practice (the Dao's) insubstantial science? If one is able to comprehend the Dao and cultivate it, then how can the Dao be far to reach?"[2]

It is the same when ruling a country with the Dao. As a ruler, you must have a kind, gentle, open, and humble heart. With this heart, the country will be ruled by itself without tough and harsh laws. The book *Shang Shu* (《尚書·湯誥》) said: "Those myriad faults are all because of me; however, when I have faults, I cannot blame myriad others."[3] This is how the temperament of a leader should be. The book *Shuo Yuan* (《說苑·君道》) says: "Yu (禹) (i.e., Xia emperor) was out and saw that a criminal was being punished; (he) got out of the carriage, asked (the reason), and sobbed. His accompanying officers said: 'This criminal is being punished because he does not follow the Dao (i.e., law). Why is the king so sad with grief?' Yu said: 'Yao (堯) and Shun (舜) (i.e., ancient emperors) always used their hearts (i.e., feeling) to understand other people's hearts (i.e., feeling); that is why it is painful.'"[4] From this you can see that to be a great ruler, you must always put your heart into people's hearts and feel their feeling. This is using the soft to lead the country.

Even though we know what is true, in reality, not too many people or rulers are able to follow that truth. They will just say all these sayings are absurd. He Shang Gong (河上公) said: "Though these are upstanding and upright words, most laymen do not know and just think the reverse."[5]

Qigong Interpretation

Qi is soft like water that can only be led and not pushed. Though qi is soft, its influence on your health, longevity, and spirit is powerful. The mind is just like a king who governs the qi (people). If a king is able to use the soft way to lead the people and educate them with right manners, the country will be peaceful, prosperous, and harmonious. As long as a person is able to keep his mind humble and willing to put his feeling into the body's feeling, then he will be able to regulate the body's function and achieve health. Feeling is a language that allows your mind and body to communicate. Pain or discomfort means the body is complaining that there is a qi stagnation or some problem. Ignoring it will lead to sickness.

Conclusions

This chapter has pointed out two important things: qi can be led but not pushed, and deep feeling is the key to correcting problems. This feeling is called "the gongfu of internal vision" (nei shi gongfu, 內視功夫) in qigong practice. It is called "gong fu" because it takes a lot of time and effort to develop deep feeling. Internal vision means to investigate or to observe internally. Through deep feeling, the body can be healthy and the spirit can be cultivated to a higher level.

1. 杜光庭說："水雖柔而能穴石，石雖堅而不能損水。若以堅攻堅，則彼此俱損；以水攻石，則石損而水全。"
2. 杜光庭說："柔弱之勝剛強，人皆知矣。雖知其事，誰能體柔修性，用道移心，挫其剛強，習其虛寂耶？有能體道而修者，道何遠哉？"
3. 《尚書·湯誥》："其爾萬方有罪，在于一人；予一人有罪，無以爾萬方。"
4. 《說苑·君道》："禹出見罪人，下車問而泣之。左右曰：'夫罪人不順道，故使然焉。君王何為痛之至于此也？'禹曰：'堯舜之人，皆以堯舜之心為心，是以痛之也。'"
5. 河上公說："此乃正直之言，世人不知，以為反言。"

CHAPTER 79

Keep Obligations—Fluent Communications

第七十九章
任契—疏通

和大怨，
　　必有餘怨；
　　安可以為善？
是以『聖人』執左契，
　　而不責於人。
有『德』司契，
　　無『德』司徹。
天道無親，
　　常與善人。

After reconciling a great dispute,
  there must be some resentments remaining.
  How can this be considered adequate?
Thus, the sages hold the left part of the contracts,
  but do not demand debits from others.
Those who have virtue hold the contracts,
  while those without virtue hold the collections.
The Dao of heaven does not have favor,
  but it always gives to kind persons.

General Interpretation

When there is a dispute, it does not matter how you reconcile it; there will always be some remaining resentment. This is because, no matter what, both sides will always think they are right and the other side is wrong. There is no perfect reconciliation that will satisfy both sides.

That is why sages will just give favors to others and never ask for a favor in return. The Chinese have a proverb, "What you don't want to have, you should not give to others."[1] Another proverb is, "You should not remember what favor you have given, but should not forget what you have received from others."[2] If you have this character trait, you will be peaceful and harmonious with others.

This chapter says that is why those sages would keep the left part of the contract so they will not collect debits. In ancient times, since paper was not available, the contract was carved on a piece of wood. After splitting it in half, the creditor kept the right part and the debtor kept the left. Since sages kept the left part, they did not demand the return of the debt. But whoever held the right part and demanded repayment of the debt, the sages would give it to them without question. Wei, Yuan (魏源) said:

"What is called 'goodness' means to those who are good, I am good to them. Those who are not good, I am also good to them. Then you are like sages who hold the left contracts. The wood contract has two parts. I keep the left. Whoever comes with the right part of the contract, I will repay him with money and goods. In this case, I will never receive blame from others. Those sages treat matters lightly, follow situations and give to others without hesitation. He will just receive whatever comes. Those who pay back the debt will not have resentment, and those whom I give and offer will not see my virtuous deed. When virtue and resentment both are obliterated, there is no difference between objects and me; then this is the true indisputable virtue."[3]

If you are able to achieve this stage of virtuous cultivation, then heaven will always be on your side and help you. In the book, *Shang Shu* (《尚書·伊訓》) it is said, "The actions (i.e., deeds) those holy sages have conducted through their profound pondering (i.e., planning) are as wide and great as an ocean and the edifying words they have spoken are very obvious and clear. Heaven does not go against natural rules. Those who have conducted good deeds will receive a hundred blessings and those who have done bad deeds will receive a hundred misfortunes."[4] It is again said in *Shang Shu* (《尚書·蔡仲》): "Heaven does not have intimates; it only helps those who have virtuous deeds."[5] This means Nature does not have favorite persons but stays neutral. Only those who have done good deeds will receive special attention from it. It is said in *Zuo Zhuan* (《左傳·僖五年》): "Those ghosts or spiritual divines do not have special intimate persons, but follow the virtuous deeds."[6] This means that whatever good deeds you have done, you will be blessed by spirits in the yin world.

Qigong Interpretation

As we have seen, *The Book of Changes* (*Yi Jing*, 易經) has influenced Chinese culture since the beginning of history. It has especially influenced Chinese thinking about qigong practice. As we have also seen, it is believed that there are two worlds coexisting in reality. One is the spiritual world (yin world) (陰間) and the other is the material world (yang world) (陽間). Although there are two worlds, they cannot be separated. One is yin and the other is yang, and each influences the other. Although there are two worlds in reality, they are actually only one in function. The spirit that is related to our mind or thinking is considered as yin and is the Dao (道) of a human body. When this Dao has manifested into actions or behaviors, it is called the De (德). Thus, the De is the manifestation of the Dao. When a person has good morality in both mind and action, the Chinese say he has good "Dao-De" (道德).

It is also believed the energy of the spiritual world (the yin world) can be influenced by the yang world, and vice versa. If you have done good deeds in the yang world, you will accumulate credit in the yin world. Naturally, if you have done evil deeds, the bad spiritual energy will also accumulate in the yin world. Eventually, this energy or qi will be manifested in the yang world. This redistribution is your karma or destiny.

In qigong practice, you are conditioning your physical life (the yang material world) while you are cultivating your spiritual life (the yin virtue world). Your thinking and deeds will be recorded in the yin world. If you are able to regulate your mind and treat all material attractions lightly, your heart will be wide open, and naturally your mind will always be in a peaceful and harmonious state. Accordingly, the qi circulating in your physical and spiritual bodies will be smooth, abundant, and harmonious. Therefore, having followed the Dao (Nature), Nature will accord with you and help you. You will feel that there is an angel always around you, protecting you.

Conclusions

Having a benevolent heart to serve and help others is the best way of cultivating your good deeds. The Chinese have a saying: "being taken advantage of by others is better than taking advantage of others."[7] See through the material world so you are not enslaved by material things. Keep your mind simple and not allured by desire so you can set yourself free from emotional bondage.

1. "己所不欲，勿施於人。"
2. "施人甚勿念，受施甚勿忘。"
3. 魏源說："善所謂德善者，善者吾善之，不善者吾亦善之，則聖人之執左契者是己。券契有二，我執其左，但有執右以來責取者，吾即以財物與之，而未嘗有所責取于人。聖人之于物，順應無心，來無不受，亦若是而已。來者不見其為怨，與者不自以為德，德怨兩泯，物我渾化，是則真能體我不爭之德矣。"
4. 《尚書·伊訓》："聖謨洋洋，嘉言孔彰；唯上帝不常，作善降之百祥；作不善降之百殃。"
5. 《尚書·蔡仲》："皇天無親，唯德是輔。"
6. 《左傳·僖五年》："鬼神非人實親，唯德是從。"
7. "被人欺，勝於欺人。"

CHAPTER 80

Independence—Return to Origin (Return to Simplicity)

第八十章
獨立—返元（返樸）

小國寡民，
　　使有什伯之器而不用，
　　使民重死而不遠徙。
雖有舟輿，
　　無所乘之；
雖有甲兵，
　　無所陳之。
　　使民復結繩而用之。
甘其食，
　　美其服；
安其居，
　　樂其俗。
鄰國相望，
　　雞犬之聲相聞，
　　民至老死，不相往來。

Be a small country with few people,
   though there are hundreds of weapons, none are used,
   let people regard death seriously and do not travel far.
Although boats and chariots are available,
   there is no need to use them.
Although armor and weapons are possessed,
   there is no place to utilize them.
   Let people return to the time with tying knots for counting.
Savor their food,
   and beautify their clothes.
Content in their living,
   and happy in their customs.
Even though neighboring countries are able to see each other (i.e., near),
   sounds of roosters and dogs can be heard,
   people do not communicate even till death.

General Interpretation

When a country is small with only a few people, the people know each other and live harmoniously and peacefully. Even though there are weapons, they are never used.

When people treat their life preciously, they will not travel too far from home and encounter dangers. Though there are boats and carriages, there is no need for them. Even though there are armories, there is no use for them. If all people are simple and so innocent as in the old times when they used tying knots for counting, then there is no sneakiness or tricks bing played. *Yi Jing, Xi-Ci* (《易‧繫辭》) said: "In ancient times, people used tying knots for counting and ruling; later those sages replaced them with bamboo tablets." "Ancient people lived in caves and the wild, and later those sages replaced them with houses."[1]

Let people enjoy and appreciate delicious food and comfortable clothes and follow their traditions and customs. Even if neighboring countries are close, people are happy to stay in their homes. The book *Huai Na Zi* (《淮南子‧齊俗訓》) says: "Thus, though neighboring counties can see each other, and the sounds of chickens and dogs can mutually be heard, there are no traces of steps that have reached the neighboring kingdoms and the rail carriages do not connect more than a thousand miles. Therefore, all the people are peaceful and happy with where they are."[2]

This whole chapter can be compared with what it says in *Zhuang Zi* (《莊子‧馬蹄》):

> *"Thus, in the era of high morality, people's behavior is solemn and serious, their minds pure and simple. During this time, there is no small path in the mountains, there is no boat for lakes, myriad objects are blooming, villages are connected with each other, animals are grouping together, and all plants are growing. Therefore, animals are able to roam around freely, and the bird nests can be peeked at after climbing. When it is the high morality era, people live together with animals and share nature with myriad objects. How can people know the differences*

between a gentleman and a small person (i.e., bad person)? When innocent, morality will not depart. When there is no desire, it means simplicity. If there is simplicity, then people have acquired the quality of nature."[3]

Qigong Interpretation

When you practice qigong, you should begin with regulating your body. Your body is so small compared with the Great Nature; however, it is just like a small independent kingdom where there is a king (mind) and people (qi). Therefore, when you begin to train qigong, start with yourself.

Though you have arms, legs, and all the organs of sense, you should know how to keep them calm and relaxed, especially when you are cultivating your mind during meditation. Not only that, you should always monitor your qi at the qi center (qi residence, 氣舍) so the qi circulation is not wasted, imbalanced, or randomly manifested. When this happens, the qi will be conserved and accumulated to an abundant level at the lower real dan tian. To keep the mind at the lower real dan tian (yi shou dan tian, 意守丹田) is a crucial key of preserving qi.

Even when there are temptations or distractions around you, your mind should not move away from the qi center. Once you are able to bring your mind to the center and keep the qi there, you will have reached the goal of embryonic breathing meditation; you have gone back to your childhood: innocent, simple, and pure. When you have achieved this level, you will feel everything return to its origin. This is the "scene of returning to origin."[4]

When you are in this simple, innocent, and pure state, your conscious mind will be downplayed—the mask will have dropped from your face—and the subconscious mind will be awakened. When this happens, you will be in a semisleeping state. Your spirit will reconnect and communicate with the natural spirit. This is the "scene of spiritual communication."[5] qigong embryonic breathing meditation will help lead you through the gate of this spiritual garden. Once you enter the spiritual garden, you will be able to feel and sense scenery other people cannot experience. It is so natural and peaceful. This is the stage of "unification of human and heaven" (天人合一).

Conclusions

Keep your mind simple without too much desire. Always appreciate what you have already acquired and do not be allured by temptation. Bring your spirit (son) to the lower real dan tian and unite with the qi (mother) at the qi residence. This practice is called "unification of mother and son."[6]

1. 《易‧繫辭》：“上古結繩而治，后世聖人易之以書契。”“上古穴居而野處，后世聖人易之以宮室。”
2. 《淮南子‧齊俗訓》：“是故鄰國相望，雞狗之音相聞，而足跡不接諸侯之境，車軌不結千里之外者，皆各得其所安。”
3. 《莊子‧馬蹄》：“故至德之世，其行填填，其視顛顛。當此之時，山無蹊隧，澤無舟梁，萬物群生，連屬其鄉，禽獸成群，草木遂長。是故禽獸可系羈而游，鳥鵲之巢可攀援而窺。夫至德之世，同與禽獸居，族與萬物并，惡知乎君子小人哉？同乎無知，其德不離；同乎無欲，是謂素朴；素朴則民性得矣。”
4. “返元之景。”
5. “神交之景。”
6. “母子相和。”

CHAPTER 81

The Manifestation of Simplicity—Seek for Truth

第八十一章
顯質—求真

信言不美，
　　美言不信。
善者不辯，
　　辯者不善。
知者不博，
　　博者不知。
『聖人』不積，
　　既已為人己愈有，
　　既已與人己愈多。
天之『道』，
　　利而不害；
『聖人』之『道』，
　　為而不爭。

True words may not be beautiful,
  beautiful words may not be truthful.
Those who are good do not have to debate,
  those who debate may not be good.
Those who (really) know may not have broad knowledge,
  those who have broad knowledge may not (really) know.
Those sages do not accumulate (things) for themselves,
  the more they serve others, the more they gain,
  the more they give to others, the more they receive.
The Dao of heaven,
  benefits (others) without harm.
The Dao of sages,
  does it without contending.

General Interpretation

First, this chapter talks about the true and the false. Often, honest talk is not light and pleasant. However, we should also know that light and pleasant talk is usually not truthful. If we are able to treat others with a truthful heart and express our real feelings, then we will have established a truthful world. As such, we will all really know each other and will not have to hide our real emotions and real selves behind our masks. Can we take the masks down and face our real selves? Those who have a good heart and do good deeds do not feel compelled to boast about how good they are or what they have done. On the other hand, those who often boast about their attainments may not actually have a good or truthful heart. Wang Bi (王弼) said: "Truth is built upon inner quality and originates from simplicity of mind."[1] He Shang Gong (河上公) also said: "People are trusted due to their truthfulness, and though they are not beautiful, they have a simplicity and pure quality (of mind)."[2] He Shang Gong (河上公) again said: "Those good people who cultivate themselves with the Dao do not express themselves with embellished speech. However, the tongues of those good at debating and skillful in tricky talk will eventually cause disaster. If there is jade in the mountain, the mountain will be dug up and destroyed; when there are pearls in the water, the depths will be contaminated. Those who are good at debating and talk too much will cause the death of their body.[3] In Chinese society, it is said: "Disasters are originated from the mouth (i.e., talking)."[4] Thus, it is better to keep silent; "silence is gold."[5]

Then this chapter mentions that those who really have comprehended the Dao and the meaning of life are usually humble and believe they know nothing. This is because they know the Dao is so great that it is impossible to understand the depth of it. On the contrary, those who always talk about how much they know may know nothing or just what is on the surface. Du, Guang Ting (杜光庭) said: "Those who have grasped the importance of the Dao, though they have acquired the meaning of the Dao, they forget to talk about it. They know the Dao and are able to act from it in their life. They gain by acting from it and forget it after teaching it. Keep singularity (i.e., keep consistent) so there is nothing bothered. Do nothing so there is nothing disordered. Those who are experts in talking and teaching are too far from the Dao. Because this is so, how can they really comprehend the marvelousness of the Dao?"[6]

Next, the chapter reminds us that those who have a good heart like the sages will keep nothing, neither material things nor knowledge, to themselves. The more they serve and share with others, the more they understand the "Dao," and the more they gain. Du, Guang Ting (杜光庭) again said: "(This chapter) says though those sages do not hesitate to talk and teach, the wisdom heart (i.e., mind) of those laymen has already emerged and is eager to learn and understand. They need sages to guide them. Thus, sages will teach them tranquility and rationality without bias, and it does not matter if they are normal or dull. To those sages, their comprehension of humanity and temperament will never be reduced or wasted. Thus, it is said: 'the more they receive' and 'the more they gain.'"[7]

Finally, this final chapter concludes with the thought that the "Heaven Dao" gives and benefits all lives without bringing them harm. Therefore, those sages will work to benefit others and all things without hesitation or difficulty. They have regulated their heart and mind without effort. Eventually, they don't have to try and make things happen (wuwei, 無為). Du, Guang Ting (杜光庭) said: "The Heaven Dao gives lives, nourishes, and grows myriad objects; it is beneficial. There is no killing and cutting; there is no harm. Sages have comprehended the Dao and respond with heaven (i.e., Nature) so to share (their understanding) with the public. The wider they have shared with and benefited others the more their minds are humble. The more they have accomplished the more their merits are hidden. Therefore, they benefit all things without harm and respond to all things without struggling."[8] Gao Heng (高亨) said: "The Dao of heaven benefits but is not harmful; the Dao of sages gives to people without struggling."[9]

Qigong Interpretation

To be a spiritual qigong practitioner, you must be truthful to yourself and others. Without a truthful mind, your "heaven eye" (tian yan, 天眼) (the third eye) will remain closed since you will not wish others to know your false and untruthful thinking. Daoists call themselves "zhen ren" (真人) which means "truthful person." This is because without the truthful heart, they must continue to hide their secret behind the third eye.

In order to be truthful, you must first be truthful to yourself. To do that, you must know how to use your rational and wisdom mind to subdue emotional and irrational thinking. Once you have cultivated your inner spiritual being, you can open your truthful heart to others.

In addition, in order to reach to a profound level of qigong practice, the mere collection of knowledge is not crucial. The most important key to reaching a high level of practice is cultivating your inner self and feeling. To be truthful, you must develop your subconscious mind that is more truthful and subdue your conscious mind that is untruthful. Remember, your subconscious mind always leads you to the truthful path of cultivation. This is the first step of embryonic breathing.

Next, you must learn how to cultivate your qi at the real lower dan tian (zhen xia dan tian, 真下丹田). The more you want the qi to accumulate in the dan tian, the harder it will be. This is because when you focus your mind on accumulating qi, your qi will actually be more disturbed and dispersed. The way of leading the qi to the real lower dan tian is through "thinking of no thinking" (wuwei, 無為). It is the same if you try very hard to fall sleep; eventually, you will be more awake than if you hadn't tried. The key is "be natural." Once your mind has reached the semisleeping state, the qi can be led and made to stay at the real lower dan tian. This is the stage of "regulating without regulating" (bu tiao er tiao, 不調而調) and the semisleeping state of "mind of no mind."

In qigong practice, you should not hesitate to share your knowledge and qi with other practitioners. This is called "dual-cultivation" (shuang xiu, 雙修). Eventually, the more you share, the more you will know how to build qi. This is because the body is alive and can be gradually conditioned. Teaching is the best way of learning. In Chinese society, it is said: "Teaching and learning help each other to grow mutually."[10]

Finally, this chapter mentions that when you practice, you should be "natural." When the conditions are in place and the time is right, everything you want to cultivate will happen naturally. The more you try to make it happen, the harder it will be.

Conclusions

To reach spiritual enlightenment, you must first reopen your third eye. In order to reopen your third eye, you must be truthful to yourself and others. In addition, you must learn the way to lead qi to the limbic system (the quality of qi's manifestation). When this happens, the conscious mind will be minimized and the subconscious mind will be enlivened. You also need to build up an abundant qi storage in your lower real dan tian (i.e., quantity of qi's storage). Embryonic breathing meditation is able to direct you to the correct path of this practice.

In addition, you should not hesitate to share both your knowledge and qi. The more you share, the more you will gain.

1. 王弼說："實在質也,本在朴也。"
2. 河上公說："信者如其實,不美者朴且質也。"
3. 河上公說："善者以道修身,不綵文也。辯者謂巧言也,不善者舌致患也。山有玉,掘其山;水有珠,濁其淵。辯口多言亡其身。"
4. "禍從口出。"
5. "沈默是金。"
6. 杜光庭說："道之要者,在乎得言而忘言,知道而行道。行之既得,教亦俱忘,守一則不煩,無為則不亂。故摶于言教者,去道遠矣,豈能得玄妙之道哉?"
7. 杜光庭說："言聖人雖不積滯言教,然眾生發明慧心,必資聖人誘導,故聖人以清靜理性,盡與凡愚而教導之,于聖人慧解之性,曾不減耗,故云'愈有','愈多'。"
8. 杜光庭說："天道施生,長養萬物,利也;無所宰割,不害也。聖人體道應天,以濟于群生,澤欲廣而志欲謙,化愈彰而功愈晦,故利物而不害,應物而不爭。"
9. 高亨說："天之道利而不害物;聖人之道,有施于民,無爭于民也。"
10. "教學相長。"

Acknowledgements

First, I thank Mr. Bob Brennan who spent a great deal of time correcting my Chinglish and editing this book. Without his effort, this book would not be as idiomatic as it could be. Next, I also thank Dr. Robert J. Woodbine who put a lot of effort into double-checking the English and grammar of this book after its first editing.

I express my deep appreciation to Dr. Gutheil, Mr. Charles Green, and Dr. Woodbine, who each wrote a foreword for this book.

I also thank Mr. Piper Chan and Mr. Quentin Lopes for drawing all the illustrations. Finally, I express my gratitude to the following proofreaders: Mr. Jamie Urquhart, Mr. Enrico Tomei, Mr. Declan King, and Mr. Garrett Mason.

Translation and Glossary of Chinese Terms

ai (哀).   Sorrow.

ai (愛).   Love, kindness.

ao (奧).   Abstruse, mysterious, profound, obscure, or difficult to understand. As used in this book, it implies concealment.

ba duan jin (八段錦).   Eight pieces of brocade. A wai dan qigong (外丹氣功) practice said to have been created by Marshal Yue, Fei (岳飛) during the Southern Song dynasty (1127–1280 CE, 南宋).

ba mai (八脈).   The eight extraordinary vessels. These are considered to be qi reservoirs, which regulate the qi in the twelve primary qi channels.

bagua (八卦).   Eight divinations, also called eight trigrams. In Chinese philosophy, the eight basic variations in the *Yi Jing* (易經, *The Book of Changes*) designated as groups of solid and broken lines.

bai (白).   White. As used in this book, it implies the origin of the mind that exists with purity.

baihui (Gv-20) (百會).   Hundred meetings. An important acupuncture cavity located on top of the head. It belongs to the governing vessel (du mai, 督脈).

bao yi (抱一).   Embracing the state of oneness. To keep the spirit (or mind) and qi at the central energy line and unify spirit and qi at the real lower dan tian (zhen xia dan tian, 真下丹田).

bao ying (報應).   Retribution or karma.

Bian Que (扁鵲).   A well-known physician who wrote the book *Nan Jing* (難經, *Classic on Disorders*) during the Chinese Qin and Han dynasties (255 BCE–220 CE, 秦漢).

Bo Yang (伯陽).   One of Lao Zi's nicknames. He also had nicknames Lao Dan (老聃) and Chong Er (重耳).

Bohai (渤海).   An inner sea on the east coast of China connecting with the west Pacific Ocean. Bohai is located between Liaodong Peninsula (遼東半島) and Shandong Peninsula (山東半島). Bohai was also called Changhai (滄海) or Beihai (北海) in ancient time.

bu (補).   Nourishment.

bu tiao er tiao (不調而調).   Regulating without regulating. The stage of doing nothing (wuwei, 無為), when regulating is no longer necessary and all regulating processes cease.

Cai Huan Gong (蔡桓公).   The lord of a feudal kingdom Cai (蔡) in the Spring and Autumn period (春秋時代). He was in position from 714 BCE to 695 BCE.

chang (常).   Often, frequent, or constant. As used in this book, it means constant, natural routine.

cheng fo (成佛).   Achieving Buddhahood.

cheng xian (成仙).   Achieving Immortality.

Cheng, Hao (1032–1085 CE) (程顥).   A philosopher who, along with his brother Cheng, Yi (程頤), developed the ideas of neo-Confucianism. They were commonly called "two Cheng" (二程). Cheng, Hao was also known by the names Bochun (伯淳) or Mingdao (明道), often called Mr. Mingdao (明道先生). He was a resident of Yichuan (伊川) or Luo city (洛城) during the Northern Song dynasty (北宋) (960–1127 CE).

Cheng, Yi (1033–1107 CE) (程頤).   A philosopher who, along with his brother Cheng, Hao (程顥), developed the ideas of neo-Confucianism. They were commonly called "two Cheng" (二程). Cheng, Yi was also known by the names Zhengshu (正叔) or Mr. Yichuan. He was from Yichuan (伊川) or Luo city (洛城) during the Northern Song dynasty (北宋) (960–1127 CE).

Cheng, Yi-Ning (程以寧).   A Daoist scholar who lived during the Ming dynasty (明朝) (1368–1644 CE). He is the author of the well-known book *Interpretation of Dao De Jing* (道德經注). The details of his personal information are unknown.

chong (沖).   Rinse or wash out. As used in this book, chong means insubstantial.

Chong Er (重耳).   One of Lao Zi's nicknames. He also had the nicknames Lao Dan (老聃) and Boyang (伯陽).

chong mai (衝脈).   Thrusting vessel. One of the eight extraordinary vessels.

Chu (1115–223 BCE) (楚).   A feudal kingdom existing during the Qin (先秦) period. The kingdom was located near Yangzi River (長江).

chu gou (芻狗).   A ceremonial dog made from straw and sacrificed in ceremonies of worship in ancient China.

Chun Qiu Zhan Guo (770–221 BCE) (春秋戰國).   Spring and Autumn Warring period. China was divided into different countries during this time and was later unified by Duke Huan of Qi (秦).

Confucius (Kong Zi) (551–479 BCE) (孔子).   A Chinese scholar who lived during the Spring and Autumn period (770–476/453 BCE) (春秋時代) and whose philosophy significantly influenced Chinese culture.

Cui, Zi-Yu (崔子玉).   A scholar of Eastern Han (東漢) (25–220 CE). He was born in Anping (安平) of Zuo County (涿郡). Also known as Yuan (瑗).

da shun (大順).   Great smooth. As used in this book, it refers to the Dao (i.e., great nature).

da si ma (大司馬).   Ancient title of a high-ranking officer.

da tian di (大天地).   The great nature is considered the "grand universe" or "grand nature" (da tian di, 大天地). The human body is considered a small universe or small nature (xiao tian di, 小天地).

da xiang (大象).   Great image. It implies "the Dao."

Dai He (代和).   Name of a territory in Yue (越) country (2032–222 BCE).

dai mai (帶脈).   Girdle vessel. One of the eight extraordinary vessels.

dan tian (丹田).   Elixir field. Locations in the body that store and generate qi. The upper, middle, and lower dan tians are located respectively in the brain, at the sternum (jiuwei, Co-15, 鳩尾), and just below the navel.

Dao (道).   The Way, or natural way.

Dao de (道德).   Human morality. When Dao de is applied to a human, the Dao means the mind, and the de is the manifestation (i.e., behavior) of the Dao. Combined, the term means the morality of a human.

Dao De Jing (道德經).   *Classic on the Virtue of the Dao.* Written by Lao Zi (老子) during the Zhou dynasty (1122–255 BCE, 周朝).

Dao Jiao (道教).   Daoism. During the Han dynasty (58 CE, 漢朝), Zhang, Dao-Ling (張道陵) mixed scholar Daoism (道學) with Buddhism (佛學) and created the Daoist religion.

Dao Xue (道學).   Scholar Daoism. Created by Lao Zi (老子) during the Zhou dynasty (1122–255 BCE, 周朝).

de (德).   The manifestation of the Dao or the activities of nature. When de is applied to a human, it is the behavior or manifestation of the mind.

de Dao (得道).   Those who have acquired and comprehended the Dao are called de Dao.

di (地).   The earth. Earth (di, 地), heaven (tian, 天), and man (ren, 人) are the "three natural powers" (san cai, 三才).

Ding, Fu-Bao (1874–1952 CE) (丁福保).   A Buddhist scholar, born in Wuxi, Jiangsu Province (無錫，江蘇省), also nicknamed Zhongyou (仲祐) and Chouyin hermit (疇隱居士).

Dong Guo Shun Zi (東郭順子).   Named Xi, Shun Zi (夕順子), a citizen of Wei (魏). He lived on the east side of the city (Dong Guo, 東郭) and was therefore called Dong Guo Shun Zi.

Dong Han (25–220 CE) (東漢).   Eastern Han, also called Late Han (Hou Han, 後漢). Commonly called Han dynasty together with Western Han (Xi Han, 西漢). A great dynasty after Qin (秦) and Western Han (西漢). The Eastern Han dynasty lasted 195 years.

Dong, Si-Jing (董思靖).   Author of the book *Gathering Interpretation of Dao De Real Classic* (道德真經集解). The book was written around the sixth year of Song Li Zong Chun You (宋理宗淳祐六年) (1246 CE).

du mai (督脈).   Governing vessel. One of the eight extraordinary vessels.

Du, Guang-Ting (850–933 CE) (杜光庭).   A famous Shang Qing Division Daoist (上清派著名道士) who lived during the Tang dynasty (618–907 CE). Also known by the names Binzhi (賓至) or Binsheng (賓聖), or the nickname Dong Ying Zi (東瀛子).

Eastern Zhou (Dong Zhou) (770–256 BCE) (東周). The dynasty after Zhou moved its capital to the east, Luoyi (雒邑) (Luoyang, 洛陽), was called Eastern Zhou (東周). The dynasty before the movement of the old capital, Haojing (鎬京), was called Western Zhou (西周).

ezhong (M-HN-2) (額中). Name of an acupuncture cavity that is located at the central area of the forehead, above the midpoint of the line connecting two eyebrows, where the spiritual light is emitted. Also named "heaven eye" (tian mu, 天目).

Fan, Ying-Yuan (范應元). A Daoist scholar of the Southern Song dynasty (1127–1279 CE) (南宋) who wrote a book *The Gathering Interpretation of the Old Copy of Dao De Jing* (老子道德經古本集注).

fang (方). Square. Implies the human society (matrix) created by emotions and desires.

fang wai zhi ren (方外之人). Person outside the square. Those who are able to jump out of the human matrix or square (fang).

feng (風). Wind. One of the four great emptinesses (si da jie kong, 四大皆空).

Gao, Heng (1900–1986 CE) (高亨). A renowned scholar of pre-Qin (先秦) Chinese literature. He is recognized for his modern interpretation of the *Dao de Jing*. Also known as Jinsheng (晉生).

ge (戈). An ancient weapon.

gong (宮). One of the five music tones. The five tones (wu yin, 五音) are gong (宮), shang (商), jiao (角), zheng (徵), and yu (羽). From these tones, all Chinese music is constructed.

Gong Zhi-Qi (宮之奇). A well-known visionary politician who lived during the Spring and Autumn period (770–476 BCE) (春秋時代). He resided in Xin Gong Li (辛宮里) of Yu (虞) (today's Shanxi Province, 山西省). The exact dates of his life are unknown.

gongfu (功夫). Energy-time. Anything that takes time and energy to learn or to accomplish is called gongfu.

gu shen (谷神). The spirit that resides in spiritual valley (shen gu, 神谷).

gua ren (寡人). Means "I, being humble." This was the way an ancient ruler referred to himself.

Guan Xue Pai (關學派).   A school of scholarship founded by Zhang Zi (張子), named Zhang, Zai (張載) (1020–1077 CE), during the Chinese Northern Song dynasty (960–1127 CE) (北宋).

Guan Zi (719–645 BCE) (管子).   A representative of legalists during the Spring and Autumn period (770–476 BCE). Also known by the names Yiwu (夷吾), Zhong (仲), and Shijing (謚敬).

gui (鬼).   Ghost. When you die, if your spirit is strong, your soul's energy does not decompose and return to nature. This soul energy is a ghost.

gui hun (鬼魂).   Gui means ghost and hun means soul.

Gui, Jing-Yu (1773–1836 CE) (龜井昱).   Author of the book *Research of History Record* (史記考). He was also known by the name Gui Jing Zhao Yang (龜井昭陽).

Guo (虢).   There were two Guo countries, Western Guo (?–655 BCE) (西虢國) and Eastern Guo (?–767 BCE) (東虢國). The countries of Western Zhou (西周) (1046–771 BCE).

hai di (海底).   Sea bottom. Martial arts name for the Huiyin (Co-1, 會陰), or perineum.

Han Fei (280–233 BCE) (韓非).   A Chinese philosopher of the "Chinese legalist" school (法家) during the Warring States period (476–221 BCE) (戰國時代). He is often considered to be the greatest representative of Chinese legalism for his eponymous work *Han Fei Zi* (韓非子). Han Fei was also known as Han Fei Zi (韓非子).

Hangu Pass (函谷關).   Hangu Fortress was build by Qi (秦) during the Spring and Autumn Warring period (770–221 BCE) (春秋戰國). It is one of the earliest established fortresses in China's history. Fortified by natural barriers, it was a strategic military pass and is noted as the pass Lao Zi used on his flight from the state of Qin.

He (河).   Name of a territory during the Chu Zhuang Wang (楚莊王) period (?–591 BCE).

He Dao Quan (河道全).   An ancient Daoist scholar.

He Shang Gong (河上公).   A true hermit in Chinese history. His book *He Shang Gong's Chapters of Lao Zi* (河上公章句) was the earliest, most widespread, and most influential book in Chinese scholar society, but no one knew his name or place of birth. Most of historical researchers believe he was the hermit of Eastern Han (25–220 CE) (東漢).

he shi bi (和氏璧). A famous jade stone in ancient China. According to legend, it was discovered by Bianhe (卞和) of Chu (1115–223 BCE) (楚).

hen (恨). Hate.

hou wang (侯王). Noble man or high official.

houtian qi (後天氣). Post-birth qi or post-heaven qi. This is converted from the essence of food and air and classified as fire qi, as it makes your body yang.

hu huang (惚恍). The state of existing but not existing and is there but not there. It is the state of semi-existing or indistinction.

huang ting (黃庭). Yellow yard. The area at the solar plexus, called jade ring (yu huan, 玉環) in Daoist society. It is the place where fire and water qi blend to generate a spiritual embryo (shen tai, 神胎). Huang ting can also refer to the middle dan tian.

huang ting gong (黃庭宮). Yellow yard palace. The area at the solar plexus, called jade ring (yu huan, 玉環) in Daoist society. It is the place where fire and water qi blend to generate a spiritual embryo (shen tai, 神胎). Huang ting gong can also refer to the middle dan tian.

Huang, Shang (黃裳). A famous politician, philosopher, and scientist of the southern Song dynasty (1127–1279 CE) (南宋).

Hui (回). Nickname of a Confucius disciple, Yan Yuan (顏淵).

Hui-Neng (慧能). Sixth Chan (禪) ancestor during the Tang dynasty (713–907 CE) (唐朝). He changed some meditation methods and philosophy and was long considered a traitor.

huiyin (Co-1) (會陰). Meet yin. The perineum, an acupuncture cavity on the conception vessel (任脈).

hun (魂). The soul. Commonly used with the word "ling" (靈), which means spirit. Daoists believe one's hun (魂) and po (魄) originate with his original qi (yuan qi, 元氣) and separate from the physical body at death.

hun po (魂魄). Hun (魂) means soul. Po (魄) is the "vital spirit" that is supported by vital energy (qi) when a person is alive.

huo (火). Fire. One of four emptinesses (si da, 四大).

Ji, Lu (李路).　One of Confucius's disciples. He was also named Zi Lu (子路).

jiaji (夾脊).　Squeezing spine. Daoist name for the cavity between the shoulder blades. Called lingtai (Gv-10) (靈臺) in acupuncture.

jiao (角).　One of the five music tones. The five tones (wu yin, 五音) are gong (宮), shang (商), jiao (角), zheng (徵), and yu (羽). From these tones all Chinese music is constructed.

Jie (?–1600 BCE) (桀).　A famous tyrant in Chinese history. The son of Fa (發) and the last monarch of the Xia dynasty (2070–1600 BCE) (夏朝). He was in power for fifty-two years.

jie tuo (解脫).　Liberate yourself from spiritual bondage.

Jin (1033–376 BCE) (晉).　A feudal country of the Spring and Autumn period (770–476 BCE) (春秋). Jin was one of the five most powerful countries at the time.

Jin Xian Gong (?–651 BCE) (晉獻公).　His ancestral name was Ji (姬), his given name, Guizhu (詭諸). He was the son of Jin Wu Gong (晉武公) of the Jin dynasty (晉) of the Spring and Autumn period (770–476 BCE) (春秋). He was in position for twenty-six years.

jing (經).　Channels or meridians. Twelve organ-related rivers that circulate qi throughout the body.

Jing people (Jing ren) (荊人).　People of Chu country (Chu guo, 楚國).

kan (坎).　Water. One of the eight trigrams.

King of Chu (Chu Zhuang Wang) (?–591 BCE) (楚莊王).　The monarch of Chu (楚). Chu was one of the five most powerful kingdoms at the time. Named Xiong Lü (熊旅), also called Jing Zhuang Wang (荊莊王), the son of Chu Mu Wang (楚穆王).

King Wen (Zhou Wen Wang) (1152–1056 BCE) (周文王).　His ancestral name was Ji (姬), and his given name, Chang (昌). The grandson of Zhou Tai Wang (周太王), the son of Ji Li (季歷), founder of the Zhou dynasty (周朝) (1046–256 BCE).

koan (kong) (空).　Emptiness.

kong qi (空氣).　The air is called kong qi, which means the qi in space.

Kong Zi (551–479 BCE) (孔子).   Confucius. A famous scholar and philosopher during the Spring and Autumn period (722–484 BCE) (春秋時代).

Ksitigarbha Buddha (地藏菩薩).   A bodhisattva primarily revered in East Asian Buddhism and usually depicted as a Buddhist monk. His name may be translated as "Earth Treasury," "Earth Store," "Earth Matrix," or "Earth Womb."

ku (苦).   Bitter.

Ku County (Ku Xian) (苦縣).   Name of a county in ancient time. Scholars believe it is today the place of Luyi County, Henan Province (河南省鹿邑縣). It was the home village of Lao Zi.

kun (坤).   Earth. One of the eight trigrams.

Kun Lun (崑崙).   One of the highest mountains in China, located in the west provinces, Xinjiang (新疆), Xizang (西藏) (Tibet), and Qinghai (青海).

la (辣).   Spicy hot.

Lao Dan (老聃).   One of the nicknames of Lao Zi (老子).

Lao Zi (604–531 BCE) (老子).   The creator of Daoism, also called Li Er (李耳), Lao Dan (老聃), or by his nickname, Bo Yang (伯陽).

le (樂).   Joy or happiness.

li (離).   Fire. One of the eight trigrams (bagua, 八卦).

li er (李耳).   One of the nicknames of Lao Zi (老子).

Li, Jia-Mou (李嘉謀).   Also known as Xizhai (息齋). His Daoist name is Xizhai Daoist (Xizhai Dao Ren, 息齋道人). He resided in Shuangliu of Sichuan Province (四川雙流人) during the Song dynasty (960–1279 CE) (宋朝).

Li, Rong (李榮).   A renowned philosopher during the Tang dynasty (唐朝) (618–907 CE). He wrote an interpretation of *Dao De Jing*. Details of his life are unknown.

Li, Si (284–208 BCE) (李斯).   A famous politician, writer, and calligrapher of the Qin dynasty (221–207 BCE) (秦朝). He was the left prime minister (左丞相) of Qin. He was from Shangcai (上蔡) (today's Shangcai County of Henan) (河南省上蔡縣) of Chu (楚) (1115–223 BCE).

liangyi (兩儀).   Two poles or two polarities.

Lie Zi (c. 450–375 BCE) (列子).　An outstanding representative of the Daoist school; a famous Daoist scholar, philosopher, writer, and educator. Originally named, Lie, Yu-Kou (列御寇). People commonly called him Lie Zi (列子). He resided in Putian (圃田) of Zhou (1046–256 BCE) (周朝) (today's Zhengzhou City, Henan Province) (河南鄭州市).

Lin, Zhao-En (1517–1598 CE) (林兆恩).　A religious ideologist and philosopher of the Ming dynasty (1368–1644 CE) (明朝). He was the founder of the Sanyi religion (三一教) (i.e., Three-One religion). Thus, he was also called Mr. Three Religions (三教先生) or Mr. Lin Three Religions (林三教). Lin, Zhao-En resided at Chizhu, Putian, of Fujian Province (福建莆田赤柱人). He had several nicknames, Mao Xun (懋勳), Longjiang (龍江), Ziguzi (子穀子), and Xinyinzi (心隱子). He was given the nicknames Hunxushi (混虛氏) and Wushishi (無始氏) later in his life.

liu yu (六慾).　Six desires that are generated from the six roots: eyes, ears, nose, tongue, body, and mind (xin, 心).

liu zhu (流注).　The main qi flow.

Lord of Wei (Wei Wen Hou) (472–396 BCE) (魏文侯).　Grandson of Wei Huan Zi (魏桓子) and the founder of Wei kingdom (衛國) during the Warring States period (476–221 BCE) (戰國時代). Also named Si (斯) or Du (都). He resided in Anyi (安邑) (today's Xia County, Shanxi Province) (今山西夏縣).

Lu Ding Gong (Duke Ding of Lu) (魯定公).　Surname Ji (姬), name Song (宋), one of the monarchs of Lu country (魯國). Lu country was one of the feudatory countries (諸侯國) during the Spring and Autumn period (770–476/403 BCE) (春秋時代). He was the brother of Lu Zhao Gong (魯昭公) and was in position for fifteen years.

Lu, De-Ming (c. 550–630 CE) (陸德明).　A philosophical philologist during the Nan (420–589 CE) (南朝) and Tang dynasties (618–907 CE) (唐朝). Also known as Yuanlang (元朗), he was a resident of Suzhouwu (蘇州吳) (today's Wu County of Jiangsu Province) (今江蘇吳縣).

luo (絡).　The small qi channels that branch out from the primary channels (jing, 經) and connect to the skin and bone marrow.

Luo Yi (洛邑).　The name of an ancient city (today's Luoyang City) (洛陽). Also called Chengzhou (成周).

Lv Yan (呂岩).　A famous Daoist, also named Dongpin (洞賓) and Chun Yang Zi (純陽子). He resided in Jingzao (京兆) during the Tang dynasty (618–907 CE) (唐朝).

Ma, Qi-Chang (1855–1930 CE) (馬其昶).　He was a historian, famous writer, and scholar. Also named Tongbo (通伯) and called Baorunweng (抱潤翁) later in his life. He lived at Tongcheng Village of Anhui Province (安徽桐城鄉) (today's Chengguan Town) (今城關鎮) from the end of the Qing dynasty (1644–1911 CE) (清朝) to the early period of the Republic of China (1911–) (中華民國).

Mencius (Meng Zi) (377–289 BCE) (孟子).　A famous follower of Confucius during the Chinese Warring States period (403–222 BCE) (戰國).

ming (明).　Shining or bright. As used in this book, it means the inner light of the heart (i.e., mind) is clearly shining with wisdom.

mingtang (明堂).　The space between the two eyebrows, one inch inward.

mu zi xiang he (母子相合).　Mutual harmonization of mother and son. Qi is referred to as mother and the spirit as the son. When the spirit is led down to unite with the qi at the real lower dan tian, it is called mu zi xiang he, the state of embryonic breathing.

nei dan (內丹).　Internal elixir. A form of qigong in which qi (elixir) is built up in the body and spread out to the limbs.

nei shi gongfu (內視功夫).　To look inside to determine your state of health and the condition of your qi.

ni wan (泥丸).　Mud pills. This refers to the pineal and pituitary glands. A Daoist name for the crown, brain, or upper dan tian (上丹田).

ni wan gong (泥丸宮).　Mud-pill palace. Qigong term for the brain or upper dan tian. Mud pills refer to the pineal and pituitary glands.

Ni, Yuan-Tan (倪元坦).　Famous scholar during Qing Daoguang period (1821–1850 CE) (清道光) who was the author of *The Interpretation of Lao Zi* (老子參註). He lived at Songjiang of Shanghai (上海松江人).

Northern Song (Bei Song) (960–1127 CE) (北宋).　A dynasty in Chinese history. Included nine emperors and lasted 167 years. Together with Southern Song (南宋), called Song dynasty (宋朝).

nu (怒).　Anger.

Pang, Ming (龐明).　A famous qigong scholar, doctor, and professor. Also known as Pang, Heming (龐鶴鳴), he was born in Dingxing County, Hebei Province (河北定興縣), in September 1940.

pin (牝).　Female animals, or mothers.

ping tian xia (平天下).　To bring peace and harmony to the world. Tian-xia (天下) literally translates as "under heaven." It implies the world.

po (魄).　Vigorous life force. The po is considered to be the inferior animal soul. It is the sentient animal life that is an innate part of the body. At death, it returns to the earth with the rest of the body. When someone is in high spirits and gets vigorously involved in some activity, it is said he has po li (魄力), which means he has vigorous strength or power.

pu (朴).　Simplicity, innocence, and purity. As used in this book, it implies the virtue of the Dao.

qi (氣).　The general definition of qi is universal energy, including heat, light, and electromagnetic energy. A narrower definition refers to the energy circulating in human or animal bodies. A current popular model is that qi in the body is bioelectricity.

qi ba (氣壩).　Qi reservoirs. The eight vessels are the qi reservoirs, like lakes, swamps, or dams, that accumulate the qi and regulate the qi's quantity in the rivers.

qi jia (齊家).　To manage the family to a peaceful and harmonious state.

qi qing (七情).　The seven passions: happiness (xi, 喜), anger (nu, 怒), sorrow (ai, 哀), joy (le, 樂), love (ai, 愛), hate (hen, 恨), and desire (yu, 慾).

qi qing liu yu (七情六慾).　The seven passions and six desires. The seven passions are happiness (Xi, 喜), anger (nu, 怒), sorrow (ai, 哀), joy (le, 樂), love (ai, 愛), hate (hen, 恨), and desire (yu, 慾). The six desires are the six sensory pleasures derived from the eyes, ears, nose, tongue, body, and mind.

qi she (氣舍).　Qi dwelling.

qi xue (氣穴).　Qi cavity.

qian (乾).　Heaven. One of the eight trigrams.

qian yi shi (潛意識).   Hidden consciousness. It means subconscious mind.

qigong (氣功).   Gong (功) means gongfu (功夫). Qigong is the study and training of qi.

Qin (221–207 BCE) (秦).   The first empire of centralized power in Chinese history. The Qin dynasty imperial family surname was Ying (嬴), so it was Ying Qin (嬴秦). The Qin dynasty originated from the feudal country of Zhou.

Qing Jing Jing (清靜經).   One of the well-known Daoist classics. The whole name is *Grand Extreme Laojun's Description, Qing Jing Jing* (太上老君說常清靜經). It was passed down orally until the Eastern Han (25–220 CE) (東漢) period, when Gexuan (164–244 CE) (葛玄) recorded the book.

Qinghai (青海).   A province of China.

Qinqiu (寢丘).   The name of a place in Chu (1115–223 BCE) (楚) during the Spring and Autumn period (770–476 BCE) (春秋時代). It is the place between Gushi (固始) and Shenqiu (沈丘) Counties today, Henan Province (河南省).

qu qing yu (去情慾).   To eliminate the desires of emotional temptations such as love, hate, sadness, and happiness.

qu wu yu (去物慾).   To avoid the temptations of material attraction and ownership.

qu xin yu (去心慾).   To regulate the emotional mind and free yourself from the bondage of glory, reputation, greed, wealth, and dignity.

Qun Jing Zhi Shou (群經之首).   The leader of all classics. *The Book of Changes* has been considered the preeminent document of all ancient Chinese classics in Chinese history.

ren mai (任脈).   Conception vessel. One of the eight extraordinary vessels.

san gong (散功).   Energy dispersion. Premature degeneration of the body where qi cannot effectively energize it, generally caused by excessive training.

san guan (三關).   Three gates in small circulation. They are weilu (尾閭), jiaji (夾脊), and yuzhen (玉枕).

san nian bu ru (三年哺乳).   Three years of nursing. One of the Buddhist and Daoist meditation processes to reach the goal of Buddhahood (成佛) or immortality (成仙).

shang (商).   One of the five music tones. The five tones (wu yin, 五音) are gong (宮), shang (商), jiao (角), zheng (徵), and yu (羽). It is from these five tones that all Chinese music is constructed.

shang dan tian (上丹田).   Upper dan tian in the brain at the third eye, the residence of shen (神).

Shang, Yang (c. 395–338 BCE) (商鞅).   A famous politician, reformer, thinker, and representative of the legalist school (法家). He was a citizen of Wei (403–225 BCE) (魏) during the Warring States period (476–221 BCE) (戰國時代).

Shaolin (少林).   Young woods. A Buddhist temple in Henan (河南), famous for its martial arts.

shen gu (神谷).   Spirit valley. Formed by the two hemispheres of the brain.

shen shi (神室).   Spiritual residence. Located in the limbic system, the center of the head.

shen tai (神胎).   Spiritual embryo. Also called ling tai (靈胎).

shen tong (神通).   Spiritual transportation. This implies that those who have become enlightened will be able to communicate with the natural spirit through the third eye.

Shen-Xiu (606–706 CE) (神秀).   A great master of Chan (禪) (i.e., Zen, 忍). His surname was Li (李), and he was born in Luoyang City (洛陽) during the late Sui dynasty (581–619 CE) (隋). He was the first disciple of Hongren (弘忍), the fifth leader of Chan Buddhism (禪宗). Later, he founded the Northern School of Chan and was considered the sixth ancestor of Chan (禪宗六祖).

Shen, Yi-Guan (1531–1617 CE) (沈一貫).   A scholar, poet, historian, and diplomat. He was also known by the names Jianwu (肩吾), Buyi (不疑), Ziwei (子維), Long Jiang (龍江), and Jiaomen (蛟門). He was born in Yin County (鄞縣) (today's Ningbo City of Zhejiang Province) (浙江寧波) during the Ming dynasty (1366–1644 CE) (明朝).

sheng ying (聖嬰).   Spiritual baby or spiritual embryo. It means the qi is gathered at the real lower dan tian to an abundant level that can be led upward to nourish the brain for the third eye's opening (i.e., enlightenment).

shi er jing (十二經).   The twelve primary qi channels, also called meridians in Chinese medicine. The twelve channels are considered qi rivers that circulate qi in the twelve organs.

Shi Ji (史記).   *Historical Records,* one of the oldest historical books. Original name: *Tai Shi Gong Shu* (太史公書). It was compiled and written by Si, Ma-Qian (司馬遷), the officer Taishiling (太史令) (Taishigong, 太史公) of Western Han (202 BCE–8 CE) (漢). This book had recorded the history from the Yellow Emperor (黃帝) to the Han Wu Emperor (157–87 BCE) (漢武帝), a total of 2,500 years of history.

shi nian mian bi (十年面壁).   Ten years facing the wall. This is the final meditation process to reach Buddhahood after the third eye has been reopened.

Shi, De-Qing (釋得清).   An ancient Daoist. Details unknown.

Shi, Xiang-Zi (師襄子).   A music officer of Lu (1043–249 BCE) (魯) during the Spring and Autumn period (770–476/403 BCE) (春秋時代). He was an expert in playing the music stone (qing, 磬), also called qingxiang (磬襄). He was Confucius's music teacher and taught him the music "Wen Wan Cao" ("King Wen's Practice") (文王操). Later he resigned and became a hermit.

shou yi (守一).   Keep at singularity.

Shou Zang Shi (守藏史).   Curator of the library. Lao Zi (老子) was a curator of the library (守藏史) at the capital (Luo Yi, 洛邑) of Eastern Zhou's (770–256 BCE) (東周) royal court.

shou zhong (守中).   Keep at center.

Shu, Zhan (叔瞻).   An officer in Zheng's court. Zheng (806–375 BCE) (鄭) was a feudal country during the Western Zhou (1046–771 BCE) (西周) and Spring and Autumn Warring period (770–221 BCE) (春秋戰國).

shuang xiu (雙修).   Double cultivation. A qigong training method in which qi is exchanged with a partner to balance the qi of both. It also means dual cultivation of the body and the spirit.

shui (水).   Water.

shui jing gong (水精宮).   Water and essence palace. It means the kidneys.

Shun (c. 2277–2178 BCE) (舜).   Shun is a posthumous title of a leader of an ancient Chinese tribe. His names were Chonghua (重華) or Dujun (都君). He was respected as an emperor and recognized as one of the five ancient emperors (五帝).

Si (賜).   A student of Confucius. His nickname was Zi gong (子貢).

si da (四大).   Four greatnesses or four larges. These are the earth (di, 地), water (shui, 水), fire (huo, 火), and wind (feng, 風) (i.e., air).

si da jie kong (四大皆空).   Four larges are empty. A stage of Buddhist training where all four elements (earth, water, fire, and air) are absent from the mind. This means one is completely indifferent to worldly temptations.

Si, Ma-Qian (145–86 BCE) (司馬遷).   A famous historian and scholar during the Western Han period (202 BCE–8 CE) (西漢). He compiled and wrote the book *Historical Records* (史記), which was recognized as a model of Chinese history books. Also known as Zichang (子長). He was born at Zuofengyi Xiayang (左馮翊夏陽人) (today's Hejin, Shanxi Province) (今山西河津).

Song (960–1279 CE) (宋).   A dynasty in Chinese history. It was divided into two periods, Northern Song (960–1127 CE) (北宋) and Southern Song (1127–1279 CE) (南宋). Song included eighteen emperors and lasted 319 years.

Song, Chang-Xing (宋長星).   An ancient Daoist. Details of his life are unknown.

Su, Che (1039–1112 CE) (蘇轍).   Also known as Ziyou (子由) or Tongshu (同叔). He called himself Yingbinyilao (穎濱遺老) later in his life. He was born at Meishan, Meizhou (眉州眉山) (today's Meishan City, Sichuan Province) (今四川省眉山市).

suan (酸).   Sour.

Sun Zi (545–470 BCE) (孫子).   A famous military strategist and politician in the Spring and Autumn period (770–476/403 BCE) (春秋時代). He is the author of the book *The Art of War* (孫子兵法). Also known as Sun, Wu (孫武) and Changqing (長卿).

Sun, Shu-Ao (c. 630–593 BCE) (孫叔敖).　　He was an officer Lingyin (令尹) of Chu (楚) during the Spring and Autumn period (770–476/453 BCE) (春秋時代). He was born at Yingdu of Chu (楚郢都人) of Jing-zhou, Hubei Province (今湖北荆州紀南城).

Sun, Yat-Sen (Sun, Yi-Xian) (1866–1925 CE) (孫逸仙).　　The father of China (國父) and the founder of Chinese Guomindang (中國國民黨). He was a medical doctor, politician, revolutionist, and philosopher. He had several names: Wen (文), Dixiang (帝象), Deming (德明), Zaizhi (載之), Yixian (逸仙), and Rixin (日新). When he was in Japan, he was also named Zhongshan Qiao (中山樵). Thus, he was commonly called "Sun, Zhong-San" (孫中山). He was born November 12, 1866, in Cuiheng Village of Xiangshan County, Canton Province (廣東省香山縣翠亨村) during the Qing dynasty (1636–1912) (清朝).

tai chu (太初).　　Grand initiation. When the original qi is not yet formed in this universe, it is called tai chu.

tai shang (太上).　　The great supreme, means Lao Zi (老子).

tai shi (太始).　　Grand beginning. When original qi just begins to initiate, it is called tai shi.

tai su (太素).　　Grand simplicity. When the shape of qi has begun to formalize, it is called tai su.

tai xi jing zuo (胎息靜坐).　　Embryonic breathing meditation. The foundation of qigong practice.

tai xu (太虛).　　Grand emptiness. The great nature of the universe (Dao, 道).

tai yi (太易).　　Grand change, extremely profound, is called tai yi.

taiji (太極).　　Grand ultimate. When the shape of qi has been formed into material, it is called taiji. Taiji is the invisible force that makes wuji (無極, no extremity) divide into yin and yang poles, and into which the two once again resolve into one. Also often called xuan pin (玄牝).

tai xi (胎息).　　Embryonic breathing. A qigong breathing technique which stores qi in the real lower dan tian (真下丹田).

Teng, Yun-Shan (滕雲山).　　An ancient Daoist. Author of the book *Brief Interpretation of Dao De Jing* (道德經淺註). Details of his life are unknown.

tian (甜).   Sweet.

tian di (天地).   Heaven and earth. It means the universe or nature.

tian gu (天谷).   Heaven valley. It means the space between two lobes of the brain.

tian ling gai (天靈蓋).   Heavenly spiritual cover. The crown, or baihui (Gv-20, 百會), in acupuncture.

stian men (天門).   Heaven gate. Also known as the third eye. It allows you to communicate with nature. In Daoist society, another place is also considered tian men. It is located at the crown (baihui, 百會), where the spirit enters and exits.

tian mu (天目).   Heavenly eye. Called the third eye by Western society. The Chinese believe that prior to our evolution into humans, our race possessed an additional sense organ in our forehead. This third eye provided a means of spiritual communication between one another and with the natural world. As we evolved and developed means to protect ourselves from the environment, and as societies became more complex and human vices developed, this third eye gradually closed and disappeared.

tian ren he yi (天人合一).   Heaven and man unified as one. A high level of qigong meditation in which one can communicate with the qi of heaven.

Tian Tai Mountain (Tian Tai Shan) (天台山).   Name of a mountain that is located in the north of Tiantai County, Zhejiang Province (浙江省天台縣), with Xianxialing (仙霞岭) in the southeast and Zhoushan islands (舟山群島) in the northeast. It is the watershed between Caoer River (曹娥江) and Yongjiang (甬江). The main peak, Huadiing Mountain (華頂山), is located in the northeast of Tiantai County (天台縣) and is 1,098 meters above sea level.

tian yan (天眼).   Heaven eye. The third eye or yintang (M-HN-3) cavity in acupuncture.

tian-xia (天下).   Under the heaven. It means the world.

Tian, Zi-Fang (田子方).   A Daoist scholar. He was a student of Confucius's student, Dan, Mu-Si (端木賜) (Zigong, 子貢). He became famous for his Daoist scholarship. Also named Wuze (無擇). A resident of Wei (1116–209 BCE) (魏國) and the friend of Lord Wei Wen Hou (魏文侯).

tiao er wu tiao (調而無調).   Regulating of no regulating. It means the work is done subconsciously without the mind's attention.

tiao qi (調氣).   To regulate the qi.

tiao shen (調神).   To regulate the spirit.

tiao shen (調身).   To regulate the body.

tiao xi (調息).   To regulate the breathing.

tiao xin (調心).   To regulate the emotional mind.

tuo yue (橐籥).   Bellows. A tube used to fan the fire in a furnace.

wai dan (外丹).   External elixir. External qigong exercises to build up qi in the limbs and lead it into the center of the body for nourishment.

Wang, An-Shi (1021–1086 CE) (王安石).   A famous politician, scholar, writer, and philosopher during the Northern Song dynasty (960–1127 CE) (北宋). Also named Jiefu (介甫) and Banxian (半仙).

Wang, Chong (c. 27–97 CE) (王充).   A famous philosopher of Eastern Han (25–220 CE) (東漢). He wrote a few books; unfortunately, only *Discussing Balance* (論衡) was preserved. Also named Zhongren (仲任). He was a resident of Shangyu, Kuaiji (會稽上虞人).

Wang, Dao (王道).   An ancient Daoist. Details unknown.

Wang, Li (王力).   An ancient Daoist. Details unknown.

Wang, Yu-Qi (王于期).   A skillful horseman who lived during the Spring and Autumn period (770–476/453 BCE) (春秋時代). The lord of Yue (越襄子) asked Wang to teach him driving skills.

Wang, Zong-Yue (王宗岳).   A famous internal style martial artist of the Wanli period, Ming dynasty (1573–1620 CE) (明朝萬曆). He mastered bare-hand arts, sword, and spear, and he was considered one of the most skilled martial artists of the time. He wrote a few books, such as *Yinfu Spear* (陰符槍譜) and *The Theory of Taijiquan* (太極拳論). The book *The Theory of Taijiquan* is one of the highest regarded theoretic classics in taijiquan society.

wei (微).   Small or weak.

Wei (衛).   One of the kingdoms of the Zhou dynasty (1046–256 BCE) (周朝). Surname Ji (姬), the descendant of the brother of Zhou Wu emperor (周武王), Kangshu (康叔). The capitals were, Chaoge (朝歌),

Chuqiu (楚丘), Diqiu (帝丘), and Yewang (野王) (today's northern Henan and south Hebei Provinces).

wei er wu wei (為而無為).　Doing of no doing. It means the work is done subconsciously without the conscious mind's attention.

wei huang wei hu (惟恍惟惚).　The state of existing but not existing and is there but not there. It is the state of semi-existing or indistinction.

wei qi (衛氣).　Protective qi or guardian qi. The qi at the surface of the body forms a shield to protect the body from negative external influences such as cold.

Wei, Yuan (1794–1857 CE) (魏源).　A philosopher and ideologist who lived during the late Qing dynasty (1644–1912 CE) (清朝). Original name was Yuanda (遠達), also named Moshen (默深), Mosheng (默生), Hanshi (漢士), and Liangtu (良圖). He was a resident of Jintan, Shaoyang County, Hunan Province (湖南省邵陽縣金潭人) (today's Jintan, Longhui County, Shaoyang city (今邵陽市隆回縣金潭).

weilv (尾閭).　Coccyx. Called changqiang (Gv-1, 長強, long strength) in Chinese medical society.

Western Han (Xi Han) (202 BCE–8 CE) (西漢).　A great dynasty after Qin dynasty (221–207 BCE) (秦朝) with a total of twelve emperors. It is commonly called Qian Han (前漢). Together with Eastern Han (25–220 CE) (東漢), it is called Han dynasty (漢朝).

wo gu (握固).　To hold and firm.

wu (午).　Noon (11 a.m. to 1 p.m.). One of the twelve terrestrial branches.

wu (悟).　To comprehend the temperament. One requirement for spiritual cultivation.

wu (武).　Martial. Martial arts is called "wuyi" (武藝) or wushu (武術).

Wu Ling Wang (340–295 BCE) (武靈王).　A monarch of Yue country (越國) during the late Warring States period (476–221 BCE) (戰國時代). Surname, Ying (嬴) and given name, Yong (雍). He was in position for twenty-seven years. He was given a title of Wuling (武靈王) after his death.

Wu Qin Xi (五禽戲).　Five Animal Sports. An important traditional health qigong (氣功) (also called daoyin, 導引) exercise, created by Hua

Tuo (c. 145–208 CE) (華佗). Huo Tuo was born at Qiao County, Pei-guo, (沛國譙縣) of the Eastern Han dynasty (25–220 CE) (東漢) (today's Hao County of Anhui Province) (今安徽亳州).

wu se (五色).　The five colors: red, yellow, blue, white, and black. From these, all the different colors are constructed.

wu wei (五味).　The five flavors: sour (suan, 酸), sweet (tian, 甜), bitter (ku, 苦), pungent (la, 辣), and salty (xian, 鹹).

wu wei er wu bu wei (無為而無不為).　Doing nothing, yet nothing is left undone. Once you have reached a state of "regulating without regulating" (tiao er wu tiao, 調而無調) or "doing without doing" (wei er wuwei, 為而無為), your mind will be neutral and peaceful.

wu yin (五音).　The five music tones: gong (宮), shang (商), jiao (角), zheng (徵), and yu (羽). From these tones, all Chinese music is constructed.

Wu, Cheng (1249–1333 CE) (吳澄).　An outstanding scholar, philosopher, and educator during the Yuan dynasty (1271–1368 CE) (元朝). Also named Youqing (幼清) and called Boqing (伯清) later in his life. He was a resident of Xiankou, Chongren Fenggang, Rao County (撫州崇仁風崗咸口) (today's Xiaokou Village, Biexi town, Dongan County, Jiangxi Province) (今江西省東安縣鱉溪鎮咸口村人).

wuji (無極).　No extremity. The state of undifferentiated emptiness before beginning.

wuwei (無為).　Doing nothing. Regulating without regulating.

xi (喜).　Joy, delight, and happiness.

xi (希).　Sparse or faint.

Xi Shan (西山).　West Mountains. It implies those high mountains located on the west of China.

Xi, Gong (谿工).　A person who was living in the village of Tian, Zi-Fang (田子方). Details unknown.

Xi, Tong (1878–1939 CE) (奚侗).　Author of the book *Collective Interpretations of Lao Zi* (老子集解). Also named Duqing (度青) and Wushi (無識). He was a resident of Huoli town, Maanshan town (馬鞍山市霍里鎮人) in the late Qing dynasty (1644–1912 CE) (清朝).

xian (鹹).　Salty.

Xiang, Yu (232–202 BCE) (項羽).   Grandson of the famous Chu general, Xiang, Yan (項燕). Also named Ji (籍). He was a resident of Xiaxiang (下相) in Chu country (1115–223 BCE) (楚國) (today's Suqian, Jiangsu Province) (今江蘇宿遷人).

xiantian qi (先天氣).   Pre-birth qi or pre-heaven qi. Also called dan tian qi (丹田氣). The qi that is converted from original essence and stored in the lower dan tian. Considered to be water qi, it calms the body.

xiao tian di (小天地).   Small heaven and earth. The human body is called a "small heaven and earth" (small universe).

Xiao, Tian-Shi (1908–1986 CE) (蕭天石).   A Daoist scholar. He devoted his lifetime to studying and promoting Daoism. He was born in Wenshan Village, Longshan town, Shaoyang County, Hunan Province (湖南邵陽縣龍山鄉文山村). He referred to himself as Wenshan Dunsao (文山遁叟) (Wenshan hermit) later in his life.

xin (心).   Heart. The mind generated from emotional disturbance, desire.

xin yuan yi ma (心猿意馬).   Heart monkey mind horse. Xin (heart) represents the emotional mind, which acts like a monkey, unsteady and disturbing. Yi is the wisdom mind generated from calm, clear thinking, and judgment. The yi is like a horse, calm and powerful.

Xinjiang (新疆).   A province in west China.

xiu shen (修身).   Cultivating the physical body.

Xizang (西藏).   Tibet. A province in west China.

Xu, You (許由).   A legendary sage and hermit during the Yao period (堯). Details unknown.

xuan (玄).   Marvelous, incredible, or mysterious. It also means original (yuan, 元).

xuan de (玄德).   Profound natural virtue.

xuan lan (玄覽).   As used in this book, it means the idea or thought.

Xuan Pin (玄牝).   The marvelous and mysterious Dao, mother of creation of millions of objects.

Xue, Hui (薛惠).   A Daoist. Details unknown.

Xun Dao She (尋道者).   Dao searcher. One who studies the truth of the Dao.

Xuan Emperor (Han Xuan Di) (94–48 BCE) (漢宣帝). The tenth emperor of Western Han (202 BCE–8 CE) (西漢). His formal official name was Han Xiaoxuan emperor (漢孝宣皇帝) and later simplified as Han Xuan Di (漢宣帝). Named Liu, Xun (劉詢), Liu, Bingyi (劉病已), and Ciqing (次卿).

Xun Zi (c. 313–238 BCE) (荀子). One of the most important books of Confucian scholarship (儒家著作), authored by Xun Zi (荀子). Xun Zi, also named Kuang (況), was the resident of Yue country (2032–222 BCE) (越國) during the late Warring States period (476–221 BCE) (戰國時代). He was commonly called Xunqing (荀卿).

Yan, Jun-Ping (86 BCE–10 CE) (嚴君平). A Daoist scholar, thinker, and philosopher, one of the legendary Eight Immortals (八仙) and the author of *Interpretation of Lao Zi* (老子注) and *Important Conclusion of Dao De Real Classic* (道德真經指歸). Also named Yan, Zun (嚴遵). He was a hermit of Chengdu, Shu (蜀，成都) (i.e. Sichuan, 四川) during the Western Han dynasty (202 BCE– 8 CE) (西漢).

Yan, Yuan (521–481 BCE) (顏淵). A prominent student of Confucius. He began his studies with Confucius at the age of fourteen. Also named Yan Hui (顏回) and Ziyuan (子淵), a resident of Lu country (1043–249 BCE) (魯國).

Yan, Zun (86 BCE–10 CE) (嚴遵). A Daoist scholar, thinker, and philosopher, one of the legendary "eight immortals" (八仙), and the author of *Interpretation of Lao Zi* (老子注) and *Important Conclusion of Dao De Real Classic* (道德真經指歸). Also named Junping (君平). He was a hermit of Chengdu, Shu (蜀，成都) (i.e. Sichuan, 四川) during the Western Han dynasty (202 BCE– 8 CE) (西漢).

Yang (卬). Prince of Wei (衛).

yang (陽). One of the two poles (liang yi, 兩儀). The other is yin (陰). In Chinese philosophy, the active, positive, masculine polarity is classified as yang. In Chinese medicine, yang means excessive, overactive, or overheated. The yang (or outer) organs are the gall bladder, small intestine, large intestine, stomach, bladder, and triple burner.

yang jian (陽間). Yang world. The material world in which we live.

yang qiao mai (陽蹻脈). Yang heel vessel. One of the eight extraordinary qi vessels.

yang wei mai (陽維脈).   Yang linking vessel. One of the eight extraordinary qi vessels.

Yang, Jwing-Ming (楊俊敏).   Author of this book.

Yao (2379–2318 BCE) (堯).   Yao is a historical, mythological emperor and considered one of the ancient Five Emperors (五帝). His capital was in Tang (唐) (Pingyang, 平陽) (today's southwest of Linfen, Shanxi Province) (今山西臨汾西南). He was also commonly called Tangyao (唐堯) or Diyao (帝堯). His name was Fangxun (放勳).

yi (夷).   Flat or extinguished. Implies emptiness or nothingness.

yi (意).   Mind. Specifically, the mind generated by clear thinking and judgment, which can make you calm, peaceful, and wise.

yi (易).   Changes.

yi (義).   Justice, righteousness.

Yi Jing (易經).   *The Book of Changes.* A book of divination written during the Zhou dynasty (1122–255 BCE, 周).

yi shi (意識).   Conscious mind.

yi shou dan tian (意守丹田).   Keep your yi at your lower dan tian (xia dan tian, 下丹田). In qigong training, you keep your mind at the lower dan tian to accumulate qi. When you circulate it, you always lead it back to your lower dan tian at the end of practice.

yin (陰).   In Chinese philosophy, this is the passive, negative, feminine polarity. In Chinese medicine, yin means deficient. The yin organs are the heart, lungs, liver, kidneys, spleen, and pericardium.

yin jian (陰間).   Yin world. The spirit world after death is considered yin.

yin qiao mai (陰蹻脈).   Yin heel vessel. One of the eight extraordinary qi vessels.

yin wei mai (陰維脈).   Yin linking vessel. One of the eight extraordinary qi vessels.

Yin, Xi (1301 BCE–?) (尹喜).   The doctor of the Zhou dynasty (1046–256 BCE) (周朝大夫), a general, philosopher, and educator. He was considered one of the ten heroes (天下十豪) at the beginning of the Qi dynasty (221–207 BCE) (秦朝). He was also named Wengong (文公), Mr. Wenshi (文始先生), Wenshi Zhenren (文始真人), or Guanyin (關尹), and was a resident of Tianshui, Gansu Province (甘肅天水). He studied ancient books from an early age and was knowledgeable about astronomy.

In the twenty-third year of Zhou Jing Wang (周敬王), the country was devolving into disorder. He resigned his position in Zhou's court and was in charge of the Hangu Pass (函谷關). He met Lao Zi at the pass and received the *Dao De Jing* from him.

ying (盈).   Full or surplus.

yinguo (因果).   Cause and consequence. It is called karma in Hinduism.

yintang (M-HN-3) (印堂).   Seal hall. Name of an acupuncture cavity located at the third eye.

Yong (雍).   Name of a territory during Chu Zhuang Wang (楚莊王) period (?–591 BCE).

You (由).   One of Confucius's disciples. Nicknamed Zi Lu (子路).

youwei (有為).   Intention of doing things.

yu (慾).   Desire or lust.

Yu (禹).   Yu is a mythological person. He was commonly called Dayu (大禹). He is widely known for his success in resolving the flood problems caused by the Yellow River (黃河). He was the first emperor of the Xia dynasty (c. 2070–1600 BCE) (夏朝) with the capital at Anyi (安邑) (today's Xia County of Shanxi Province) (今山西夏縣). Yu was given the name Xiabo (夏伯) by Yao (堯). Thus, he was also called Boyu (伯禹) or Xiayu (夏禹).

yu (羽).   One of the five music tones. The five tones are gong (宮), shang (商), jiao (角), zheng (徵), and yu (羽).

Yu (?–655 BCE) (虞).   A kingdom of the Zhou dynasty (1046–256 BCE) (周朝). It was located in today's northeast Pinglu County, Shanxi Province (山西省平陸縣東北).

yu men (玉門).   Jade gate. The third eye.

Yuan (元).   Origin.

Yuan (淵).   Profound. As used in this book, it means calm and deep without movement.

yuan pin (元牝).   The female animal (mother) that gives birth to new life.

yuan qi (元氣).   Original qi. Created from the original essence (yuan jing, 元精) inherited from your parents.

yuan shen (元神).   Original spirit. The spirit you already had when you were born.

Yue (2032–222 BCE) (越).   Yue country was a kingdom in southeast China during the Xia, Shang, Western Zhou, and Spring and Autumn Warring periods (c. 2070–221 BCE) (夏商、西周以及春秋戰國時期).

Yue people (Yue ren) (越人).   People of Yue country (越國).

Yun Zhong (雲中).   Name of a territory in Yue country (2032–222 BCE) (越).

yuzhen (玉枕).   Jade pillow. The Daoist name for the acupuncture cavity naohu (Gv-17, 腦戶, brain's household). This cavity is the third gate of small circulation.

zan xuan (贊玄).   Praise the marvelousness. The title of *Dao De Jing*, chapter 14.

Zeng, Jin-Zao (1911–1976) (曾金灶).   Dr. Yang, Jwing-Ming's White Crane master.

Zeng, Shen (505–435 CE) (曾參).   One of the representatives of Confucius's school (儒家). He was a disciple of Confucius. Zi Si was his disciple. He was commonly called "Zeng Zi" (曾子). Also named Ziyu (子輿). He was a resident of Nanwu City (南武城) in Lu country (1043–249 BCE) (魯國) (today's Jiaxiang, Shangdong Province) (山東嘉祥).

Zhan, Zai (張載).   Zhang Zi (張子), named Zhang, Zai (張載) (1020–1077 CE), was a founder of the Guan Xue school (關學派) of scholarship during the Chinese Northern Song dynasty (960–1127 CE) (北宋).

Zhang Zi (張子).   Zhang Zai (張載), the founder of the Guan Xue school (關學派) of scholarship during the Chinese Northern Song dynasty (960–1127 CE) (北宋).

Zhang, Dao-Ling (張道陵).   A Daoist who combined scholarly Daoism with Buddhist philosophies to create religious Daoism (Dao Jiao, 道教) during the Chinese Eastern Han dynasty (25–220 CE) (東漢).

Zhang, Er-Qi (1612–1678 CE) (張爾歧).   A famous writer. Also named Jirou (稷若) and Haoan (蒿庵). He was a resident of Jiyang, Shangdong

Province (山東省濟陽人) during the late Ming dynasty (1368–1644 CE) (明朝).

Zhang, Qi-Gan (1859–1946 CE) (張其淦).   An official and scholar of the late Qing dynasty (1644–1912 CE) (清朝). Nicknamed Yuquan (豫泉), he was a resident of Dongwan, Canton Province (廣東東莞人).

zhen dan tian (真丹田).   Real lower dan tian, the main qi reservoir or bioelectric battery in the body.

zhen ren (真人).   Truthful person. Daoists often called themselves zhen ren.

zhen xia dan tian (真下丹田).   Real lower dan tian, the main qi reservoir or bioelectric battery in the body.

Zheng (徵).   One of the five music tones. The five tones are gong (宮), shang (商), jiao (角), zheng (徵), and yu (羽).

Zheng (806–375 BCE) (鄭).   Zheng was a kingdom of Western Zhou (1046–771 BCE) (西周) and the Spring and Autumn Warring period (770–221 BCE) (春秋戰國). It is famous for its commercial development, fair legal system, democratic politics, and poetry and music culture.

zheng qi (正氣).   Righteous qi. When one is righteous, he is said to have righteous qi that evil qi cannot overcome.

zhi (止).   Stop.

zhi (執).   To keep or to hold.

zhi guo (治國).   To govern or to rule a country.

zhong yong zhi Dao (中庸之道).   The Dao of moderation.

zhong zheng zhi Dao (中正之道).   The Dao of the center.

Zhou (c. 1105–1045 BCE) (紂).   Emperor Xing (帝辛) also named Shou (受). He was a resident of Moyi (沬邑) (today's Nanqi County, Henan Province) (今河南淇縣). He was a tyrant and the last monarch of Shang dynasty (c. 1600–1046 BCE) (商朝). He was the son of Emperor Yi (帝乙) with the posthumous title of Zhou (紂). He was often called Yin Zhou King (殷紂王) or Shang Zhou King (商紂王) in history.

Zhou dynasty (Zhou Chao) (1046–256 BCE) (周朝).   A dynasty after Shang dynasty (商朝) (c. 1600–1046 BCE). It was divided into two periods, Western Zhou (1046–771 BCE) (西周) and Eastern Zhou (770–256 BCE) (東周).

Zhu Zhen Ren (朱真人).   Zhu Zhen Ren was his Daoist name. His real name is unknown. He was a resident of Ying County (郢縣) (today's Jiang Ling Dong Nan, Hubei Province) (今湖北江陵東南). He entered the Daoist monastery when he was nine years old. It was known that he lived in two caves, Lengrang (冷然) and Changdong (長東), in seclusion at Hualong Mountain, Neijiang (內江化龍山), around the time of the Song Du Emperor Ninth Year (宋度宗咸淳九年) (1273 CE).

Zhuang Zi (莊子).   Named Zhuang Zhou (莊周). A Daoist scholar during the Warring States period (403–222 BCE). He wrote a book called *Zhuang Zi* (莊子).

zi (子).   Midnight (11 p.m. to 1 a.m.). One of the twelve terrestrial branches.

Zi Gong (520–446 BCE) (子貢).   He was one of the ten most famous disciples of Confucius (孔門十哲). His surname was Duanmu (端木), and his name was Si (賜). He was a resident of Wei country (?–209 BCE) (衛國). Zi Gong was his nickname.

Zi Han (子罕).   Named Dong, Xi (東喜). A prime minister (正卿) of Song (宋) (1114–286 BCE). Details unknown. Zi Han was also the name of one of the chapters of *Lun Yu* (論語).

zi jue (自覺).   Self-awareness.

Zi Lu (542–480 BCE) (子路).   He was one of the ten most famous disciples of Confucius (孔門十哲). He was nine years younger than Confucius and also the person who served Confucius the longest. Also called Ji Lu (季路). A resident of Lu country (1043–249 BCE) (魯國).

zi shi (自識).   Self-recognition.

Zi Si (483–402 BCE) (子思).   One of the representatives of Confucian scholarship (Rujia, 儒家). He was the grandson of Confucius and son of Kong, Li (孔鯉). He received his education from Confucius's top disciple, Zeng, Shen (曾參) (also called Zeng Zi, 曾子). Zi Si was the nickname of Kong, Ji (孔伋). He resided at Lu country (1043–249 BCE) (魯國) at the beginning of the Warring States period (476–221 BCE) (戰國時代).

zi wu / zi xing (自悟／自醒).   Self-awakening.

zizhong (輜重).   Heaviness. It means the luggage carriage that travels with a traveler.

zong (宗).   Origin or root. As used in this book, it means "return and belong to."

zou huo ru mo (走火入魔).   Walk into the fire and enter the devil. If you lead your qi into the wrong path, it is called walking into the fire. If your mind has been led into confusion, it is called entering the devil.

About the Author

Yang, Jwing-Ming, PhD (楊俊敏博士)

Dr. Yang, Jwing-Ming was born on August 11, 1946, in Xinzhu Xian (新竹縣), Taiwan (台灣), Republic of China (中華民國). He started his wushu (武術) (gongfu or kung fu, 功夫) train-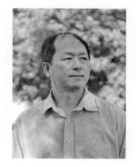ing at the age of fifteen under Shaolin White Crane (Shaolin Bai He, 少林白鶴) Master Cheng, Gin-Gsao (曾金灶). Master Cheng originally learned taizuquan (太祖拳) from his grandfather when he was a child. When Master Cheng was fifteen years old, he started learning White Crane from Master Jin, Shao-Feng (金紹峰) and followed him for twenty-three years until Master Jin's death.

In thirteen years of study (1961–1974) under Master Cheng, Dr. Yang became an expert in the White Crane style of Chinese martial arts, which includes both the use of bare hands and various weapons, such as saber, staff, spear, trident, two short rods, and many others. With the same master he also studied White Crane qigong (氣功), qin na or chin na (擒拿), tui na (推拿), and dian xue massage (點穴按摩) and herbal treatment.

At sixteen, Dr. Yang began the study of Yang-tyle taijiquan (楊氏太極拳) under Master Kao Tao (高濤). He later continued his study of taijiquan under Master Li, Mao-Ching (李茂清). Master Li learned his taijiquan from the well-known Master Han, Ching-Tang (韓慶堂). From this further practice, Dr. Yang was able to master the taiji bare-hand sequence, pushing hands, the two-man fighting sequence, taiji sword, taiji saber, and taiji qigong.

When Dr. Yang was eighteen years old, he entered Tamkang College (淡江學院) in Taipei Xian to study physics. In college, he began the study of traditional Shaolin Long Fist (Changquan or Chang Chuan, 少林長拳) with Master Li, Mao-Ching at the Tamkang College Guoshu Club (淡江國術社), 1964–1968, and eventually became an assistant instructor under Master Li. In 1971, he completed his MS degree in physics at the National Taiwan University (台灣大學) and then served in the Chinese Air Force from 1971 to 1972. In the service, Dr. Yang taught physics at the Junior Academy of the Chinese Air Force (空軍幼校) while also teaching wushu. After being honorably discharged in 1972, he returned to Tamkang College to teach physics and resumed study under Master Li, Mao-Ching. From Master Li, Dr. Yang learned Northern Style Wushu, which includes both bare hand and kicking techniques, and numerous weapons.

In 1974, Dr. Yang came to the United States to study mechanical engineering at Purdue University. At the request of a few students, Dr. Yang began to teach gongfu, which resulted in the establishment of the Purdue University Chinese Kung Fu Research Club in the spring of 1975. While at Purdue, Dr. Yang also taught college-credit courses in taijiquan. In May of 1978, he was awarded a PhD in mechanical engineering by Purdue.

In 1980, Dr. Yang moved to Houston to work for Texas Instruments. While in Houston, he founded Yang's Shaolin Kung Fu Academy, which was eventually taken over by his disciple, Mr. Jeffery Bolt, after Dr. Yang moved to Boston in 1982. Dr. Yang founded Yang's Martial Arts Academy in Boston on October 1, 1982.

In January of 1984, he gave up his engineering career to devote more time to research, writing, and teaching. In March of 1986, he purchased property in the Jamaica Plain area of Boston to be used as the headquarters of the new organization, Yang's Martial Arts Association (YMAA). The organization expanded to become a division of Yang's Oriental Arts Association, Inc. (YOAA).

In 2008, Dr. Yang began the nonprofit YMAA California Retreat Center. This training facility in rural California is where selected students enroll in a five-year residency to learn Chinese martial arts.

Dr. Yang has been involved in traditional Chinese wushu since 1961, studying Shaolin White Crane (Bai He), Shaolin Long Fist (Changquan), and taijiquan under several different masters. He has taught for more than forty-six years: seven years in Taiwan, five years at Purdue University, two years in Houston, twenty-six years in Boston, and more than eight years at the YMAA California Retreat Center. He has taught seminars all around the world, sharing his knowledge of

Chinese martial arts and qigong in Argentina, Austria, Barbados, Botswana, Belgium, Bermuda, Brazil, Canada, China, Chile, England, Egypt, France, Germany, Holland, Hungary, Iceland, Iran, Ireland, Italy, Latvia, Mexico, New Zealand, Poland, Portugal, Saudi Arabia, Spain, South Africa, Switzerland, and Venezuela.

Since 1986, YMAA has become an international organization, which currently includes more than fifty schools located in Argentina, Belgium, Canada, Chile, France, Hungary, Ireland, Italy, New Zealand, Poland, Portugal, South Africa, Sweden, the United Kingdom, Venezuela, and the United States.

Many of Dr. Yang's books and videos have been translated into many languages, including French, Italian, Spanish, Polish, Czech, Bulgarian, Russian, German, and Hungarian.

Books and videos by Dr. Yang, Jwing-Ming

Books

Analysis of Shaolin Chin Na, 2nd ed. YMAA Publication Center, 1987, 2004

Ancient Chinese Weapons: A Martial Artist's Guide, 2nd ed. YMAA Publication Center, 1985, 1999

Arthritis Relief: Chinese Qigong for Healing & Prevention, 2nd ed. YMAA Publication Center, 1991, 2005

Back Pain Relief: Chinese Qigong for Healing and Prevention, 2nd ed. YMAA Publication Center, 1997, 2004

Baguazhang: Theory and Applications, 2nd ed. YMAA Publication Center, 1994, 2008

Comprehensive Applications of Shaolin Chin Na: The Practical Defense of Chinese Seizing Arts. YMAA Publication Center, 1995

Essence of Shaolin White Crane: Martial Power and Qigong. YMAA Publication Center, 1996

How to Defend Yourself. YMAA Publication Center, 1992

Introduction to Ancient Chinese Weapons. Unique Publications, Inc., 1985

Meridian Qigong, YMAA Publication Center, 2016

Northern Shaolin Sword 2nd ed. YMAA Publication Center, 1985, 2000

Qigong for Health and Martial Arts, **2nd ed.** YMAA Publication Center, 1995, 1998

Qigong Massage: Fundamental Techniques for Health and Relaxation, 2nd ed. YMAA Publication Center, 1992, 2005

Qigong Meditation: Embryonic Breathing. YMAA Publication Center, 2003

Qigong Meditation: Small Circulation, YMAA Publication Center, 2006

Qigong, the Secret of Youth: Da Mo's Muscle/Tendon Changing and Marrow/Brain Washing Qigong, 2nd ed. YMAA Publication Center, 1989, 2000

Root of Chinese qigong: Secrets of qigong Training, 2nd ed. YMAA Publication Center, 1989, 1997

Shaolin Chin Na. Unique Publications, Inc., 1980

Shaolin Long Fist Kung Fu. Unique Publications, Inc., 1981

Simple Qigong Exercises for Health: The Eight Pieces of Brocade, 3rd ed. YMAA Publication Center, 1988, 1997, 2013

Tai Chi Ball Qigong: For Health and Martial Arts. YMAA Publication Center, 2010

Tai Chi Chuan Classical Yang Style: The Complete Long Form and Qigong, 2nd ed. YMAA Publication Center, 1999, 2010

Tai Chi Chuan Martial Applications, **2nd ed.** YMAA Publication Center, 1986, 1996

Tai Chi Chuan Martial Power, 3rd ed. YMAA Publication Center, 1986, 1996, 2015

Tai Chi Chuan: Classical Yang Style, 2nd ed. YMAA Publication Center, 1999, 2010

Tai Chi qigong: The Internal Foundation of Tai Chi Chuan, 2nd ed. rev. YMAA Publication Center, 1997, 1990, 2013

Tai Chi Secrets of the Ancient Masters: Selected Readings with Commentary. YMAA Publication Center, 1999

Tai Chi Secrets of the Wŭ and Li Styles: Chinese Classics, Translation, Commentary. YMAA Publication Center, 2001

Tai Chi Secrets of the Wu Style: Chinese Classics, Translation, Commentary. YMAA Publication Center, 2002

Tai Chi Secrets of the Yang Style: Chinese Classics, Translation, Commentary. YMAA Publication Center, 2001

Tai Chi Sword Classical Yang Style: The Complete Long Form, qigong, and Applications, 2nd ed. YMAA Publication Center, 1999, 2014

Taiji Chin Na: The Seizing Art of Taijiquan, 2nd ed. YMAA Publication Center, 1995, 2014

Taijiquan Theory of Dr. Yang, Jwing-Ming: The Root of Taijiquan. YMAA Publication Center, 2003

Xingyiquan: Theory and Applications, 2nd ed. YMAA Publication Center, 1990, 2003

Yang Style Tai Chi Chuan. Unique Publications, Inc., 1981

Videos alphabetical

Advanced Practical Chin Na in Depth, YMAA Publication Center, 2010

Analysis of Shaolin Chin Na. YMAA Publication Center, 2004

Baguazhang (Eight Trigrams Palm Kung Fu). YMAA Publication Center, 2005

Chin Na in Depth: Courses 1–4. YMAA Publication Center, 2003

Chin Na in Depth: Courses 5–8. YMAA Publication Center, 2003

Chin Na in Depth: Courses 9–12. YMAA Publication Center, 2003

Five Animal Sports Qigong. YMAA Publication Center, 2008

Knife Defense: Traditional Techniques. YMAA Publication Center, 2011

Meridian Qigong, YMAA Publication Center, 2015

Neigong, YMAA Publication Center, 2015

Northern Shaolin Sword. YMAA Publication Center, 2009

Qigong Massage. YMAA Publication Center, 2005

Saber Fundamental Training. YMAA Publication Center, 2008

Shaolin Kung Fu Fundamental Training. YMAA Publication Center, 2004

Shaolin Long Fist Kung Fu: Basic Sequences. YMAA Publication Center, 2005

Shaolin Saber Basic Sequences. YMAA Publication Center, 2007

Shaolin Staff Basic Sequences. YMAA Publication Center, 2007

Shaolin White Crane Gong Fu Basic Training: Courses 1 & 2. YMAA Publication Center, 2003

Shaolin White Crane Gong Fu Basic Training: Courses 3 & 4. YMAA Publication Center, 2008

Shaolin White Crane Hard and Soft Qigong. YMAA Publication Center, 2003

Shuai Jiao: Kung Fu Wrestling. YMAA Publication Center, 2010

Simple Qigong Exercises for Arthritis Relief. YMAA Publication Center, 2007

Simple Qigong Exercises for Back Pain Relief. YMAA Publication Center, 2007

Simple Qigong Exercises for Health: The Eight Pieces of Brocade. YMAA Publication Center, 2003

Staff Fundamental Training: Solo Drills and Matching Practice. YMAA Publication Center, 2007

Sword Fundamental Training. YMAA Publication Center, 2009

Tai Chi Ball Qigong: Courses 1 & 2. YMAA Publication Center, 2006

Tai Chi Ball Qigong: Courses 3 & 4. YMAA Publication Center, 2007

Tai Chi Chuan: Classical Yang Style. YMAA Publication Center, 2003

Tai Chi Fighting Set: 2-Person Matching Set. YMAA Publication Center, 2006

Tai Chi Pushing Hands: Courses 1 & 2. YMAA Publication Center, 2005

Tai Chi Pushing Hands: Courses 3 & 4. YMAA Publication Center, 2006

Tai Chi Qigong. YMAA Publication Center, 2005

Tai Chi Sword, Classical Yang Style. YMAA Publication Center, 2005

Tai Chi Symbol: Yin/Yang Sticking Hands. YMAA Publication Center, 2008

Taiji 37 Postures Martial Applications. YMAA Publication Center, 2008

Taiji Chin Na in Depth. YMAA Publication Center, 2009

Taiji Saber: Classical Yang Style. YMAA Publication Center, 2008

Taiji Wrestling: Advanced Takedown Techniques. YMAA Publication Center, 2008

Understanding Qigong, DVD 1: What is Qigong? The Human Qi Circulatory System. YMAA Publication Center, 2006

Understanding Qigong, DVD 2: Key Points of Qigong & Qigong Breathing. YMAA Publication Center, 2006

Understanding Qigong, DVD 3: Embryonic Breathing. YMAA Publication Center, 2007

Understanding Qigong, DVD 4: Four Seasons Qigong. YMAA Publication Center, 2007

Understanding Qigong, DVD 5: Small Circulation. YMAA Publication Center, 2007

Understanding Qigong, DVD 6: Martial Arts Qigong Breathing. YMAA Publication Center, 2007

Xingyiquan: Twelve Animals Kung Fu and Applications. YMAA Publication Center, 2008

Yang Tai Chi for Beginners. YMAA Publication Center, 2012

YMAA 25-Year Anniversary. YMAA Publication Center, 2009